Brain Tumor Targeting Drug Delivery Systems: Advanced Nanoscience for Theranostics Applications

Edited by

Ram Kumar Sahu

Department of Pharmaceutical Sciences
Hemvati Nandan Bahuguna Garhwal University (A Central University)
Chauras Campus, Tehri Garhwal-249161, Uttarakhand, India

Brain Tumor Targeting Drug Delivery Systems:
Advanced Nanoscience for Theranostics Applications

Editor: Ram Kumar Sahu

ISBN (Online): 978-981-5079-72-2

ISBN (Print): 978-981-5079-73-9

ISBN (Paperback): 978-981-5079-74-6

Published by Bentham Science Publishers Pte. Ltd. Singapore. All Rights Reserved.

First published in 2023.

need for a court order if at any point you breach any terms of this License Agreement. In no event will any delay or failure by Bentham Science Publishers in enforcing your compliance with this License Agreement constitute a waiver of any of its rights.

3. You acknowledge that you have read this License Agreement, and agree to be bound by its terms and conditions. To the extent that any other terms and conditions presented on any website of Bentham Science Publishers conflict with, or are inconsistent with, the terms and conditions set out in this License Agreement, you acknowledge that the terms and conditions set out in this License Agreement shall prevail.

Bentham Science Publishers Pte. Ltd.
80 Robinson Road #02-00
Singapore 068898
Singapore
Email: subscriptions@benthamscience.net

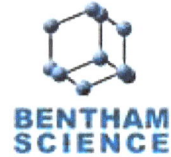

CONTENTS

PREFACE

There are still many unmet medical requirements, including brain tumours. Brain tumours can now be treated with considerably less toxicity and better pharmacokinetics and pharmacodynamics because of recent nano-drug delivery technologies. It is still difficult to treat brain tumours due to their rapid growth and poor prognoses, even with surgery, radiation, and chemotherapies. To combat the disease, therapeutic delivery methods that maximise drug accumulation in the tumour location and decrease toxicity in normal brain and peripheral tissue are a potential new strategy. The fact that brain tumours differ in many ways from tumours in other tissues means that drug delivery to brain tumours can take advantage of the constantly changing vascular characteristics and microenvironment. For brain tumour theranostics, nanocarrier-based delivery methods address brain architecture and tumours in addition to the advances and problems in delivering medicines across the blood brain barrier. Theranostics combines diagnostics and therapeutics. A growing number of people are becoming interested in individualised therapy and diagnostics approaches. As well as conserving money, this method also limits the negative effects of a specific goal.

This book contains several sections on nanotechnology, including the most recent developments in the field and practical advice on how to build more effective nanocarriers for medication and gene delivery. There is much helpful information in this book that will help readers to create innovative drug delivery systems for brain tumour therapy that will help to boost nanomedical technology. The key features highlighted in this book are various theranostic-based delivery systems for brain tumour diagnosis and treatment. This book will be of interest to many academicians, scientists, and researchers. It will enable them to understand the possible prospects of nanotechnology for delivering nanocarriers that can better diagnose and cure brain tumours in the future.

Ram Kumar Sahu
Department of Pharmaceutical Sciences
Hemvati Nandan Bahuguna Garhwal University (A Central University), Chauras Campus
Tehri Garhwal-249161, Uttarakhand, India

List of Contributors

Amitha Muraleedharan Shraga Segal Department of Microbiology, Immunology, and Genetics, Faculty of Health Sciences, Ben-Gurion University of the Negev, Beer Sheva, Israel

Ardra Thottarath Prasanthan Department of Pharmaceutics, Amrita School of Pharmacy, Amrita Vishwa Vidyapeetham, AIMS Health Science Campus, Kochi, Kerala, India

Aseem Setia Department of Pharmacy, Shri Rawatpura Sarkar University, Raipur, (C.G) - 492015, India

Ayodeji Folorunsho Ajayi Reproductive Physiology and Bioinformatics Research Unit, Department of Physiology, Ladoke Akintola University of Technology, Ogbomoso, Oyo state, Nigeria

Devesh Kapoor Dr. Dayaram Patel Pharmacy College, Bardoli, Surat, Gujarat, India

Deepak Prashar KC Institute of Pharmaceutical Sciences, Una-177207, H.P., India

Emmanuel Tayo Adebayo Reproductive Physiology and Bioinformatics Research Unit, Department of Physiology, Ladoke Akintola University of Technology, Ogbomoso, Oyo state, Nigeria

Grace Fumilayo Adigun Reproductive Physiology and Bioinformatics Research Unit, Department of Physiology, Ladoke Akintola University of Technology, Ogbomoso, Oyo state, Nigeria

Geetika Sharma Department of Pharmacy, Indira Gandhi National Tribal University, Amarkantak, Madhya Pradesh, 484887, India

Jiyauddin Khan School of Pharmacy, Management and Science University, 40100 Shah Alam, Selangor, Malaysia

Kajal Kumari Department of Pharmacy, Banasthali Vidyapith, Banasthali, P.O. Rajasthan, India

Krishna Yadav University Institute of Pharmacy, Pt. Ravishankar Shukla University, Raipur, Chhattisgarh 492010, India

Manish Philip Department of Pharmaceutics, Amrita School of Pharmacy, Amrita Vishwa Vidyapeetham, AIMS Health Science Campus, Kochi, Kerala, India

Madhulika Pradhan Rungta College of Pharmaceutical Sciences and Research, Kohka, Kurud Road, Bhilai, Chhattisgarh, 490024, India

Nikhil Ponnoor Anto Shraga Segal Department of Microbiology, Immunology, and Genetics, Faculty of Health Sciences, Ben-Gurion University of the Negev, Beer Sheva, Israel

Nirdesh Salim Kumar Department of Pharmaceutics, Amrita School of Pharmacy, Amrita Vishwa Vidyapeetham, AIMS Health Science Campus, Kochi, Kerala, India

Nidhal Khazaal Maraie Department of pharmaceutics, college of pharmacy, Al-Farahidi University, Baghdad, Iraq

Narayana Subbiah Hari Narayana Moorthy Department of Pharmacy, Indira Gandhi National Tribal University, Amarkantak, Madhya Pradesh, 484887, India

Oluwadunsin Iyanuoluwa Adebayo	Reproductive Physiology and Bioinformatics Research Unit, Department of Physiology, Ladoke Akintola University of Technology, Ogbomoso, Oyo state, Nigeria
Payal Kesharwani	Department of Pharmacy, Banasthali Vidyapith, Banasthali, Rajasthan, India Rameesh Institute of Vocational and Technical Education, Greater Noida, India
Ram Kumar Sahu	Department of Pharmaceutical Sciences, Hemvati Nandan Bahuguna Garhwal University (A Central University), Chauras Campus, Tehri Garhwal-249161, Uttarakhand, India
Sivadas Swathi Krishna	Department of Pharmaceutics, Amrita School of Pharmacy, Amrita Vishwa Vidyapeetham, AIMS Health Science Campus, Kochi, Kerala, India
Shiv Kumar Prajapati	Institute of Pharmaceutical Research, GLA University, Mathura, Uttar Pradesh, India
Smita Jain	Department of Pharmacy, Banasthali Vidyapith, Banasthali, Rajasthan, India
Swapnil Sharma	Department of Pharmacy, Banasthali Vidyapith, Banasthali, Rajasthan, India
Swati Dubey	Department of Pharmacy, Indira Gandhi National Tribal University, Amarkantak, Madhya Pradesh, 484887, India
Shalini Singh	Department of Pharmacy, Indira Gandhi National Tribal University, Amarkantak, Madhya Pradesh, 484887, India
Sunita Minz	Department of Pharmacy, Indira Gandhi National Tribal University, Amarkantak, Madhya Pradesh, 484887, India
Tayo Adebayo	Reproductive Physiology and Bioinformatics Research Unit, Department of Physiology, Ladoke Akintola University of Technology, Ogbomoso, Oyo state, Nigeria
Vidya Viswanad	Department of Pharmaceutics, Amrita School of Pharmacy, Amrita Vishwa Vidyapeetham, AIMS Health Science Campus, Kochi, Kerala, India
Zainab H. Mahdi	Department of pharmaceutics, college of pharmacy, Applied Science Private University, Amman, Jordan
Zahraa Amer Al-Juboori	Department of Pharmaceutics, College of Pharmacy, Mustansiriyah University, Baghdad, Iraq

CHAPTER 1

Anatomy and Physiology of the Brain: Pathophysiology of Brain Tumor

Amitha Muraleedharan[1,*] and **Nikhil Ponnoor Anto**[1]

[1] *Shraga Segal Department of Microbiology, Immunology, and Genetics, Faculty of Health Sciences, Ben-Gurion University of the Negev, Beer Sheva, Israel*

Abstract: The brain is an efficient processor of information. It is the most complex and sensitive organ in the body and is responsible for all functions of the body, including serving as the coordinating center for all sensations, mobility, emotions, and intellect. The magnitude of its myriad function is often realized usually when there is a disruption of the nervous system due to injury, disease, or inherited predispositions. Neuroscience is the field of study that endeavors to make sense of such diverse questions; at the same time, it points the way toward the effective treatment of dysfunctions. The two-way channel of information: findings from the laboratory leading towards stricter criteria for diagnosing brain disorders and more effective methods for treating them and in turn, the clinician's increasingly acute skills of diagnosis and observation that supply the research scientist with more precise data for study in the lab diligently expands the field of neuroscience. Tumors of the brain produce neurological manifestations through several mechanisms. Stronger hypotheses about the mechanism of a disease can point the way toward more effective treatments and new possibilities for a cure. In highly complex disorders of the brain, in which many factors genetic, environmental, epidemiological, even social and psychological—play a part, broadly based hypotheses are exceedingly useful. With the advancements in technology and a better understanding of brain anatomy and physiology, the quest to discover an efficient cure for life-threatening tumors of the brain is underway.

Keywords: Blood brain barrier, Brain, Brain tumor, Glia, Nervous system, Neuron, Synapse.

INTRODUCTION

The nervous system is a very complex structure that can be divided into two major regions: the central nervous system (CNS) which consists of the brain and spinal cord and the peripheral nervous system (PNS) which is an extensive net-

* **Corresponding Author Amitha Muraleedharan:** Shraga Segal Department of Microbiology, Immunology, and Genetics, Faculty of Health Sciences, Ben-Gurion University of the Negev, Beer Sheva, Israel; E-mail: prashardeepak99@yahoo.in

Ram Kumar Sahu (Ed.)

work of nerves that consists of (i) Craniospinal nerves having 12 pairs of cranial nerves and 31 pairs of spinal nerves, (ii) Visceral nervous system comprising the sympathetic nervous system and parasympathetic nervous system connecting the CNS to the muscles and sensory structures [1, 2]. The spinal cord is a single structure, whereas the adult brain is divided into four major regions: (i) The cerebral hemispheres, comprised of the cerebral cortex, basal ganglia, white matter, hippocampi, and amygdalae; (ii) The diencephalon, with the thalamus and hypothalamus; (iii) The brain stem, consisting of the medulla, pons, and midbrain; and (iv) The cerebellum. The brain is the central control module of the body and coordinates activities like task-evoked responses, senses, movement, emotions, language, communication, thinking, and memory [3, 4]. In this book chapter, we discuss the anatomy of the brain, its functions, development, and pathology with a special focus on brain carcinogenesis.

THE ANATOMY OF THE HUMAN BRAIN

The brain is protected by the skull (cranium) which is in turn covered by the scalp. The scalp is composed of an outer layer of skin, which is loosely attached to the aponeurosis, a flat, broad tendon layer that anchors the superficial layers of the skin. The periosteum, below the aponeurosis, firmly encases the bones of the skull and provides protection, nutrition to the bone, and the capacity for bone repair. Below the skull are three layers of protective covering called the meninges that surround the brain and the spinal cord. The meningeal layer closest to the bones of the skull called the dura mater (meaning *tough mother*) is thick and tough and includes two layers; the periosteal layer lines the inner dome of the skull followed by the meningeal layer below. The space between the layers allows the passage of veins and arteries that supply blood to the brain. Below the dura mater lies the arachnoid mater (*spider-like mother*) which is comprised of a thin web-like connective tissue called arachnoid trabeculae and is devoid of nerves or blood vessels. The innermost meningeal layer is a delicate membrane called the pia mater (*tender mother*). The pia mater firmly adheres to the convoluted surface of the CNS, lining the inside of the sulci in the cerebral and cerebellar cortices, and is rich in veins and arteries. Between the arachnoid mater and pia mater is the subarachnoid space which is filled with cerebrospinal fluid (CSF), produced by the cells of the choroid plexus—areas in each ventricle of the brain (discussed further below). The CSF serves to deliver nutrients and removes waste from neural tissues and also provides a liquid cushion to the brain and spinal cord (Fig. 1) [5, 6].

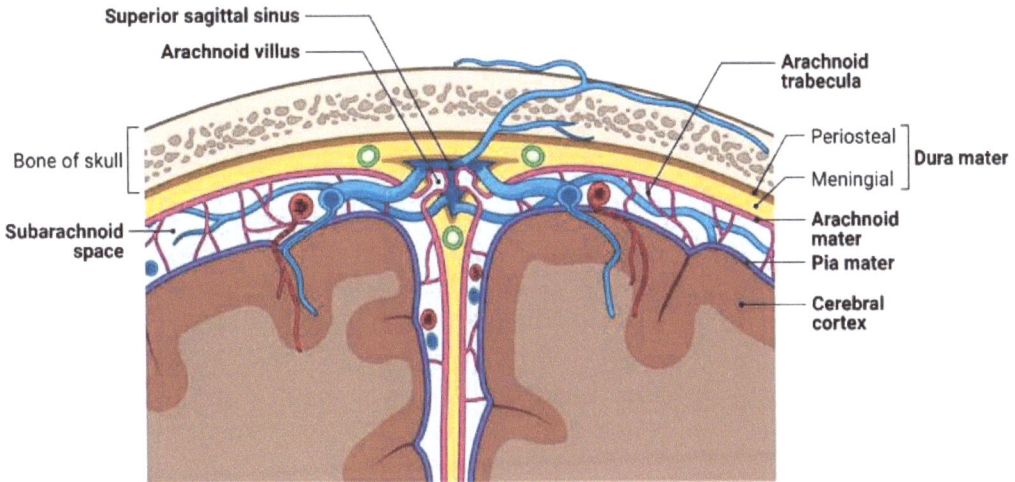

Fig. (1). The layers of the tissue surrounding the human brain including three meningeal membranes: the dura mater, the arachnoid mater, and pia mater.

Cerebrum

The cerebrum, which appears to make up most of the brain mass, consists of two cerebral hemispheres demarked by a large separation called the longitudinal fissure. Each hemisphere has an inner core composed of white matter-the corpus callosum-and and an outer surface-the cerebral cortex- composed of gray matter. The corpus callosum, the largest of the five commissural nerve tracts, provides the major pathway for communication between the two hemispheres. According to the concept known as localization of function, different regions of the cerebral cortex can be associated with particular functions. In the early 1900s, an extensive study of the microscopic anatomy—the cytoarchitecture—of the cerebral cortex was undertaken by a German neuroscientist named Korbinian Brodmann who divided the cortex into 52 separate regions based on the histology of the cortex. The results from Brodmann's work on the anatomy align very well with the functional differences within the cortex and resulted in a system of classification known as Brodmann's areas, which is still used today to describe the anatomical distinctions within the cortex [7]. Each hemisphere is conventionally divided into four lobes namely the frontal lobe, temporal lobe, occipital lobe, and parietal lobe (Fig. **2**).

- **Frontal lobe:** positioned at the front of the brain, the lobe is associated with executive functions. Containing a majority of dopamine-sensitive neurons, the region is responsible for self-control, planning, reasoning, motivation, and abstract thinking. Broca's area is responsible for the production of language, or controlling movements responsible for speech; in the vast majority of people, it is located only on the left side [4, 8, 9].

- **Temporal lobe:** It processes sensory information for the retention of memories, language, and emotions. The presence of olfactory nerves and auditory nerves makes it a major player in the sensations of smell and hearing [10].
- **Occipital lobe:** housing the visual cortex, the lobe is dedicated to vision [4].
- **Parietal lobe:** The main sensation associated with the parietal lobe is somatosensation. It integrates and interprets sensory information including vision, hearing, motor, sensory, spatial awareness, navigation, and memory function. Wernicke's area is located here, which is responsible for understanding spoken and written language [9].
- Anterior to these regions is the prefrontal lobe, which serves cognitive functions that can be the basis of personality, short-term memory, and consciousness.

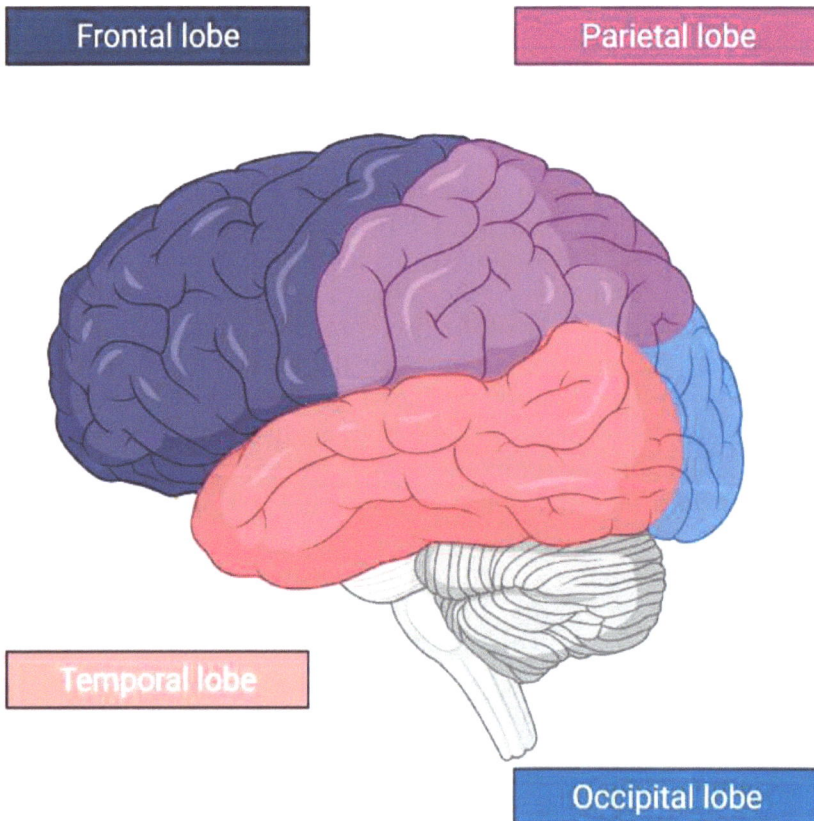

Fig. (2). Lobes of the Cerebral Cortex: The cerebral cortex is divided into four lobes. Extensive folding increases the surface area available for cerebral functions.

Subcortical Structures

Beneath the cerebral cortex lies a set of nuclei called the subcortical nuclei deep within the hemispheres that augment cortical processes (Fig. **3**). The nuclei of the basal forebrain structures serve as the primary location for the production of acetylcholine which is then distributed throughout the cortex possibly leading to greater attention to sensory stimuli. Alzheimer's disease is associated with the loss of neurons in these nuclei. The hippocampus and amygdala are medial-lobe structures that are involved in long-term memory formation and emotional responses. The basal ganglia or basal nuclei which include structures like the striatum, substantia nigra, and the subthalamic nucleus are involved in the control of voluntary motor movements, procedural learning, and influence the likelihood of movements taking place [7].

The Diencephalon

Diencephalon (*through the brain*) connects the cerebrum and the rest of the nervous system. The thalamus is a major processing region for sensory information and relays impulses between the cerebral cortex and the periphery, the spinal cord, or brain stem. Positioned in the center of the brain, the thalamus is involved in the regulation of consciousness, sleep, awareness, and alertness. The hypothalamus is largely involved in the regulation of homeostasis. It controls the autonomic nervous system and endocrine system by regulating the anterior pituitary secretions (*e.g.* LH) by releasing stimulating hormones (*e.g.* GnRH) into the hypophysial portal blood [11]. The secretions of the posterior pituitary (antidiuretic hormone, oxytocin) are also controlled by the hypothalamus. As part of the limbic system, certain parts of the hypothalamus are also involved in memory and emotion (Fig. **3**) [7].

Brain Stem

The brain stem which includes the midbrain and hindbrain (pons and medulla) connects the cerebrum to the spinal cord (Fig. **3**). The midbrain is a complex structure with a range of neuronal clusters that coordinate sensory representations of the visual, auditory, and somatosensory perceptual spaces. The pons is the main connection with the cerebellum. The pons and the medulla regulate several crucial functions, including the cardiovascular and respiratory systems and rates. The brain stem continues below the large opening in the occipital bone, called the foramen magnum, as the spinal cord and is protected by the vertebral column. A diffuse region of gray matter throughout the brain stem, known as the reticular formation, is related to sleep and wakefulness, such as general brain activity and attention [7, 12].

Cerebellum

The cerebellum (*little brain*) is largely responsible for comparing information from the cerebrum with the sensory feedback from the periphery through the spinal cord to fine-tune the precision and accuracy of motor activity. The cerebellum lies in the back of the cranial cavity, lying beneath the occipital lobes, separated by the cerebellar tentorium (Fig. **3**). It is divided into three lobes; anterior lobe, posterior lobe, and floccondular lobe which function to coordinate voluntary muscle movements, maintain posture, balance, and equilibrium. The output of the cerebellum reaches the midbrain, which then sends a descending input to the spinal cord to correct the messages going to the skeletal muscles [7, 13].

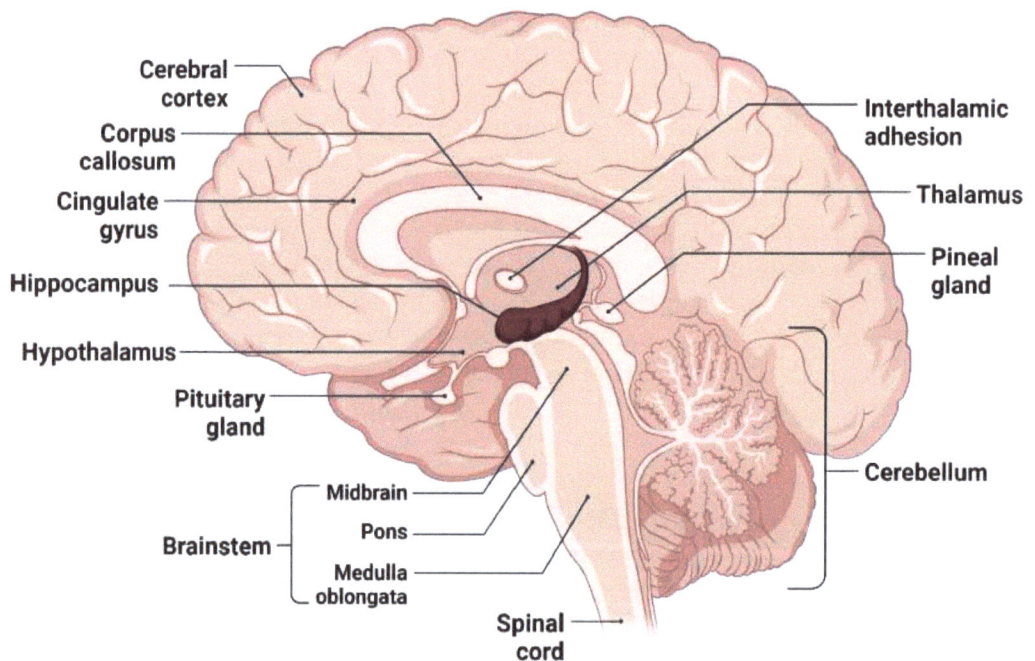

Fig. (3). Anatomy of the human brain (sagittal)

Circulation and CSF

Blood is carried to the brain by two sets of arteries; the internal carotid arteries which enter the cranium through the carotid canal in the temporal bone and vertebral arteries which enter through the foramen magnum of the occipital bone. The internal carotid artery supplies most of the cerebrum, while the vertebral arteries supply the cerebellum, brainstem, and underside of the cerebrum. The two vertebral arteries then merge into the basilar artery, which gives rise to branches to the brain stem and cerebellum. The left and right internal carotid arteries and branches of the basilar artery all become the circle of Willis, a confluence of arteries that can maintain perfusion of the brain even if narrowing or a blockage limits flow through one part thus preventing brain damage. The external carotid arteries supply blood to the tissues on the surface of the cranium [14, 15].

The venous circulation of the brain is very different from the body. After passing through the CNS, blood returns to the circulation through a series of dural sinuses and veins. The superior sagittal sinus runs in the groove of the longitudinal fissure, where it absorbs CSF from the meninges. The superior sagittal sinus drains to the confluence of sinuses, along with the occipital sinuses and straight sinus, to then drain into the transverse sinuses. The transverse sinuses connect to the sigmoid sinuses, which then connect to the jugular veins. From there, the blood continues toward the heart to be pumped to the lungs for reoxygenation. The two jugular veins are the only drainage of the brain [15, 16].

The cerebrospinal fluid (CSF) is a modified transcellular fluid that circulates throughout and around the CNS. The ventricles are the open spaces within the brain where CSF is produced by filtering of the blood that is performed by a specialized membrane known as a choroid plexus which are networks of blood capillaries lined by ependymal cells in the walls of the ventricles. Specifically, CSF circulates through all of the ventricles to remove metabolic wastes from the interstitial fluids of nervous tissues to eventually emerge into the subarachnoid space where it is reabsorbed into the blood. The CSF also acts as a mechanical buffer; by remaining inside and outside the CNS, it equalizes mechanical pressure thus acting as a cushion between the soft and delicate tissues of the brain and the rigid cranium [6, 14].

There are four ventricles within the brain, all of which developed from the original hollow space within the neural tube, the central canal. The first two are named the lateral ventricles and are deep within the cerebrum. These ventricles are connected to the third ventricle by two openings called the interventricular foramina. The third ventricle is the space between the left and right sides of the diencephalon, which opens into the cerebral aqueduct that passes through the midbrain. The aqueduct opens into the fourth ventricle, which is the space between the cerebellum and the pons and upper medulla. Three separate openings, the middle and two lateral apertures, drain the cerebrospinal fluid from the fourth ventricle to the cisterna magna one of the major cisterns. From the fourth ventricle, the CSF flows into the subarachnoid space where it bathes and cushions the brain. The single median aperture and the pair of lateral apertures connect to the subarachnoid space so that CSF can flow through the ventricles and around the CNS [14, 17].

The tissues of the CNS have extra protection in that they are not exposed to blood or the immune system in the same way as other tissues. The blood vessels that supply the brain with nutrients and other chemical substances lie on top of the pia mater. The capillary endothelial cells joined by tight junctions control the transfer of blood components to the brain. In addition, cranial capillaries have far fewer fenestra (pore-like structures that are sealed by a membrane) and pinocytotic vesicles than other capillaries. As a result, materials in the circulatory system have a very limited ability to interact with the CNS directly. This phenomenon is referred to as the *blood-brain barrier (BBB)* [5, 14]. The barrier is less permeable to larger molecules but is still permeable to water, carbon dioxide, oxygen, and most fat-soluble substances (including anesthetics and alcohol). The blood-brain barrier is not present in the circumventricular organs—which are structures in the brain that may need to respond to changes in body fluids—such as the pineal gland, area postrema, and some areas of the hypothalamus. There is a similar blood-cerebrospinal fluid barrier, which serves the same purpose as the blood-brain barrier, but facilitates the transport of different substances into the brain due to the distinct structural characteristics between the two barrier systems. Morphological characteristics of the blood-brain barrier show; a) The high electron density of endothelial cytoplasm, b) Thicker basement membrane, c) Absence of perivascular connective tissue, d) Complete covering of the endothelial processes by astrocytic processes, and e) Small number or absence of cytoplasmic vesicles in endothelial cells. Lateral zonulae occludens of the capillary endothelium force solutes to pass through the cytoplasm of astrocytes which restrains the passage of molecule through its plasma membrane [18]. The blood-brain barrier maintains the constancy of the environment of the neurons in the CNS in such a way that the multiple homeostatic mechanisms of the ionic transfer during neuronal activity is maintained. While nutrient molecules, such as glucose or amino acids, can pass through the BBB, it is impermeable to larger molecules causing problems with drug delivery to the CNS. Pharmaceutical companies are thus challenged to design drugs that can cross the BBB as well as have an effect on the nervous system to treat conditions like neurodegenerative diseases and intracranial brain tumors [5]. Recently, a paravascular pathway, also known as the "glymphatic" pathway, has been described as a system for waste clearance in the brain. According to this model, cerebrospinal fluid (CSF) enters the paravascular spaces surrounding penetrating arteries of the brain, mixes with interstitial fluid (ISF) and solutes in the parenchyma, and exits along the paravascular spaces of draining veins [19].

MICROANATOMY

The human brain is primarily composed of neurons, glial cells, neural stem cells, and blood vessels. Neurons are the structural and functional unit of the nervous system. They are responsible for the computation and communication that the nervous system provides. They are electrically active and release chemical signals to target cells *via* specialized connections called synapses [20]. Glial cells, or glia, are known to play a supporting role in the nervous tissue. Ongoing research pursues an expanded role for glial cells in signalling, but neurons are still considered the basis of this function. Neurons are important, but without glial support, they would not be able to perform their function.

The first way to classify a neuron is by the number of processes attached to the cell body. Using the standard model of neurons, one of these processes is the axon, and the rest are dendrites. Because information flows through the neuron from dendrites or cell bodies toward the axon, these names are based on the neuron's polarity. Axon is the process of a nerve cell that carries impulse away from it. Nerve fibers that carry impulses to the CNS are termed afferent and those carrying impulses from the CNS to the periphery are known as efferent. It arises from the part of the cell called the axon hillock. It is generally long with few branches and contains no Nissl granules. The axon hillock also has the greatest density of voltage-dependent sodium channels which makes it the most easily excited part of the neuron and the spike initiation zone for the axon. In electrophysiological terms, it has the most negative threshold potential. Dendrites collect impulses from other neurons and carry them to the cell body. The short cellular extensions with specific branching patterns resemble a dendritic tree, hence the name [21] (Fig. **4**).

Neurons are typically classified into three types based on their function; i.) Sensory neurons respond to stimuli such as touch, sound, or light that affect the cells of the sensory organs, and they send signals to the spinal cord or brain, ii.) Motor neurons receive signals from the brain and spinal cord to control everything from muscle contractions to glandular output, iii.) Interneurons connect neurons to other neurons within the same region of the brain or spinal cord. A group of connected neurons is called a neural circuit [22]. Neurons can also be classified according to the number of their processes: 1) Unipolar cells have only one process emerging from the cell. True unipolar cells are only found in invertebrate animals, so the unipolar cells in humans are more appropriately called "pseudo-unipolar" cells. All developing neuroblasts pass through a stage when they have only one process-the axon. Human unipolar cells have an axon that emerges from the cell body, but it splits so that the axon can extend over a very long distance. At one end of the axon are dendrites, and at the other end, the axon forms synaptic connections with a target. Unipolar cells are exclusively sensory neurons and have two unique characteristics.

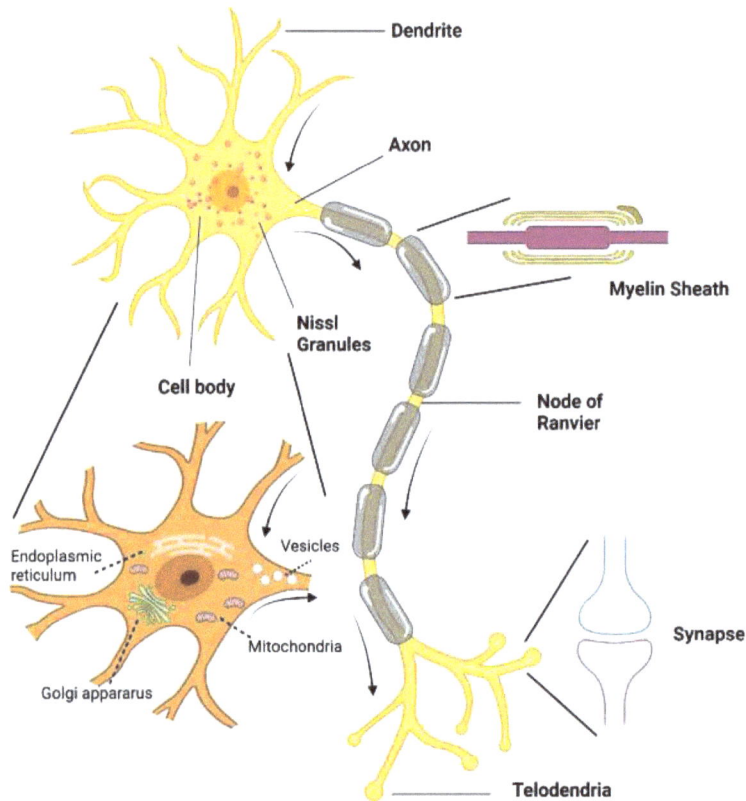

Fig. (4). Parts of a Neuron: The major parts of the neuron are labelled on a multipolar neuron from the CNS.

First, their dendrites are receiving sensory information, sometimes directly from the stimulus itself. Secondly, the cell bodies of unipolar neurons are always found in ganglia. Sensory reception is a peripheral function (those dendrites are in the periphery, perhaps in the skin) so the cell body is in the periphery, though closer to the CNS in a ganglion. The axon projects from the dendrite endings, past the cell body in a ganglion, and into the central nervous system; 2) Bipolar cells have two processes, which extend from each end of the cell body, opposite to each other. One is the axon and one the dendrite. Bipolar cells are not very common. They are found mainly in the olfactory neuro-epithelium (where smell stimuli are sensed), in the vestibular ganglion, in the spiral ganglion of the cochlea, and as part of the retina; 3) Multipolar neurons are all of the neurons that are not unipolar or bipolar. They have one axon and two or more dendrites (usually many more). Except for the unipolar sensory ganglion cells, and the specific bipolar cells mentioned above, all other neurons are multipolar. A few of the common types of multipolar neurons are the Purkinje cell of the cerebellar cortex, pyramidal cell of the motor cortex, small neuron from the spinal nucleus of the trigeminal nerve, and motor neuron from the ventral horn of the spinal cord [20, 22]. Some sources describe a fourth type of neuron, called an anaxonic neuron. Anaxonic neurons are very small, and if looked through a microscope at the standard resolution used in histology (approximately 400X to 1000X total magnification), one will not be able to distinguish process specifically as an axon or a dendrite. Any of those processes can function as an axon depending on the conditions at any given time and are therefore multipolar [20].

An alternate classification also exists where neurons are classified based on the length of their axon. (i) Golgi type I neuron has a very long axon that has an extensive course outside the gray matter of the CNS and passes the white matter. These cells form the bulk of the neurons which constitute the peripheral nerves and main fiber tracts of the brain and spinal cord. *e.g.*, Pyramidal cell and Purkinje cell. (ii) Golgi type II neuron is stellate and has a short axon that does not leave the gray matter. These cells are found in the retina, the cerebellar, and the cerebral cortices. *e.g.*, granule cell.

Glia (glial cells or neuroglia) are the non-neuronal cells in the nervous tissue and were first described by a German pathologist Rudolf Virchow in 1856. They maintain homeostasis, form myelin, and provide support and protection to neurons. In the central nervous system, glial cells include oligodendrocytes, astrocytes, ependymal cells, and microglia, and in the peripheral nervous system; glial cells include Schwann cells and satellite cells [23]. They have four main functions: (1) To surround neurons and hold them in place; (2) To supply nutrients and oxygen to neurons; (3) To insulate one neuron from another; (4) To destroy pathogens and remove dead neurons. Astrocytes are the most abundant type of glial cells in the CNS. In general, there are two types of astrocytes, protoplasmic and fibrous, similar in function but distinct in morphology and distribution. Protoplasmic astrocytes have short, thick, highly branched processes and are typically found in gray matter. Fibrous astrocytes have long, thin, less branched processes and are more commonly found in white matter. Some ways in which they support neurons in the central nervous system are by maintaining the concentration of chemicals in the extracellular space, removing excess signalling molecules, reacting to tissue damage, and contributing to the blood-brain barrier [20, 23 - 25]. Oligodendrocytes sometimes called just "oligo," are the glial cells that coat the axon in the CNS. The few processes that extend from the cell body reach out and surround an axon to insulate it in myelin. One oligodendrocyte will provide the myelin for multiple axon segments, either for the same axon or for separate axons. The myelin sheath provides insulation to the axon that allows electrical signals to propagate more efficiently [23]. Ependymal cells are involved in the creation and secretion of cerebrospinal fluid (CSF) and beat their cilia on their apical surface to help circulate the CSF through the ventricular space and make up the blood-CSF barrier [23]. Microglia are specialized macrophages capable of phagocytosis. They are derived from the earliest wave of mononuclear cells that originate in the yolk sac and colonize the brain shortly after the neural precursors begin to differentiate. These cells are found in all regions of the brain and spinal cord. They are mobile within the brain and multiply when there is damage. In the healthy central nervous system, microglia processes constantly sample all aspects of their environment (neurons, other glial cells, and blood vessels). In a healthy brain, microglia direct the immune response to brain damage and play an important role in the inflammation that accompanies the damage [23, 26].

DEVELOPMENT

According to developmental neuroscientists, the essential stages in the development and shaping of the human brain are (i) Proliferation of a vast number of undifferentiated brain cells; (ii) Migration of the cells toward a predetermined location in the brain and the beginning of their differentiation into the specific type of cell appropriate to that location; (iii) Aggregation of similar types of cells into distinct regions; (iv) Formation of innumerable connections among neurons, both within and across regions; and (v) Competition among these connections, which results in the selective elimination of many and the stabilization of the 100 trillion or so that remain. These events do not occur in rigid sequence but overlap in time, from about 5 weeks after conception onward. After about 18 months of age, no more neurons are added, and the aggregation of cell types into distinct regions is roughly complete. But the pruning of excess connections—clearly a process of great importance for the shape of the mature brain—continues for years [27].

The formation of the nervous system begins with the process called neurulation which follows gastrulation and results in the formation of the neural tube. As the embryo develops, a portion of the ectoderm differentiates into a specialized region of neuroectoderm, which is the precursor for the tissue of the nervous system. Molecular signals induce cells in this region to differentiate into the neuroepithelium, forming a neural plate. Shortly after the neural plate has formed, its edges thicken and move upward to form the neural folds. A neural groove forms, visible as a line along the dorsal surface of the embryo. As the neural folds come together and converge, the underlying structure forms into a tube just beneath the ectoderm called the neural tube. This entire process leading up to the formation of the neural tube is called primary neurulation [28, 29]. Cells from the neural folds at the dorsal most portion of the neural tube then separate from the ectoderm to form a cluster of cells referred to as the neural crest, which runs lateral to the neural tube. The anterior end of the neural tube develops into the brain and the posterior portion forms the spinal cord. The neural crest migrates away from the nascent, or embryonic central nervous system that will form along the neural groove and develops into several parts of the peripheral nervous system, including the enteric nervous tissue. Many tissues that are not part of the nervous system also arise from the neural crest, such as craniofacial cartilage and bone, and melanocytes. The two open ends of the neural tube are called the anterior neuropore and the posterior neuropore. Different neural tube defects are caused when various parts of the neural tube fail to close. Failure to close the human posterior neural tube regions results in a condition called spina bifida, the severity of which depends on how much of the spinal cord remains exposed. Failure to close the anterior neural tube regions results in a lethal condition, anencephaly, where the forebrain remains in contact with the amniotic fluid and subsequently degenerates. The failure of the entire neural tube to close over the entire body axis is called craniorachischisis [29].

In secondary neurulation, the differentiation of the neural tube into various regions of the central nervous system takes place simultaneously. On the gross anatomical level, the neural tube and its lumen bulge and constrict to form the chambers of the brain and the spinal cord. At the tissue level, the cell populations within the wall of the neural tube rearrange themselves to form the different functional regions of the brain and the spinal cord. Finally, on the cellular level, the neuroepithelial cells themselves differentiate into the numerous types of nerve cells (neurons) and supportive cells (glia) present in the body. As the anterior end of the neural tube starts to develop into the brain, it undergoes a couple of enlargements; the result is the production of sac-like vesicles. Three primary vesicles form the forebrain (prosencephalon), midbrain (mesencephalon), and hindbrain (rhombencephalon). The three vesicles further differentiate into five secondary vesicles. The prosencephalon enlarges into two new vesicles called the telencephalon and the diencephalon. The telencephalon will eventually form the cerebral hemispheres. The diencephalon gives rise to several adult structures like the thalamus and the hypothalamus. In the embryonic diencephalon, a structure known as the optic vesicles or eye cup develops, which will eventually become the nervous tissue of the eye called the retina. This is a rare example of nervous tissue developing as part of the CNS structures in the embryo, but becoming a peripheral structure in the fully formed nervous system. The mesencephalon does not differentiate into any finer divisions and its lumen eventually becomes the cerebral aqueduct. The midbrain is an established region of the brain at the primary vesicle stage of development and remains that way. The rest of the brain develops around it and constitutes a large percentage of the mass of the brain. The rhombencephalon develops into an anterior metencephalon and posterior myelencephalon. The metencephalon corresponds to the adult structure known as the pons and also gives rise to the cerebellum, the part of the brain responsible for coordinating movements, posture, and balance. The most significant connection between the cerebellum and the rest of the brain is at the pons because the pons and cerebellum develop out of the same vesicle. The myelencephalon corresponds to the adult structure known as the medulla oblongata whose neurons generate the nerves that regulate respiratory, gastrointestinal, and cardiovascular movements. The structures that come from the mesencephalon and rhombencephalon, except for the cerebellum, are collectively considered the brain stem, which specifically includes the midbrain, pons, and medulla. The rhombencephalon develops a segmental pattern that specifies the places where certain nerves originate. Periodic swellings called rhombomeres divide the rhombencephalon into smaller compartments and will form ganglia clusters of neuronal cell bodies whose axons form a cranial nerve [28, 29].

The neurons of the brain are divided into cortices (layers) and nuclei (clusters). New neurons are formed by mitosis in the neural tube. The neural precursors can migrate away from the neural tube and form a new layer. Neurons forming later have to migrate through the existing layers. This forms the cortical layers. The germinal zone at the lumen of the neural tube is called the ventricular zone. The new layer is called the mantle zone (gray matter). The cerebral cortex in humans has six layers, and the mantle zone is called the neocortex. Cell fates are often fixed as they undergo their last division. Neurons derived from the same stem cell may end up in different functional regions of the brain. Neural stem cells have been observed in the adult human brain. We now believe humans can continue making neurons throughout life, although at nowhere near the fetal rate [29].

PHYSIOLOGY

Neurons are electrically excitable. To understand how neurons communicate it is necessary to describe the role of an excitable membrane. In neurons and other excitable cells, regulation of the ionic environment is crucial for the development and maintenance of the specific signalling pathway for these cells, known as the *electrical signalling system*. This system is composed of two basic elements: i) A lipid bimolecular diffusion barrier, termed *lipid bilayer*, that separates cells from their environment, and ii) Two classes of macromolecule proteins, known as *ion channels* and *ion carriers*, that actively regulate the movement and distribution of ions across the lipid barrier in the plasma membrane, as well as in the endoplasmic reticulum (ER) and nuclear membranes; of special interest is the carrier protein referred to as the sodium/potassium pump that moves sodium ions (Na^+) out of a cell and potassium ions (K^+) into a cell, thus regulating ion concentration on both sides of the cell membrane [30, 31]. Neurons communicate with each other through two types of electrical signals: 1) Graded potential for short-distance communication and 2) Action potential for communication over long-distance. Graded potentials and action potentials occur because the membranes of neurons contain many different kinds of ion channels that allow specific charged particles to cross the membrane in response to an existing concentration gradient termed electrochemical gradient [32]. The ion channels can be classified based on the charge of the ions they transport; (1) *Cation channels* that most often allow sodium ions (Na^+) to pass when opened, but sometimes allow potassium (K^+) and/or calcium (Ca^{2+}) ions as well, and (2) *Anion channels* that allow mainly chloride ions (Cl^-) to pass but also minute quantities of other anions. Based on the mechanism of activation, ion channels are classified into four types: (1) A *ligand-gated channel* opens and closes in response to a specific chemical stimulus. A wide variety of chemical ligands including neurotransmitters, hormones, and particular ions can open or close ligand-gated channels. The neurotransmitter acetylcholine, for example, opens cation channels that allow Na^+ and Ca^{2+} to diffuse inward and K^+ to diffuse outward; (2) A *mechanically-gated channel* opens in response to a physical distortion of the cell membrane. Many channels associated with the sense of touch (somatosensation) are mechanically gated. Examples of mechanically gated channels are those found in auditory receptors in the ears, in receptors that monitor the stretching of internal organs, and in touch receptors and pressure receptors in the skin. (3) A *voltage-gated channel* is a channel that responds to changes in the electrical properties of the membrane in which it is embedded. Voltage-gated channels participate in the generation and conduction of action potentials. (4) A *leakage channel* is randomly gated. There is no actual event that opens the channel; instead, it has an intrinsic rate of switching between the open and closed states. Plasma membranes have many more K^+ leakage channels than Na^+ leakage channels, and the potassium ion leakage channels are leakier than the sodium ion leakage channels. Thus, the membrane's permeability to K^+ is much higher than its permeability to Na^+. Leakage channels contribute to the resting transmembrane voltage of the excitable membrane. The *resting membrane potential* of a neuron is -70mV which describes the steady-state of a cell which is a dynamic process that is balanced by ion transport across the membrane [30, 33].

Action Potential

An action potential or impulse is a sequence of rapidly occurring events that lead to depolarization and subsequent repolarization of the neuronal membrane (Fig. 5). In the presence of a stimulus, the voltage-gated Na^+ channels open and the ions rush into the cell driven by the concentration gradient. The potential difference rises from -70mV to 0mV to +30mV and is called the *depolarization phase*. This increase in voltage causes the opening of voltage-gated K^+ channels and ions to accelerate out of the cell and the simultaneous closure of Na^+. This causes the voltage to revert to -70mV and is called *repolarization*. Sometimes the K^+

channels open for a prolonged period leading to the plunge of the voltage to -90mV called the after-hyperpolarization phase. The voltage returns to -70mV resting potential once the K^+ channels close. An action potential occurs in the membrane of the axon of a neuron when depolarization reaches a certain level termed the *threshold* (about -55 mV) and the stimulus is termed threshold stimulus. While an action potential is in progress, another one cannot be initiated. That effect is referred to as the *refractory period*. There are two phases of the refractory period: the absolute refractory period and the relative refractory period. During the absolute phase, another action potential will not start. Once that channel is back to its resting conformation (less than -55 mV), a new action potential could be started, but only by a stronger stimulus than the one that initiated the current action potential. This is because of the flow of K^+ out of the cell. Because that ion is rushing out, any Na^+ that tries to enter will not depolarize the cell, but will only keep the cell from hyperpolarizing. This is termed as the *relative refractory period*. Action potentials maintain the strength of the signal by using positive feedback. This is called propagation. There are two types of propagation: continuous conduction and saltatory conduction. The type of action potential propagation described so far is continuous conduction, which involves step-by-step depolarization and repolarization of each adjacent segment of the plasma membrane. Action potential transmits more rapidly in myelinated axons because of the uneven distribution of voltage-gated Na^+/K^+ channels in the nodes of Ranvier where the signal jumps between the nodes due to resistance by myelin sheath. This mode of propagation is called saltatory conduction [30, 34].

Graded Potential

A graded potential is a small deviation from the membrane potential that makes the membrane either more polarized (hyperpolarizing graded potential) or less polarized (depolarizing graded potential). A graded potential is when ligand-gated or mechanically-gated ion channels open or close, hence they occur mainly in the dendrites and cell body of neurons where these channels are abundant. For the unipolar cells of sensory neurons, graded potentials develop in the dendrites that influence the generation of an action potential in the axon of the same cell and is called a generator potential. For other sensory receptor cells, such as taste cells or photoreceptors of the retina, graded potentials in their membranes result in the release of neurotransmitters at synapses with sensory neurons. This is called a receptor potential.

A postsynaptic potential (PSP) is the graded potential in the dendrites of a neuron that is receiving synapses from other cells. Postsynaptic potentials can be depolarizing or hyperpolarizing. Depolarization in a postsynaptic potential is called an excitatory postsynaptic potential (EPSP) because it causes the membrane potential to move towards the threshold. Hyperpolarization in a postsynaptic potential is an inhibitory postsynaptic potential (IPSP) because it causes the membrane potential to move away from the threshold. The graded potential can combine resulting in an additive effect or cancel each other in a process called summation. Graded potentials summate at a specific location at the beginning of the axon to initiate the action potential, namely the initial segment. For sensory neurons, which do not have a cell body between the dendrites and the axon, the initial segment is directly adjacent to the dendritic endings. For all other neurons, the axon hillock is essentially the initial segment of the axon, and it is where summation takes place. These locations have a high density of voltage-gated Na^+ channels that initiate the depolarizing phase of the action potential. A graded potential is decremental as the signal dies within a few of its point of origin making it useful for short communications only. In contrast to action potentials, graded potentials do not exhibit a refractory period [35].

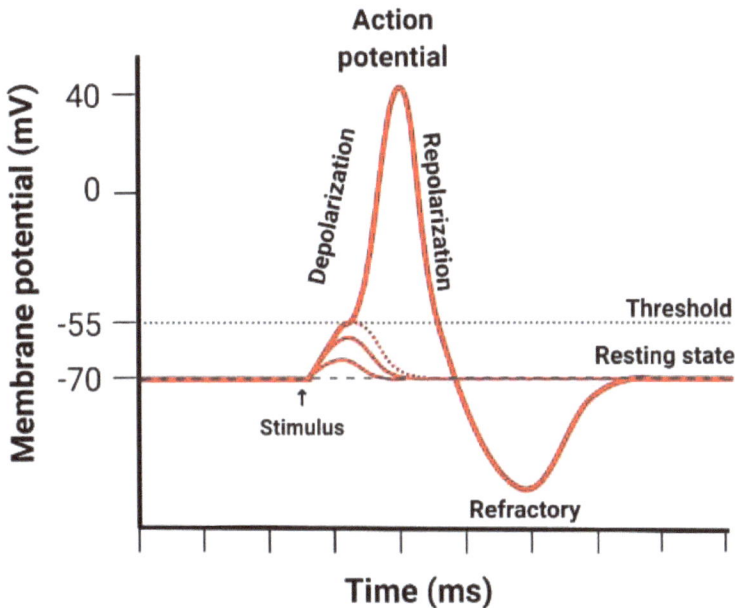

Fig. (5). Graph of Action Potential: Plotting voltage measured across the cell membrane against time, the action potential begins with depolarization, followed by repolarization, which goes past the resting potential into hyperpolarization, and finally the membrane returns to rest

Synapse

There are two types of synapses between electrically active cells: (1) Chemical synapses, (2) Electrical synapses.

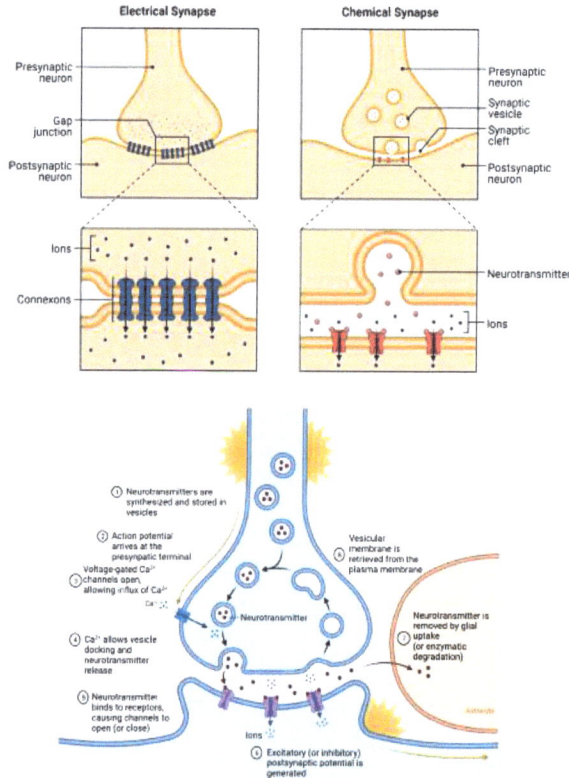

Fig. (6). The Synapse The synapse is a connection between a neuron and its target cell (which is not necessarily a neuron). Panel A (i) electrical synapse, (ii) Chemical synapse. Panel B The presynaptic element is the synaptic end bulb of the axon where Ca^{2+} enters the bulb to cause vesicle fusion and neurotransmitter release. The neurotransmitter diffuses across the synaptic cleft to bind to its receptor. The neurotransmitter is cleared from the synapse either by enzymatic degradation, neuronal reuptake, or glial reuptake.

Almost all synapses used for signal transduction in the CNS are chemical synapses. In chemical synapses, nerve impulses are transmitted between neurons by the release and binding of neurotransmitters to ligand-gated ion channels. The neurotransmitters can excite, inhibit or modify the target neuron depending on its functional activity. Some well-defined neurotransmitters are acetylcholine, serotonin, dopamine, GABA (Table **1**). At an electrical synapse, action potentials directly traverse the adjacent neuron through gap junctions. Electrical synapses lead to faster communication and synchronization [36].

Physiological Anatomy of A Synapse

The structure of a chemical synapse has been elucidated over many years of research and is considered a standard model of what defines a synapse (Fig. **6**). At a chemical synapse, the presynaptic neuron converts a nerve impulse into a chemical signal and the postsynaptic neuron converts this signal back to an electrical signal. The presynaptic terminal is separated from the postsynaptic membrane by a synaptic cleft of width 200-300 angstroms and is filled with interstitial fluid. These structures can be excitatory or inhibitory based on the neurotransmitters the presynaptic neurons synthesize and release. A typical chemical synapse transmits nerve impulses as follows: (1) A nerve impulse arrives at the presynaptic neuron, (2) The depolarization opens voltage-gated Ca^{2+} channels at the synaptic bulb, (3) The increase in intracellular Ca^{2+} triggers the exocytosis of synaptic vesicles harbouring neurotransmitters, (4) The neurotransmitters diffuse across the synaptic cleft and bind to the receptors on the postsynaptic membrane, (5) Ligand-gated ion channels open and the flow of ions changes the voltage across the membrane called postsynaptic potential (6) when the depolarizing potential reaches the threshold it activates action potential in the postsynaptic neuron [36, 37].

Table 1. Key central nervous system Neurotransmitters [38]

Classical	Amino Acids	Glutamate Glycine Aspartate GABA(γ-aminobutyric acid)
	Monoamines	Acetylcholine Dopamine Epinephrine Norepinephrine Serotonin
Neuropeptides	Opioids	Dynorphins Endorphins Enkephalins
	Tachykinins	Substance P
	Hormones	Cholecystokinin Somatostatin

BRAIN TUMOR (BT)

A brain tumor, known as intracranial tumor, occurs when an abnormal mass of cells forms within the brain. Brain tumors originate from the elements within the brain called *primary* or represent the spread of distant cancers called *metastatic*. Primary tumors arise from the CNS and account for roughly half of the intracranial tumors. Primary tumors are classified as glia (called gliomas which include astrocytomas, oligodendrogliomas, ependymomas, and medulloblastomas) or non- glial (from extraneural structures which include meningiomas, acoustic neuromas, and other schwannomas) as well as benign or malignant [39,

40]. Secondary brain tumors or metastatic tumors arise elsewhere in the body and migrate to the brain *via* the hematogenous dissemination through the arterial system and are ten times more common than primary tumors. About two-thirds of BT in children arise in the cerebellum and brainstem (infratentorial) and most BT in adults arise in the cerebrum (supratentorial) [41]. Most CNS tumors are thought to arise from individual cell mutations and transformations. Recent studies suggest that most gliomas and other tumors of the neural elements arise from the neural stem cells (NSCs). The genetic aberrations observed in brain tumors are the ones that regulate neurogenesis and gliogenesis (*e.g.* Nestin, EGFR, PTEN) hence suggesting a dysregulation in NSCs maintenance and renewal. Other factors include age; young children show a higher incidence of BT, radiation exposure; exposure of the head to radiation increases the predisposition to BT, Epstein-Barr virus, chemical carcinogenesis; most potent neurocarcinogens are nitroso compounds and vinyl chloride, and immunosuppression; cerebral lymphoma is common in individuals with a suppressed immune system like patients with HIV, renal transplants, congenital immunodeficiency syndrome. Inherited syndromes like neurofibromatosis, and tuberous sclerosis also increase the risk for the development of BT. Lung cancer is the most common solid tumor that causes brain metastases making up about half of the metastatic BT followed by breast, melanoma, and colon cancers [42, 43]. The World Health Organization (WHO) has developed a grading system to indicate malignancy or benignity of a tumor based on its histological features using four grades with grade I being the least malignant and grade IV the most malignant (Table **2**).

Table 2. World Health Organization (WHO) Brain Tumor Grades [44]

	Grade	Characteristics	Tumor Types
Low Grade	WHO Grade I	• Benign • Slow-growing • Non-infiltrative • Long-term survival • Curable *via* surgical resection	• Pilocytic astrocytoma • Craniopharyngioma
	WHO Grade II	• Relatively slow-growing • Mildly invasive • May recur as high grade	• Diffuse Astrocytoma • Oligodendroglioma
High Grade	WHO Grade III	• Malignant • Invasive • Aggressive • Recur as high grade	• Anaplastic astrocytoma • Anaplastic ependymoma • Anaplastic oligodendroglioma
	WHO Grade IV	• Highly malignant • Aggressive • Widely invasive • Rapid recurrence • Necrosis prone	• Glioblastoma multiforme • Medulloblastoma

Gliomas are the most prevalent type of adult brain tumor referring to all glial tumors in general (primarily glioblastoma, astrocytoma, oligodendroglioma, and ependymoma) [39, 45]. Some commonly occurring BT are discussed below:

- Astrocytomas are the most common gliomas comprising half of the reported cases of primary tumors and are most commonly observed in the cerebrum. Neoplastic astrocytes share the presence of intermediate cytoplasmic filaments, and glial fibrillary acidic protein (GFAP), with normal astrocytes the increase of which can be detected by immunohistochemistry. Astrocytomas are prevalent in adults- particularly middle-aged men. Low-grade astrocytomas are more frequent in young patients and high-grade astrocytomas in older ones. Astrocytes that develop tumorigenic alterations progress from low-grade diffuse astrocytoma (DA) to grade III anaplastic astrocytoma (AA) to secondary glioblastoma multiforme [46, 47].
- Glioblastoma multiforme (GBM) is the most invasive type of malignant BT. It accounts for 60% of all brain tumors in adults with an extremely poor prognosis of median survival of 14-15 months. Its most common sites are the frontal and temporal lobes, but it may occur at any age and involve any part of the CNS. Glioblastoma arises most commonly de novo (primary glioblastoma). Some glioblastomas arise by malignant transformation of low-grade astrocytomas (secondary glioblastoma). Ongoing and recent advances have demonstrated molecular correlates of these clinical definitions. Hallmark alterations of primary GBM include epidermal growth factor receptor (EGFR) gene mutation and amplification, overexpression of mouse double minute 2 (MDM2), deletion of p16, and loss of heterozygosity (LOH) of chromosome 10q holding phosphatase and tensin homolog (PTEN) and TERT promoter mutation. The characteristic features of secondary GBMs include overexpression of platelet-derived growth factor A, and platelet-derived growth factor receptor alpha (PDGFA/ PDGFRa), retinoblastoma (RB), LOH of 19q, and mutations of isocitrate dehydrogenase (IDH)1/2, TP53, and ATRX. Recent findings in paediatric GBM have proposed that there may exist a 3rd major category of GBM, different from primary and secondary GBM based on mutations in the histone H3F3 gene. Microscopically, glioblastoma shows high cellularity, cellular and nuclear anaplasia which is the basis of the designation "multiforme", mitoses, microvascular proliferation, and necrosis [47, 48].
- Pilocytic astrocytoma (PA) is histologically and biologically distinct astrocytoma and the most common primary BT in children. They commonly arise in the cerebellum, hypothalamus, optic chiasm, and brain stem. Pilocytic astrocytomas are circumscribed and often cystic with a solid mural nodule. Activation of BRAF and subsequent MAPK oncogenic signalling are involved

in the pathogenesis of PA. Histologically, they are sparsely cellular tumors without anaplasia or mitoses. They have a biphasic pattern, consisting of cellular and fibrillary perivascular areas, alternating with loose microcystic zones. Most PAs are biologically low grade and do not evolve into more malignant tumors. Surgical excision of cerebellar PA can sometimes result in a permanent cure [47, 49].

- Oligodendrogliomas constitute 5-6% of glioma. They are slow-growing tumors that arise usually in the cerebral hemispheres of middle-aged adults. Due to their tendency to calcify, it is helpful in radiological and histological diagnosis. Some oligodendrogliomas contain neoplastic astrocytes which are mixed with the oligodendroglial cells or grow in adjacent but separate areas. Such mixed tumors are called oligoastrocytomas. Oligodendrogliomas and oligoastrocytomas can be classified as low-grade (WHO grade II) or high-grade/anaplastic (WHO grade III) based on cellularity, anaplasia, mitotic activity, microvascular proliferation, and necrosis. The signature molecular change of oligodendroglioma is the co-deletion of entire arms of 1p and 19q caused by an unbalanced translocation. The 1p19q codeletion is specific to oligodendroglioma and serves as a diagnostic marker as well as predicts increased chemosensitivity and better prognosis [50, 51].

- Ependymoma occurs most frequently in the fourth ventricle and causes hydrocephalus by blocking the CSF flow. They are predominant in children and adolescents. Most ependymomas are well defined and grow in an exophytic fashion protruding into and out of the fourth ventricle. Ependymomas are graded as grade II or III according to the WHO system and account for 2-3% of all brain tumors. Most are low-grade (WHO grade II). Some have increased cellular density, mitoses, necrosis, and microvascular proliferation while retaining the typical ependymoma tissue pattern (anaplastic ependymoma, WHO grade III) [52].

- Choroid plexus tumors are classified as Choroid plexus carcinoma-CPC (WHO grade III) which is most common in very young children < 2 years, and choroid plexus papilloma-CPP (WHO grade I) which is seen in older patients. In children, CPP and CPC arise in both, lateral and fourth ventricles. In adults, CPP is infratentorial. CPP tumor resembles a normal choroid plexus, but is more cellular, with cuboidal and columnar epithelial cells resting on a fine fibrovascular stroma and is benign which can be cured by surgery. In CPC the tumor cells are multi-layered, atypical, and mitotic, and the papillary structure may be effaced such that the tumor appears solid and is malignant [47].

- Medulloblastomas are tumors of the cerebellum arising most frequently in the midline adjacent to the roof of the fourth ventricle and are frequent in children representing 20% of all BT. Medulloblastoma is an embryonal tumor of the brain, underlined by its high incidence in infants and children and by its undifferentiated, immature appearance, which resembles developing neural tissue. They are high-grade tumors but are usually responsive to radiation and chemotherapy. There are four histological variants of medulloblastomas: Classic, Desmoplastic/nodular (D/N), Medulloblastoma with extensive nodularity (MBEN), Large-cell/anaplastic. Medulloblastoma is highly malignant and leptomeningeal dissemination occurs more frequently than any other BT [52, 53].

- Schwannomas are commonly benign, slow-growing tumors in adults. Acoustic neuromas are the most common schwanomas (vestibular schwanoma), arise from the 8th cranial nerve root called the vestibular cochlear nerve that travels from the brain to the ear. They do not invade but rather displace the spinal cord and brain stem as they grow (extra-axial) [52].

- Meningiomas are the most common benign intracranial tumors. These tumors arise from the meninges, in particular arachnoid cells. Most meningiomas are benign and grow slowly. They are also extra-axial like schwannomas. The majority of meningiomas show complete loss of chromosome 22 or 22q which contain the tumor suppressor gene merlin. Because they are extra-axial, complete resection is possible and may be curative [52].

- Pituitary adenomas arise from the adenohypophysis and makeup about 10% of all intracranial tumors. They are mostly benign and slow-growing. Adenomas are the most common disease that affects the pituitary and is seen in individuals in their 3rd and 4th decade [52].

- Hemangioblastomas are infrequent vascular tumors of the CNS commonly seen in the cerebellum. About 75% are sporadic and the rest are familial and occur in the background of the autosomal dominant von Hippel Lindau disease. Sporadic tumors are solitary and affect most frequently middle-aged adults but may occur at any age. Typically, the cerebellar hemangioblastoma is a mural nodule within a cyst [52].

- Other less common tumors include Chondroma, Craniopharyngioma, Rhabdoid tumors [52].

Pathophysiology of BT

Tumors of the brain produce neurologic manifestations through several mechanisms. The general effects of brain tumors have to do mainly with the increased intracranial pressure (ICP) caused by the growth of the intracranial tumor with accompanying cerebral edema in the limited volume of the cranial cavity. Tumors adjacent to the ventricles may obstruct the circulation of the CSF thus causing hydrocephalus. The high vascularity of rapidly growing tumors disrupt the BBB and promote edema. ICP is life-threatening causing displacements (herniations) of brain tissue under the falx cerebri through tentorium cerebelli, or the foramen magnum. and compression of brain structures with lethal effects [47, 54, 55].

Signs and Symptoms of BT

Symptoms of a brain lesion depend on what part of the brain is affected. General symptoms of BT include [52, 54 - 56]:

- Headaches that are usually non-specific and resemble tension-type headaches. Pain is worsened in the morning and is accompanied by nausea or vomiting.
- Deterioration in the mental status like drowsiness, lethargy, personality changes, impaired cognition.
- Focal brain dysfunction: development of focal deficits often suggests the tumors' location.
- Seizures or convulsions
- Impaired consciousness

Specific Symptoms include [56]

- **Frontal lobe:** tumors may cause emotional and behavioural changes; impaired judgment; an impaired sense of smell or vision loss; speech impairment (Broca's area); partial paralysis.
- **Parietal lobe:** tumors may cause poor spatial and visual perception; poor interpretation of languages; lack of recognition; writing, drawing, naming difficulties.
- **Occipital lobe:** tumors may lead to partial or complete vision loss; visual field cuts; illusions and hallucinations.
- **Temporal lobe:** tumors may cause difficulty in language comprehension (Wernicke's area); poor memory; loss of hearing.
- **Brainstem:** tumors can cause seizures; muscle weakness on one side of the body and face; uncoordinated gait.
- **Cerebellum:** tumors may cause poor balance, muscle movements, and posture.
- **Pituitary gland:** tumors may cause increased secretion of hormones; decreased libido; abnormal menstruation and milk production.

Diagnosis Therapy

- **Neurologic exam:** to test for changes in balance, coordination, hearing, vision, mental status that can pinpoint the location of a tumor.
- **Blood test:** to check for tumor markers *e.g.*, increase in endocrine hormones caused by pituitary tumors.

- **Imaging techniques:** Diagnostic tools include computed tomography (CT) and magnetic resonance imaging (MRI). CT with contrast agent is the imaging modality of choice of emergency physicians where tumors show enhancement and appear in varying densities. Gadolinium-enhanced MRI can detect low-grade tumors like astrocytomas and oligodendrogliomas earlier than CT. MRI is also efficient in detecting tumors of the posterior fossa. Positron emission tomography (PET) can detect recurring tumors.
- **Biopsy:** A biopsy can show cancer, changes in tissues, and other conditions. It is the only way to identify details of a tumor including its pace of growth and whether it is malignant. A biopsy can be done as part of an open surgical procedure to remove a tumor or as a separate diagnostic procedure known as needle biopsy.
- Spinal tap lumbar puncture collects CSF from the spinal cord which is checked for the presence of cancer cells that can indicate malignancy in the CNS.
- Molecular testing of tumors to test for specific gene proteins or other tumor markers unique to the tumors. *e.g.*, 1p/19q co-deletion in oligodendrogliomas, IDH mutations in gliomas, MGMT mutations in glioblastomas.
- **Surgery:** Surgery is the most desired course of action for the treatment of brain tumors. The introduction of surgical navigation systems has increased the efficiency of tumor removal (resection) with reduced risks. This procedure is limited by the accessibility of the tumor and the dependence on a pre-procedure MRI/CT scan. Intraoperative language mapping is a procedure done on conscious patients having tumors affecting their language areas like large dominant-hemisphere gliomas to monitor the anatomy of their language functions. Ventriculoperitoneal shunting is opted by neurosurgeons to control hydrocephalus and resultant ICP. In this procedure, a permanent shunt is used to divert the CSF to the peritoneal cavity.
- **Radiation therapy:** Radiation therapy is opted for when the tumor is inaccessible by surgery, or when the tumor is low-grade or metastatic. The procedure employs focused high-energy X-rays to kill tumor cells by damaging the DNA. Radiation therapy is most effective in aggressive tumors. The radiation is applied to the tumors externally or internally. Standard External Beam Radiotherapy uses a variety of high-energy radiation beams to form a conformal coverage of the tumor while limiting the dosage to surrounding tissues. This treatment requires 10-30 sittings where standard-dose fractions of radiation are applied to the brain. Proton beam therapy delivers accelerated proton beams to tumors. This method is used in children as it incurs minimum damage to surrounding normal structures. Stereotactic radiosurgery methods like Gamma knife, Cyberknife, and Novalis use computerized calculations to deliver a single high-energy dose of radiation to the target tumor. Internal radiation (brachytherapy), is where radioactive implants are placed inside an empty tumor

cavity after surgery to kill any remaining malignant cells.

- **Chemotherapy:** Chemotherapy is the preferred treatment for paediatric tumors as it is less toxic to the developing brain than radiation. Chemotherapy has been proved to increase overall survival in patients with the most aggressive and malignant primary brain tumors. Chemotherapy functions by interfering with the DNA damage repair mechanisms in tumor cells (*e.g.* oral administration of temozolomide or TMZ, an alkylating agent, concomitant with radiation therapy is considered standard of care for patients of GBM) Resistance to chemotherapy occurs when the tumors are insensitive to a drug (*e.g.* TP73 AS1 promote TMZ resistance in GBM by facilitating the expression of detoxifying enzyme ALDH1A) or when the drug cannot cross the BBB which is one of the major challenges in treating intracranial brain tumors [57, 58]. Chemotherapeutic drugs are administered orally or intravenously alongside radiation therapy (Table **3**). In certain high-grade gliomas, wafers carrying the drug is implanted directly into the tumor where the drug over several weeks diffuses into the tumor. IDH1 and IDH2 mutations in gliomas, as well as deletion of chromosome arms 1p and 19q, generally indicate better prognosis and effectiveness of chemotherapy.
- **Laser Ablation Therapy:** This involves placing a tiny catheter within the tumor after biopsy by employing a real-time MRI and thermally ablating the tumor using a laser [48, 52, 54 - 56].

Some medications are used in relieving the symptoms of BT namely: corticosteroids to stabilize cell membrane and diminish the vasogenic edema associated with tumors, *e.g.*, Dexamethasone; Hyperosmolar agents reduce ICP and edema by creating an osmotic gradient across the intact BBB, *e.g.*, Mannitol [41].

Table 3. Commonly used chemotherapeutic agents in BT [48, 55]

Agents	Brain tumor type	Target	Route of Administration	Side Effects
Carmustine	Malignant Glioma	Crosslinks DNA, RNA Modifies glutathione reductase	Intravenous infusion	Nausea, myelosuppression, pulmonary fibrosis
Lomustine	Malignant Glioma, Oligodendroglioma, Adult Low-Grade Infiltrative Supratentorial Astrocytoma/Oligodendroglioma (Excluding Pilocytic Astrocytoma), Glioblastoma, Primitive neuroectodermal tumors, Adult Medulloblastoma	Crosslinks DNA, RNA	Oral	Nausea, myelosuppression, pulmonary fibrosis

(Table 3) cont.....

Agents	Brain tumor type	Target	Route of Administration	Side Effects
Temozolomide	Malignant Glioma, Adult Low-Grade Infiltrative Supratentorial Astrocytoma /Oligodendroglioma (Excluding Pilocytic Astrocytoma), Glioblastoma, Primary CNS Lymphoma.	Crosslinks DNA, RNA	Oral	Nausea, fatigue, headache, constipation, myelosuppression
Vincristine	Oligodendroglioma, Glioblastoma, Primary CNS Lymphoma, Primitive neuroectodermal tumors, Adult Medulloblastoma	Inhibits microtubule structures	Intravenous	Peripheral neuropathy, constipation
Cisplatin	Malignant Glioma, Primitive neuroectodermal tumors, Adult Low-Grade Infiltrative Supratentorial Astrocytoma /Oligodendroglioma (Excluding Pilocytic Astrocytoma), Adult Medulloblastoma.	Crosslinks DNA	Intravenous	Nausea, renal Insufficiency, peripheral Neuropathy, myelosuppression
Bevacizumab	Anaplastic Gliomas, Glioblastoma	Selectively bind VEGF	Intravenous	Bleeding gums, body pain, burning, tingling, numbness, chest pain, chills, convulsions, cough, cracks in the skin, difficult breathing, dilated neck veins
Etoposide	Adult Low-Grade Infiltrative Supratentorial Astrocytoma/Oligodendroglioma (Excluding Pilocytic Astrocytoma), Anaplastic Gliomas, Primitive neuroectodermal tumors, Adult Medulloblastoma	Crosslinks DNA and topoisomerase II	Intravenous	Cough, difficulty in swallowing, dizziness, rapid heartbeat, headache, Itching, nervousness, numbness, puffiness or swelling of the eyelids or around the eyes, face, lips, or tongue, sweating
Procarbazine	Adult Low-Grade Infiltrative Supratentorial Astrocytoma/Oligodendroglioma, Anaplastic Gliomas, Glioblastoma, Primary CNS Lymphoma	Interferes with protein translation	Oral	Confusion, convulsions, tiredness, hallucinations, shortness of breath, thick bronchial secretions

Complications

Although with modern dosing regimens and concomitant use of corticosteroids, acute radiation toxicity rarely occurs, certain delayed neurotoxic effects may occur post radiation therapy. Subacute encephalopathy or early-delayed neurotoxicity occurs 6-16 weeks after radiation. Late-delayed neurotoxicity occurs when patients have survived long enough. Chronic effects of prolonged radiation exposure can lead to intellectual disabilities to complete incapacity. The BBB hindrance on chemotherapeutic drugs can result in the circulation of the drugs in the system thereby causing non-specific cytotoxicity [54].

Investigative Therapies

Glioblastoma multiforme and anaplastic astrocytomas are aggressive and lethal cancers. They are refractory to conventional therapies such as surgical resection, radiation, and chemotherapy. Much research is being conducted to treat such cancers with a poor prognosis. Immunotherapy and gene therapy are at the forefront of investigational therapies [52]. Neuro-onco-immunotherapy includes (1) Nonspecific methods using adjuvants, lymphokine-activated killer cells, or gene-modified tumor cells; (2) Specific immunotherapy utilizing monoclonal antibodies, tumor-infiltrating lymphocytes, allogeneic reactive T cells, chimeric antigen-redirected T cells, purified and cloned tumor antigens used either alone or in combination with *in vitro* cultured dendritic cells (DCs) [59]. Transgenes under investigation for brain tumor therapy include prodrug activating genes (suicide genes), intracellular signalling molecules, immune modulators, and inhibitors of angiogenesis and cell invasion [60]. Radioimmunotherapy is another attractive strategy for targeting BT because of its potential for selective irradiation. Many studies are involved in clinical trials investigating its therapeutic potential. Monoclonal antibodies labelled with β-emitters ^{131}I, ^{90}Y, or α-emitters [211]At that specifically target BT are being developed. Tenascin C (a glycoprotein expressed by 90% of GBM extracellular matrix) is the target being studied to treat both recurring and newly diagnosed brain tumors. The initial clinical studies show promising results with the need for optimization of radionuclides, carrier molecules, and delivery methods for improved efficacy [61].

FUTURE DIRECTIONS

The challenges that BBB poses for the effective delivery of chemotherapeutic drugs to BT and non-specific cytotoxicity of circulating drugs demand the need to innovate the methods of targeting and delivery of drugs to BT [57, 62]. The 'leaky' vasculature of GBM tumors due to angiogenesis results in an enhanced permeation retention effect (EPR). Particles smaller than 100nm can cross tumor vasculature and greater than 20nm is retained within the tumor. Research in nanoparticle-mediated targeted delivery and nanomedicine exploits this feature to develop efficient therapy for BT [63]. Nanoparticle-mediated targeted delivery of drugs can significantly reduce the dosage and optimize their release properties, increase specificity and bioavailability, improve shelf-life, and reduce toxicity [64]. Recently, Lahann's team from the University of Michigan reported that synthetic human serum albumin attached the STAT3 inhibitor and a peptide called iRGD, which serves as a tumor homing device was able to eradicate recurring brain tumors in mice [65]. The future of using nanotechnology to combat brain tumors looks promising, as there are now both academic and commercial developments being made that will hopefully ensure that people with brain tumors have a better chance of survival [66, 67].

CONCLUSION

The complexity of the nervous system remains elusive and ambiguous. Although significant progress has been made in experimental techniques, the human cognition functions that emerge from neuronal networks is not entirely understood. Out of all the brain carcinogenesis, GBM remains incurable due to its heterogeneity and complex pathogenesis and no therapy has shown any promise to improve life expectancy. A priori knowledge of cytogenetic alterations in tumors is now being incorporated into therapeutic selection algorithms with treatments specific to a tumor subtype. To date, there is a relative scarcity of effective research in oncology, but this is expected to change with rising controls on healthcare expenditures. Continued focused research in developing better and efficient treatment options to combat life-threatening tumors should be promoted.

ACKNOWLEDGEMENTS

Figs. created with BioRender.com

REFERENCES

[1]   Tortora GJ, Derrickson B. Organization of the Nervous System Principles of Anatomy and Physiology. 12th ed. New Jersey: John Wiley & Sons, Inc. 2009; pp. 425-6.

[2]   Betts JG, Young KA, Wise JA, Johnson E, Poe B, Kruse DH, *et al.* Basic Structure and Function of the Nervous System 2013.https://openstax.org/books/anatomy-and-physiology/pages/12-1-b-sic-structure-and-function-of-the-nervous-system

[3]   Ludwig PE, Reddy V, Varacallo M. Neuroanatomy, Central Nervous System (CNS) StatPearls [Internet]: Treasure Island (FL): StatPearls Publishing; 2020. https://www.ncbi.nlm.nih.gov/books/ NBK442010/

[4]   Maldonado KA, Alsayouri K. Physiology, Brain StatPearls [Internet]: Treasure Island (FL): StatPearls Publishing; 2021. https://www.ncbi.nlm.nih.gov/books/NBK551718/

[5]   Tortora GJ, Derrickson B. Brain Organization, Protection, and Blood Supply Principles of Anatomy and Physiology. 12th ed. New Jersey: John Wiley and Sons, Inc. 2009; pp. 496-9.

[6]   Scanlon VC, Sanders T. Meninges and Cerebrospinal fluid Essentials of Anatomy and Physiology. 5th ed. Philadelphia: F.A. Davis Company 2007; pp. 184-5.

[7]   Betts JG, Young KA, Wise JA, Johnson E, Poe B, Kruse DH, *et al.* The Central Nervous System 2013.https://openstax.org/books/anatomy-and-physiology/pages/13-2-the-central-nervous-system

[8]   Chayer C, Freedman M. Frontal lobe functions. Curr Neurol Neurosci Rep 2001; 1(6): 547-52. [http://dx.doi.org/10.1007/s11910-001-0060-4] [PMID: 11898568]

[9]   Scanlon VC, Sanders T. The Brain Essentials of Anatomy and Physiology. 5th ed. Philadelphia: F.A. Davis Company 2007; pp. 180-1.

[10]   Scanlon VC, Sanders T. The Brain Essentials of Anatomy and Physiology. 5th ed. Philadelphia: F.A. Davis Company 2007; pp. 181-2.

[11]   Nielsen SE, Herrera AY. Sex Steroids, Learning and Memory. In: Donald W. Pfaff MJ, editor. Hormones, Brain and Behavior. 3 ed. Los Angeles: Academic Press; 2017. p. 399-422.

[12]   Tortora GJ, Derrickson B. The Brain Stem Principles of Anatomy and Physiology. 12th ed. New Jersey: John Wiley & Sons, Inc. 2009; pp. 503-7.

[13]   Tortora GJ, Derrickson B. Cerebellum Principles of Anatomy and Physiology. 12th ed. New Jersey: John Wiley & Sons, Inc. 2009; pp. 507-10.

[14]   Betts JG, Young KA, Wise JA, Johnson E, Poe B, Kruse DH, *et al.* Circulation and the Central Nervous System 2013.https://openstax.org/books/anatomy-and-physiology/pages/13-3-circula-ion-and-the-central-nervous-system

[15]   Hines T. Anatomy of the Brain: Mayfield Clinic; 2018 [Available from: https://mayfieldclinic.com/pe-anatbrain.htm]

[16]   Tortora GJ, Derrickson B. The Systemic Circulation Principles of Anatomy and Physiology. 12th ed. New Jersey: John Wiley & Sons, Inc. 2009; pp. 804-5.

[17]   Tortora GJ, Derrickson B. Cerebrospinal Fluid Principles of Anatomy and Physiology. 12th ed. New Jersey: John Wiley & Sons, Inc. 2009; pp. 499-503.

[18]   Chow BW, Gu C. The molecular constituents of the blood-brain barrier. Trends Neurosci 2015; 38(10): 598-608. [http://dx.doi.org/10.1016/j.tins.2015.08.003] [PMID: 26442694]

[19]   Bacyinski A, Xu M, Wang W, Hu J. The Paravascular Pathway for Brain Waste Clearance: Current Understanding, Significance and Controversy. Front Neuroanat 2017; 11(101): 101. [http://dx.doi.org/10.3389/fnana.2017.00101] [PMID: 29163074]

[20]   Betts JG, Young KA, Wise JA, Johnson E, Poe B, Kruse DH, *et al.* Nervous Tissue 2013.https://openstax.org/books/anatomy-and-physiology/pages/12-2-nervous-tissue

[21]   Lodish H, Berk A, Zipursky SL. Overview of Neuron Structure and Function 2000.https://www.ncbi.nlm.nih.gov/books/NBK21535/

[22]   Tortora GJ, Derrickson B. Histology of Nervous Tissue Principles of Anatomy and Physiology. 12th ed. New Jersey: John Wiley & Sons, Inc. 2009; pp. 417-21.

[23]   Tortora GJ, Derrickson B. Histology of Nervous Tissue Principles of Anatomy and Physiology. 12th ed. New Jersey: John Wiley & Sons, Inc. 2009; pp. 421-2.

[24]   Siracusa R, Fusco R, Cuzzocrea S. Astrocytes: Role and Functions in Brain Pathologies. Front Pharmacol 2019; 10(1114): 1114. [http://dx.doi.org/10.3389/fphar.2019.01114] [PMID: 31611796]

[25]   Sofroniew MV, Vinters HV. Astrocytes: biology and pathology. Acta Neuropathol 2010; 119(1): 7-35. [http://dx.doi.org/10.1007/s00401-009-0619-8] [PMID: 20012068]

[26]   Ginhoux F, Lim S, Hoeffel G, Low D, Huber T. Origin and differentiation of microglia. Front Cell

Neurosci 2013; 7: 45.
[http://dx.doi.org/10.3389/fncel.2013.00045] [PMID: 23616747]

[27]   Ackerman S. The Development and Shaping of the Brain.Discovering the Brain. Washington: National Academies Press 1992.https://www.ncbi.nlm.nih.gov/books/NBK234146/ Internet

[28]   Betts JG, Young KA, Wise JA, Johnson E, Poe B, Kruse DH, *et al.* The Embryologic Perspective 2013.https://openstax.org/books/anatomy-and-physiology/pages/13-1-the-embryologic-perspective

[29]   Gilbert SF. The central nervous system and the epidermis Developmental Biology. 6th ed., Sunderland: Sinauer Associates 2000.

[30]   Betts JG, Young KA, Wise JA, Johnson E, Poe B, Kruse DH, *et al.* The Action Potential 2013.https://openstax.org/books/anatomy-and-physiology/pages/12-4-the-action-potential

[31]   Sundberg DK, Spencer RF. Ion Channels and Electrical Signaling.Neuroscience in Medicine. 2nd ed., New Jersey: Humana Press Inc. 2003.

[32]   Tortora GJ, Derrickson B. Electrical signals in Neurons Principles of Anatomy and Physiology. 12th ed. New Jersey: John Wiley & Sons, Inc. 2009; pp. 426-8.

[33]   Tortora GJ, Derrickson B. Electrical signals in Neurons Principles of Anatomy and Physiology. 12th ed. New Jersey: John Wiley & Sons, Inc. 2009; pp. 428-31.

[34]   Tortora GJ, Derrickson B. Electrical signals in Neurons Principles of Anatomy and Physiology. 12th ed. New Jersey: John Wiley & Sons, Inc. 2009; pp. 434-9.

[35]   Tortora GJ, Derrickson B. Electrical signals in Neurons Principles of Anatomy and Physiology. 12th ed. New Jersey: John Wiley & Sons, Inc. 2009; pp. 432-4.

[36]   Betts JG, Young KA, Wise JA, Johnson E, Poe B, Kruse DH, *et al.* Communication Between Neurons 2013.https://openstax.org/books/anatomy-and-physiology/pages/12-5-communication-be-ween-neurons

[37]   Tortora GJ, Derrickson B. Signal Transmission at Synapses Principles of Anatomy and Physiology. 12th ed. New Jersey: John Wiley & Sons, Inc. 2009; pp. 441-2.

[38]   Tortora GJ, Derrickson B. Neurotransmitters Principles of Anatomy and Physiology. 12th ed. New Jersey: John Wiley & Sons, Inc. 2009; pp. 448-51.

[39]   Lapointe S, Perry A, Butowski NA. Primary brain tumours in adults. Lancet 2018; 392(10145): 432-46.
[http://dx.doi.org/10.1016/S0140-6736(18)30990-5] [PMID: 30060998]

[40]   Perkins A, Liu G. Primary Brain Tumors in Adults: Diagnosis and Treatment. Am Fam Physician 2016; 93(3): 211-7.
[PMID: 26926614]

[41]   Lo BM. Brain Neoplasms: WebMD LLC.; 2019 Jan 2 [Available from: https://emedicine.medscape.com/article/779664-overview

[42]   Focusing on brain tumours and brain metastasis. Nat Rev Cancer 2020; 20(1): 1-1.
[http://dx.doi.org/10.1038/s41568-019-0232-7] [PMID: 31863025]

[43]   Boire A, Brastianos PK, Garzia L, Valiente M. Brain metastasis. Nat Rev Cancer 2020; 20(1): 4-11.
[http://dx.doi.org/10.1038/s41568-019-0220-y] [PMID: 31780784]

[44]   Louis DN, Perry A, Reifenberger G, *et al.* The 2016 World Health Organization Classification of Tumors of the Central Nervous System: a summary. Acta Neuropathol 2016; 131(6): 803-20.
[http://dx.doi.org/10.1007/s00401-016-1545-1] [PMID: 27157931]

[45]   Weller M, Wick W, Aldape K, *et al.* Glioma. Nat Rev Dis Primers 2015; 1(1): 15017.
[http://dx.doi.org/10.1038/nrdp.2015.17] [PMID: 27188790]

[46]   Kapoor M, Gupta V. Astrocytoma StatPearls [Internet]: Treasure Island (FL): StatPearls Publishing; 2021 Jan [updated 2021 July 21. Available from: https://www.ncbi.nlm.nih.gov/books/NBK559042/

[47]   Agamanolis DP. Tumors of the Central Nervous System [updated 2021 Feb. Available from: https://neuropathology-web.org/chapter7/chapter7aTumorsgeneral.html

[48]   Hanif F, Muzaffar K, Perveen K, Malhi SM, Simjee ShU. Glioblastoma Multiforme: A Review of its Epidemiology and Pathogenesis through Clinical Presentation and Treatment. Asian Pac J Cancer Prev 2017; 18(1): 3-9.
[PMID: 28239999]

[49]   Rodriguez FJ, Lim KS, Bowers D, Eberhart CG. Pathological and molecular advances in pediatric low-grade astrocytoma. Annu Rev Pathol 2013; 8(1): 361-79.
[http://dx.doi.org/10.1146/annurev-pathol-020712-164009] [PMID: 23121055]

[50]   Rodriguez FJ, Giannini C. Oligodendroglial tumors: diagnostic and molecular pathology. Semin Diagn Pathol 2010; 27(2): 136-45.
[http://dx.doi.org/10.1053/j.semdp.2010.05.001] [PMID: 20860317]

[51]   Wesseling P, van den Bent M, Perry A. Oligodendroglioma: pathology, molecular mechanisms and markers. Acta Neuropathol 2015; 129(6): 809-27.
[http://dx.doi.org/10.1007/s00401-015-1424-1] [PMID: 25943885]

[52]   Tumors B. American Association of Neurological Surgeons. 2021. [Available from: https://www.aans.org/en/Patients/Neurosurgical-Conditions-and-Treatments/Brain-Tumors

[53]   Orr BA. Pathology, diagnostics, and classification of medulloblastoma. Brain Pathol 2020; 30(3): 664-78.
[http://dx.doi.org/10.1111/bpa.12837] [PMID: 32239782]

[54]   Goldman SA. Overview of Intracranial Tumors: Merck Sharp & Dohme Corp.; 2021 [Available from: https://www.msdmanuals.com/en-in/professional/neurologic-disorders/intracranial-and-sp-nal-tumors/overview-of-intracranial-tumors

[55]   Tumor B. American Society of Clinical Oncology 2021.https://www.cancer.net/cancer-types/brai--tumor

[56]   Brain tumors: an introduction: Mayfield Clinic; 2018 [Available from: https://mayfieldclinic.com/pe-braintumor.htm

[57]   Aldape K, Brindle KM, Chesler L, *et al.* Challenges to curing primary brain tumours. Nat Rev Clin Oncol 2019; 16(8): 509-20.
[http://dx.doi.org/10.1038/s41571-019-0177-5] [PMID: 30733593]

[58]   Mazor G, Levin L, Picard D, *et al.* The lncRNA TP73-AS1 is linked to aggressiveness in glioblastoma and promotes temozolomide resistance in glioblastoma cancer stem cells. Cell Death Dis 2019; 10(3): 246.
[http://dx.doi.org/10.1038/s41419-019-1477-5] [PMID: 30867410]

[59]   Ge L, Hoa N, Bota DA, Natividad J, Howat A, Jadus MR. Immunotherapy of brain cancers: the past, the present, and future directions. Clin Dev Immunol 2010; 2010: 1-19.
[http://dx.doi.org/10.1155/2010/296453] [PMID: 21437175]

[60]   Lawler SE, Peruzzi PP, Chiocca EA. Genetic strategies for brain tumor therapy. Cancer Gene Ther 2006; 13(3): 225-33.
[http://dx.doi.org/10.1038/sj.cgt.7700886] [PMID: 16138122]

[61]   Zalutsky MR. Current status of therapy of solid tumors: brain tumor therapy. J Nucl Med 2005; 46 (Suppl. 1): 151S-6S.
[PMID: 15653663]

[62]   Fisusi FA, Schätzlein AG, Uchegbu IF. Nanomedicines in the treatment of brain tumors. Nanomedicine (Lond) 2018; 13(6): 579-83.

[http://dx.doi.org/10.2217/nnm-2017-0378] [PMID: 29376468]

[63]   Tzeng SY, Green JJ. Therapeutic nanomedicine for brain cancer. Ther Deliv 2013; 4(6): 687-704.
        [http://dx.doi.org/10.4155/tde.13.38] [PMID: 23738667]

[64]   Cerna T, Stiborova M, Adam V, Kizek R, Eckschlager T. Nanocarrier drugs in the treatment of brain
        tumors. J Cancer Metastasis Treat 2016; 2(10): 407-16.
        [http://dx.doi.org/10.20517/2394-4722.2015.95]

[65]   Kadiyala P, Gregory JV, Lowenstein PR, Lahann J, Castro MG. Targeting gliomas with STAT3-
        silencing nanoparticles. Mol Cell Oncol 2021; 8(2): 1870647-47.
        [http://dx.doi.org/10.1080/23723556.2020.1870647] [PMID: 33855166]

[66]   Arami H, Patel CB, Madsen SJ, *et al.* Nanomedicine for Spontaneous Brain Tumors: A Companion
        Clinical Trial. ACS Nano 2019; 13(3): 2858-69.
        [http://dx.doi.org/10.1021/acsnano.8b04406] [PMID: 30714717]

[67]   Critchley L. Nanotechnology in Cancer Research: The Future of Brain Tumor Treatment.: AZoNano;
        2020 May 13 [Available from: https://www.azonano.com/article.aspx?ArticleID=5493

CHAPTER 2

Barriers to Targeted Drug Delivery Strategies in Brain

Payal Kesharwani[1,2]**, Kajal Kumari**[1]**, Smita Jain**[1] **and Swapnil Sharma**[1,*]

[1] *Department of Pharmacy, Banasthali University, P.O. Rajasthan, India*

[2] *Rameesh Institute of Vocational and Technical Education, Greater Noida, India*

Abstract: Brain tumor is considered to be the most detrimental disease found in humans. Amongst the various brain tumors, glioblastoma has emerged as a highly invasive malignant disease that has contributed to significant mortality worldwide. Despite surgical and drug innovations, most of the patients suffering from brain tumours have shown poor prognosis, with a median life span. The presence of the blood-brain barrier (BBB) acts as a protective layer outside the brain for most of the conventional, diagnostic and therapeutic agents, which in turn leads to poor diagnosis and less efficacy in most clinical subjects. In recent years, multifunctional nanotechnology systems have been employed to deliver theranostic agents to the brain, showing promising outcomes in the treatment of various forms of cancer. The present chapter provides comprehensive information on the most recent developments in BBB-crossing nanotechnology, with a slight focus on the thoughtful design of multifunctional nanoplatforms for effective BBB penetration, accurate tumor imaging, and substantial brain tumor inhibition. Besides, various physiological barriers and transportation mechanisms, different drug delivery systems for brain tumors are also highlighted. Furthermore, major advancements in brain tumor theranostics pertaining to employing different nanosystems such as liposomes, polymeric nanoparticles, bio-nano particles, and inorganic-nanoparticles for effective nano-drug delivery for theranostics in brain tumors have also been discussed.

Keywords: Blood-brain barrier, Brain tumour, Nanotechnology, Stimuli-responsive, Theranostic.

INTRODUCTION

The brain is the most sophisticated organ of the human body. Several ailments of the brain, such as encephalitis, neurological disorders, multiple sclerosis, stroke, and tumor, have no effective therapy to date [1]. Brain tumor is one of the most atrocious kinds of cancer among numerous cancer types due to its poor prognosis,

---

*[*] **Corresponding Author Swapnil Sharma:** Department of Pharmacy, Banasthali University, P.O. Rajasthan, India; E-mail: skspharmacology@gmail.com

Ram Kumar Sahu (Ed.)

aggressive nature, and large number of deaths observed among kids and adults every year. According to the latest survey by WHO, 86,000 people were diagnosed with a brain tumor, and 700,000 people are suffering from the same [2]. There are two classes of brain tumors: primary brain tumor which grows in the brain itself and secondary brain tumor which migrates to the brain from other organs of the body [1]. Among all the available treatments for a brain tumor, Radiotherapy and Chemotherapy are the most often used. However, there are significant flaws associated with chemotherapy which include poor quality of life and limited duration of response. Due to the variety of factors involved in cancer therapy, treating the tumor with an anticancer drug has become quite challenging [3, 4]. The distribution of drugs to the brain tissues is challenging due to the robust protection that exists immediately outside the brain, anatomically known as the blood-brain barrier (BBB), protecting it from shock. It restricts the passage of anticancer drugs hydrophilic in nature and diagnostic agents into the brain and shows its effectiveness. This generates the need for an effective strategy for delivery of drugs to the brain cells [5].

Recently, scientists are focused more on the development of a delivery system that effectively delivers drugs to the tumour cells and benefits the cancer patient. The nanostructured drug delivery system has recently gained attention for transporting drugs to tumour cells and tissues present at the tumour site of the brain and avoiding damage caused to the normal tissue nearby. Altogether they perform two important functions, the first is the therapy to the tumour site and the second is its diagnosis [6]. They can transport therapeutic compounds across the BBB, such as tiny chemicals, proteins, peptides, and genetic material [1]. The new drug delivery system includes a combination of drugs and molecular imagining probes such as metal nanoparticles (NPs), polymer-drug conjugates, polymer micelles, liposomes, and dendrimers [7].

Theranostic application is also used bringing a new opportunity to bridle the hurdles faced in the current treatment/therapy of brain tumors [1]. It requires the usage of molecular imagining tools along with a drug delivery system. The molecular imagining tools include computed tomography (CT), magnetic resonance imaging (MRI), optical and ultrasound (US) imaging, positron emission tomography (PET), and single-photon emission computed tomography (SPECT), which are currently under study with drug delivery system. The theranostic approach uses sensible and specific probes which help to achieve the specific therapeutic application [7]. Despite significant attempts to create diagnostic tools and therapeutic avenues in the field of brain cancer therapy and its diagnosis, researchers and scientists face significant difficulty. This Chapter aids in the comprehension of various barriers and transportation mechanisms for drug delivery to brain tumors. It also focuses on major advancement in brain tumor theranostic: A description of the creation of different nanosystems such as Liposomes, Polymeric Nanoparticles, Bio-nanoparticles, and Inorganic-nanoparticles for effective nano-drug delivery for theranostic in brain tumors.

BRAIN TUMOUR: CAUSE, SYMPTOMS, CATEGORY, AND LIMITATIONS OF CONVENTIONAL THERAPY

Brain Tumour: Cause and Symptoms

The term "Brain tumor" refers to a group of primary and metastatic neoplasms that affect the central nervous system (CNS) and have a poor prognosis and survival rate [6]. The CNS consists of the brain and spinal column, and it is here that all critical processes such as cognition, speech, and body movement are governed. This implies that as a brain tumor grows, it impairs a person's critical functions. Patients with brain tumors may have nausea, vomiting, cognitive abnormalities, hemiparesis, aphasia, urine incontinence, and headache, depending on the size, location, and pace of invasion of the tumor. At the time of diagnosis, 50% of the patient who are diagnosed with a brain tumor had a headache [8]. Genetic susceptibility could be one of the risk factors for a brain tumor as studies of syndromes, gene-linkage, mutagen sensitivity, and familial agglomeration suggest its genesis of glioma. Although brain tumor caused due to rare inherited mutations accounts for a few cases, they only provide genetic pathways for the identification of glioma [9]. Research studies have provided a piece of very clear evidence for the role of platelet-derived growth factor receptor (PDGFR) over-expression which allows cells to evade apoptosis in the pathophysiology of brain tumors [10]. Human herpesviruses (HHV), notably Cytomegalovirus (CMV), Epstein-Barr virus (EBV), and Human herpesviruses 6 (HHVs6), are thought to have an important role in brain tumor pathophysiology, according to recent research. These viruses have been found in most gliomas which facilitate its comodulation and immunomodulation and also promote tumour cell proliferation, invasion, and apoptosis. Although a direct relation between these viruses with a brain tumor is still not cleared [11]. Apart from these factors exposure to large therapeutic, high-dose radiation or impaired DNA repair plays a potential role in the development of brain tumors [12].

Classification of Brain Tumour

Brain tumor has five stages based on their progression rate (Stage-0,1,2,3 and 4). Stage-1 tumours refer to the one which do not spread to the surrounding cells, while at stage-2 and 3, tumor cells spread rapidly to the nearby cells. At stage-4, tumor cells spread throughout the body which is a devastating stage [13]. Brain tumors can be either benign or malignant. Malignant brain tumors are cancerous and originate from the brain which is the most lethal type of tumours whereas benign brain tumor is (non-cancerous) the one that grows relatively slow in the brain [14].

The brain tumor (gliomas) originates from glial cells which may be classified according to the World Health Organization (WHO) as low infiltrating to being highly aggressive. A low-grade tumor generally grows slowly as compared to a high-grade but it can turn into a high-grade tumor which can be hard or soft depending upon the number of fibers present in it [15]. Pleomorphic xanthoastrocytoma, central neurocytoma, infantile desmoplastic astrocytoma/ ganglioglioma, and dysembryoplastic neuroepithelial tumors are some of the brain tumors classified by WHO. Among them, glioblastoma is the most lethal kind of cancer [16]. Gliomas are classified into four categories by the WHO in 2007 based on histopathologic characteristics such as mitotic index, anaplasia, cytological atypia, microvascular proliferation, and necrosis. There are four grades: grade I (pilocytic astrocytoma), grade II (astrocytomas and oligodendrogliomas), grade III (anaplastic astrocytomas and oligodendrogliomas), and grade IV (anaplastic astrocytomas and oligodendrogliomas). Grade IV glioma is the most common type of primary brain tumor in humans, and it is more aggressive and fatal, with a survival rate of just 8 to 14 months when detected [6]. In 2016, the WHO updated the Gliomas classification to add molecular diagnostic criteria for invasive gliomas caused by mutations in the isocitrate dehydrogenase gene, deletion of the 1p/19q chromosome, and histone alterations. Malignant gliomas or those of high grade (III and IV) have a favorable prognosis [17]. It results in poor prognosis due to multidrug resistance, limitation in surgical abscission, residual remaining glioma cells which later develop into a new primary tumor, and the tendency of a malignant tumor to spread to a new area [6]. Furthermore, brain metastases occur in 8–10% of adult cancer patients, with the frequency changing significantly depending on the initial malignancy. Brain metastases can be caused by lung, breast, colon, kidney, or melanoma cancer, with lung and breast cancer being the most prevalent causes [17].

Limitations of Conventional Treatment

Surgical excision, radiation, and chemotherapy are the most common treatments for brain tumors, however, they all cause DNA damage with limited therapeutic efficacy, substantial adverse effects, and harm to healthy tissues, necessitating frequent intrusive dosage regimens. The patient's quality of life is harmed as a result of mental and physical imbalance [6]. A brain tumor is challenging to treat due to its exceedingly protective layer (Blood-Brain Barrier) present outside the brain, as most anti-cancer drugs are hydrophilic in nature and BBB becomes an obstacle for the drug to reach the site of the tumor [18]. Although lack of water solubility, selectivity, and the use of multidrug in traditional chemotherapy lead to drug resistance. Researchers are confronting enormous challenges in developing effective chemotherapy [19]. In conventional therapy, the drug accumulates in the healthy region of the brain along with the tumorous site, hence increasing the toxicity in normal brain and peripheral tissues [20]. The effective strategy to overcome these obstacles is brain tumor-targeting drug delivery systems.

DIFFERENT BARRIERS AND TRANSPORTATION PATHWAYS FOR THE DELIVERY OF DRUGS TO BRAIN TUMOURS

Blood-Brain Barrier (BBB)

The BBB is a highly selective semipermeable membrane of endothelial cells that inhibit the non-selective passage of solutes from the circulating blood into the extracellular fluid of the central nervous system. The BBB is made up of pericytes, astrocytes, basement membrane, and perivascular macrophages, and it acts as a physical barrier that prevents lipophobic chemicals from entering the brain (Fig. 1). Pericytes are contractile in nature that regulate the capillary blood flow and help in permeability through BBB [21]. Astrocytes protect the neurons by regulating neurotransmitter and ion concentration that maintains the neural homeostatic balance and in the development of BBB. The BBB tightness is maintained by various effector molecules released by the astrocytes such as apolipoprotein (cholesterol), and phospholipid transporter molecules [22]. Underneath the endothelium and epithelial cells of the BBB, there are two different kinds of basement membrane (BM): an endothelial BM and a parenchymal BM, are separated by pericytes [23]. Apart from neurons, basal membrane, and microglia, there are macrophages and fibroblasts also present in BBB. Moreover, many enzymes are found to be present within the endothelial cells capable of drug degradation and restriction in entry of various chemicals into the brain fluid microenvironment [24]. P-glycoprotein (Pgp), an efflux transporter found in BBB endothelial cells capable of transportation of important chemicals through the BBB, belongs to the family of ATP-binding cassette transporter. In a healthy brain, the BBB works by protecting the brain from a sensitive internal environment by preventing the invasion of microorganisms and toxins. The BBB is degraded and dysfunctional in brain tumours, resulting in a heterogeneous increase in vascular permeability all over the tumour cells and their outer environment [25]. As it progresses, the BBB gets disrupted that lead to the formation of Blood tumour barrier (BTB).

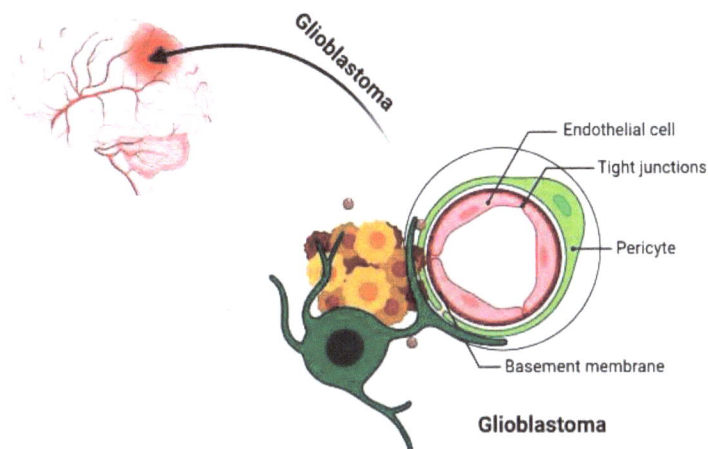

Glioblastoma

Fig. (1). Blood vessels of glioblastoma restricting the entry of drugs.

Carrier Mediated BBB Transport (CMT)

Hexose transporter, amino acid transporter, peptide transporter, amine transporter, and other transporters use BBB selective transporter mechanism to transfer chemicals from the blood to the brain. As a result, CMT transcytosis is a key route for transporting drugs across the BBB [26]. CMT has been widely employed for transporting nano-drug delivery systems to the brain *via* transporters such as glucose transporter, neutral amino acid transporter, glutathione transporter, choline transporter, and carnitine transporter.

Absorptive Mediated Transcytosis (AMT)

It is a technique that aids in the transportation of drugs across the BBB. The ligand present in AMT interacts with the moieties found on luminal surface of cerebral endothelial cells. Polycationic proteins like protamine show the ability to cross the BBB as well as bind to the endothelial cell surface due to the presence of AMT. Because AMT does not bind to the plasma membrane receptor directly, it is referred to as non-specific transcytosis. It is found that in AMT, the positively charged moieties of the protein are present which interact with the negatively charged membrane of the brain endothelial cells *via* electrostatic interactions [27]. Because these cationic targets are large therapeutic molecules, the drug-encapsulated vectors such as liposomes and NPs can easily cross BBB when coupled with AMT.

Receptor-Mediated Transcytosis (RMT)

The RMT is also referred to as selective transcytosis due to its ability to bind selectively to the plasma membrane, which has been widely utilized as a strategy for drug administration across the BBB. Many receptors such as insulin and transferrin are found to be present on the surface of BBB for binding RMT which acts as a medium for the transportation of lipoprotein to the brain. Clathrin-coated pits are a kind of endocytic vesicles (endothelial cells) that participate in transportation along with RMT. A complex of the drug and a receptor-targeted entity is formed in RMT for the transportation process [28]. There are five steps involved in this process: (i) Ligand recognition on the luminal side. (ii) Ligand binding on the luminal side. (iii) Receptor-mediated endocytosis at the brain capillary endothelium's luminal side. (iv) Recycling of receptors to the brain capillary endothelium's luminal side. (v) Ligand exocytosis through albumin transport protein present on the brain capillary endothelium [29]. Transferrin receptor, insulin receptor, nicotinic acetylcholine receptor, and low-density lipoprotein receptor (LDLR) are expressed on the surface of BBB. Angiopep-conjugated poly (ethylene glycol)-co-poly(epsilon-caprolactone) ANG-PEG NPs are also transported across the BBB *via* RMT [30].

Blood-Brain-Tumor Barrier (BBTB)

In brain tumours and other neurological diseases including multiple sclerosis, epilepsy, and dementia, the function, and organization of the BBB are interrupted. The BBB is damaged when brain tumour progresses, resulting in the development of the blood brain tumour barrier (BBTB). The extent of damage to BBB is unaffected by tumour size or its type [31]. Vascular endothelial growth factor (VEGF), is an important factor in BBTB. The increased metabolic rate of high-grade gliomas generates a state of hypoxia in the surrounding area that encourages the production of VEGF resulting in the breakdown of rent BBB structure [32]. Furthermore, VEGF suppresses the production of a critical structural component of BBB, tight junction protein, resulting in increased junctional permeability in brain tumours [33]. The neurovascular unit controls the permeability of BBB under normal physiological conditions which change in tumour due to the large size of endothelial clefts and transendothelial fenestration [34]. Consequently, the BBB becomes leaky in brain tumours leading to cerebral edema due to the accumulation of water and metabolic protein waste in brain parenchyma. Various studies examined BBB permeability during various stages of tumour progression and it has been found that the BBB remains undamaged at early stages of tumour. However, it becomes leaky when the mass of the tumour is increased up to 10 mm^3 [25]. The BBTB blood arteries helps to supply nutrition and oxygen to tumour cells, nourishing them and allowing its movement to different regions of the brain.

Tumour Microenvironment

The tumour microenvironment plays a critical role in tumour genesis, growth, and treatment response [35]. Tumours are made up of stromal cells and extracellular matrix (ECM) that form tumour microenvironment. The stromal cells enhance the tumour growth, and are also responsible for tumour growth inhibition. The interactions between the tumour cells and their surrounding microenvironment govern the pathological behavior of tumour cells [36]. Experimental research demonstrated that tumours originating from the same cancerous cells show higher blood vessel density during their growing phase. Over expressions of VEGF in tumour cells are responsible for "angiogenesis" only in brain tumour but not tumours which originate from the same cancerous cells [37]. Endothelial cells associated with tumours play an important role in the development of tumour microenvironment (Fig. **2**) [38]. Endothelial cells line the vascular system and regulate tumour initiation. Tumour endothelial cells secrete cytokines that help to activate receptors present in tumour cells and suppress the antitumour immune reactions by reducing the cytotoxic responses of the immune cells [39]. A recent study shows that when normal cells come in contact with tumour cells, astrocytes protect normal cells from the chemo resistance of gliomas. Resistance to inhibition of the colony-stimulating factor-1-receptor (CSF-1R), which targets macrophages, accumulates in glioma development due to the tumour microenvironment. The tumour microenvironment enhances the malignant transition of bone marrow stromal cells into glioma tumour stem cells [40]. Exosomes are tiny vesicles generated in vesicular bodies that carry microRNAs, mRNAs, DNA fragments, and proteins. They are an essential element of the tumour microenvironment and are known as tumour-derived exosomes since they secrete cancer cells. They create a favorable environment that promotes tumour growth, angiogenesis, and invasion process of the cell by suppressing the immune responses and boosting chemoresistance by eliminating chemotherapeutic drugs [41]. ECM makes up 60% of the bulk of tumours, and ECM molecules are produced by the tumour cell itself. ECM influences tumour malignancy development by paracrine stromal cell-derived-factor-1(SDF1) and transforming growth factor-beta (TGF) regulation by intratumor signaling, transport mechanisms, metabolism, oxygenation, and immunogenicity [42]. TGFβ regulates the activity of reactive astrocytes. The expression of TGFβ by reactive astrocytes initiates an increase in the invasion of tumour cells and helps in the formation of new ECM components. TGFβ promotes tumour because it mediates several effects that support its growth such as angiogenesis, increase in ECM components, and immunosuppression. However, the TGFβ ligand also suppresses the tumour gene as it can prevent cellular proliferation and induce apoptosis in stromal cells (paracrine) and autocrine cells. The complete loss of TGFβ signal transduction to date has not been shown in brain tumour [43]. Fibroblast activation protein (FAP) also known as prolyl endopeptidase has been seen in the progression of tumour cells. FAP is expressed more in brain tumours cells. Although the mechanism that governs the FAP expression is unknown, researchers have found that TGF increases the FAP expression in transformed and stromal cells that make up the tumour microenvironment. Both FAP and TGF have been reported to be upregulated in brain tumours cells. TGF-1 promotes the production of FAP in non-stem glioma cells but not in glioma stem. It also plays a role in the transcription of the FAP gene [44]. Increased FAP expression is linked to a poorer clinical outcome across a wide range of tumour types [45]. The major component of the tumour microenvironment is cancer associated fibroblasts (CAF), which include myofibroblast and fibroblast that regulate anti-tumour immune responses. Certain CAF subsets have also been demonstrated to influence the anti-tumour immune response in the recent decade. In fact, by regulating the secretion of cytokines, chemokines, growth factors, and ECM proteins, they can enhance the amount of regulatory T lymphocytes while inhibiting the activity of effector and cytotoxic immune cells [46]. Tumour progression is influenced not just by cancer cell genetic changes or epigenetic modifications, but also by factors in the tumour microenvironment.

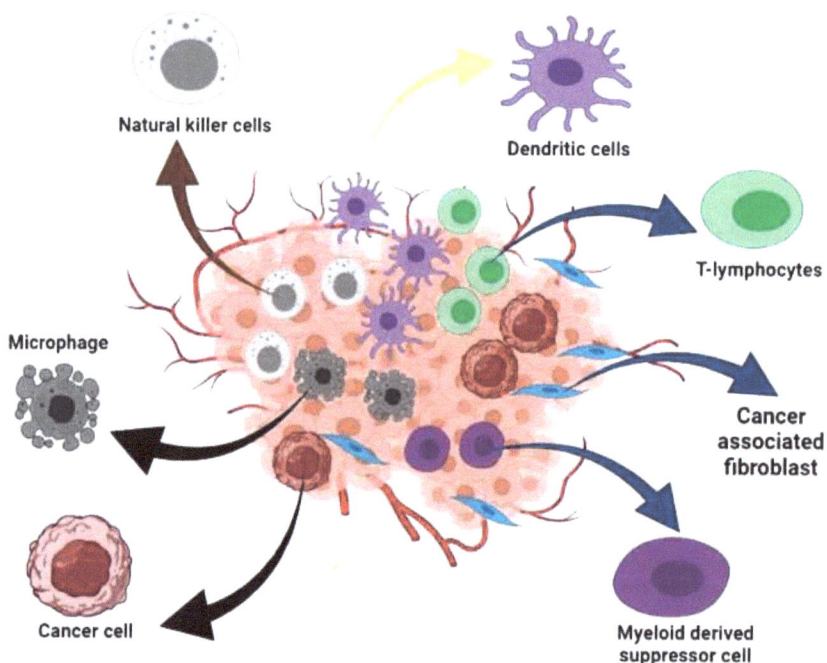

Fig. (2). Tumour microenvironment and associated cells.

APPLICATION

Vesicular Drug Delivery for Brain Tumour Theranostic

The primary constraint in the treatment of brain tumours and the administration of chemotherapeutic and imaging agents is crossing the BBB, which leads to inadequate accumulation and prevents tumour cells from being killed. Because of its efficient biodegradability, non-toxicity, good tumour targeting ability, and simplicity of surface modification, the vesicular drug delivery system is getting popular [47].

Liposomal Nanoparticles for Brain Tumour Theranostic

Liposomes are a targeted drug delivery system that constitutes one or more lipid bilayer spheres separated by water or aqueous buffer compartments made up of natural or synthesized phospholipid. Phospholipids and cholesterol are the two major components for the formation of liposomes [48]. Nanotechnology based liposomes are one of the most popularly used drug delivery system due to their biocompatibility, biodegradability, low toxicity, and surface modification. It is the first nanomedicine authorized for clinical use by the US Food and Drug Administration (USFDA) [49]. Drugs are loaded into liposomes through, (i) Organic solvents and solvent exchange mechanism, (ii) By the use of lipophilic drugs, and (iii) pH gradient methods [48]. The half-life of the liposomes can be increased by engrafting polyethylene at their surface. Apart from these advantages, liposomes also reduce the uptake of macrophages and encapsulate both hydrophilic and lipophilic drug molecules. Around sixteen drugs are available in the market for brain tumour treatment and its diagnosis. Doxil is the first liposome approved by USFDA in 1995 which contains doxorubicin and hydrochloride. Liposomes have the potential to cross the BBB through the interendothelial gaps of highly vascularized leaky BBTB in high-grade glioblastoma multiforme (GBM). It can also cross the intact BBB *via* CMT that can be utilised as an important approach to treat a variety of tumour grades [50]. There are currently very few formulations classified as theranostic for brain tumours. We present a few recent instances of liposomes for brain tumours theranostic in this chapter.

Sonali *et al.* [51] formed a theranostic liposome attached with arginyl glycyl aspartic acid (RGD) peptide for targeted co-delivery of Docetaxel and Quantam dots (QDs) into the brain cells in 2016, which enhanced brain imaging and medication targeting. Due to their enhanced pharmacokinetic characteristics, liposome NPs are employed as carriers for diagnostic imaging as they deliver the fluorescent imaging agent to the target location more efficiently. As a result, researchers created liposomal NPs to make it easier to employ IR780 (heptamethine cyanine dye) for brain tumour fluorescence imaging [51, 52]. Furthermore, scientists have created gold liposome nanoparticles (NPs) coupled with the peptides apolipoprotein E (ApoE) and rabies virus glycoprotein, which target the brain (RVG). The size, charge, encapsulation efficiency, and transport efficiency of the NPs into brain tumour cells were all measured [53]. Paclitaxel, an antitumour drug that prevents the production of microtubules, has proved to be effective against a variety of malignancies, including ovarian cancer, lung cancer, and brain tumours. However, due to its limited capacity to penetrate the BBB, the currently available paclitaxel formulation is ineffective due to less efficacy against brain tumours. Another antitumour drug, Artemether, has significant cytotoxicity against several malignant cells by inhibiting the production of vascular endothelial growth factor (VEGF). As a result, scientists have produced paclitaxel and artemether loaded liposomes that cause apoptosis in brain tumour cells [54].

Exosomes for Brain Tumour Theranostic

Exosomes are nanosized vesicular drug delivery systems with vesicles size ranging from 30 to 100 nm that has the potential to cross the BBB and transport drugs to their desired location [55]. Exosomes, which are non-immunogenic in nature, are tiny extracellular vesicles produced by cells. They are more stable in the body and have a longer circulation time. Exosomes derived from the EC of the brain help in chemical exchange across the BBB and communicate with the brain. This aids in the transportation of tiny molecules, proteins, and nucleic acids across the BBB [56]. They also have the ability to integrate therapeutic mRNAs, interfering RNAs, and compounds with chemotherapeutic properties, making it a promising approach for cancer treatment. Exosomes derived from tumour cells carry tumour antigens, and microRNA (miR)-146b-expressing MSCs aid in the decrease of glioblastoma development in primary brain tumours observed in microscopic examination. Exosomes derived from dendritic cells stimulate the immune system and aid in the therapy of primary malignancies [57]. Using an ultracentrifugation method, Zhu *et al.* [55], extracted an exosome from NK-cell culture media. Bioluminescence imaging (BLI), fluorescence-activated cell sorting (FACS), and western blotting indicated that it had an antitumor impact [57]. The anti-GBM activity of ESC-exos loaded with (RGDyK)-modified and paclitaxel (PTX), termed cRGD-Exo-PTX, was demonstrated by Zhu Q *et al.* [55] The researchers discovered that modified exosomes transported to tumour cells site efficiently and precisely [55].

Niosomes for Brain Tumour Theranostic

The primary obstacle faced in the treatment of brain tumours and the administration of chemotherapeutic and imaging agents is the blood-brain barrier, which causes inadequate accumulation and prevents tumour cell death. Due to its efficient biodegradability, nontoxicity, good tumour targeting ability, and simplicity of surface modification, the vesicular drug delivery method is gaining a lot of attention [58]. De *et al*. [59], formulated a niosome with a modified surface with chlorotoxin encapsulating temozolomide. The nanosized particle facilitates the accumulation of drugs by 3.04 folds. Quantitative tissue distribution studies suggested enhanced permeation in brain tissues [59].

Nanoparticles for Brain Tumour Theranostic

Polymeric Nanoparticles

NPs assist to accomplish the objective of treating cancer due to their tiny size, which allows them to cross BBB, the ease with which they can modify the surface, and their versatility in incorporating a large number of functional components into a single unit. They are also useful in cancer therapy for therapeutic and diagnostic purposes. The NPs have the ability to locate tumour cell and distribute around it without harming the normal cells of the brain. This helps to increase the treatment efficacy. It modifies the surface with the addition of markers, proteins, medicines, or genes to provide a stimuli-responsive activity near to the tumour's microenvironment [6].

Polymer Nanotechnologies are one of the important aspects to achieve drug delivery challenges. There are several polymers that have been used in drug delivery as they increase the therapeutic benefits with few side effects. Polymeric NPs, formed from a natural or synthetic polymer ranges in size from 1 to 1000 nm that can be utilized in nanoencapsulation of various bioactive compounds or drugs. Polymeric NPs can be prepared by two methods, the first method includes the preparation of emulsified system while the second method is the polymerization of the monomer or precipitation of a polymer. Polyalkyilcyanoacrylate (PACA) is one of the most commonly used polymers for NPs in brain tumour targeting and drug delivery. Here are a few recent examples of polymeric NPs being used to treat brain tumour.

Guanlian *et al*. [60] suggested a multistage drug delivery system in 2015, citing the fact that large NPs have poor tumour penetration while tiny NPs have poor retention. On the basis of MMP-2's size sensitivity, they developed an RGD-DOX-DGL-GNP, a multistage drug delivery method. The RGD-DOX-DGL-GNP improves treatment efficacy by delivering Doxorubicin to the site of solid tumours where tumour stem cells are often found [60]. Kah jing *et al.* [59] developed polymeric curcumin NPs that suppress the development of malignant brain tumours in 2011. The researchers analyzed apoptosis and cell cycle characteristics in vehicle-treated cells, where they discovered that curcumin NPs suppress tumour cell growth through a mechanism of programmed cell death and G2/M cell cycle arrest [59]. The impact of surface charges of poly(lactide)-poly(ethylene glycol) NPs on interaction with the surroundings of brain tumours was discovered by Brandon *et al.* [59]. The negatively charged carboxyl (COOH) and neutrally charged methoxy surface functions of polymeric NPs with identical sizes were employed (OCH_3). For all cell lines studied *in vivo*, negatively charged carboxyl NPs showed more absorption per cell than neutrally charged methoxy NPs, suggesting that NPs interactions with cells are mediated by the polymers' physiochemical characteristics [59]. Furthermore, in 2018, VJ, Muniswamy *et al.* [59] developed a novel hybrid of nanoformulation of doxorubicin and Dendrimer-cationized-Albumin (dCatAlb). Functionalization of NPs improves the drug's ability to overcome the BBB as it provides improved ligand-receptor interactions and selectivity for the target site [59]. Recently, Methotrexate-Loaded solid lipid NPs have been developed and found that endocytosis process helps NPs to have more ability to cross the BBB. Advanced nanomedicine research has focused on developing dual-coated polymeric NPs, in 2016 by jiangang *et al.* [61], pH-sensitive dual-targeting Doxorubicin was synthesized using polydopamine (PDA)-coated mesoporous silica NPs and PDA with Asn-Gly-Arg (NGR). This dual-coated polymeric NP was shown to enhance BBB permeability [61]. Polymeric NPs have always been given great importance because of their attractive features such as easy penetration through the cell membrane, protection of the drug against degradation, and enhanced site-specific delivery.

Inorganic-Nanoparticles for Brain Tumour Theranostic

After exploration by the researchers, it has been found that inorganic NPs possess unique material and size-dependent physicochemical properties which make them different from organic NPs, and hence, they are widely used for therapeutic and diagnostic purposes in brain tumour [62]. However, there are very few inorganic NPs available for brain tumour theranostics.

<u>*Gold NPs*</u>

In the field of brain tumours, gold NPs have lately emerged as a promising possibility for a targeted drug delivery system to the brain. Gold NPs are inert and non-toxic in nature and can be synthesized very easily [63]. Gold NPs have been the most commonly utilized NPs despite the availability of numerous inorganic

NPs due to their unique optical and surface Plasmon resonance properties (SPR). Several research groups utilized Gold NPs for brain tumours theranostic. For example, epidermal growth factor (EGF) modified conjugates of gold NPs have improved selectivity at the target site of brain tumours than unconjugated gold NPs [64]. Peptide-targeted gold NPs were explored for the delivery of photodynamic (treatment drugs) to brain tumours. The researchers created Transferrin peptide (Tfpep) targeted gold NPs (Tfpep—Au-NPs) loaded with photodynamic prodrug in 2015, which showed improvement in drug delivery efficiency and specificity over untargeted gold NPs [65]. Similarly, Methotrexate and Doxorubicin both drugs have shown the highest cytotoxicity for tumour cells when conjugated with gold NPs. Gold NPs have been used as photothermal therapy since it has the ability to melt tumours cells by inducing localized therapeutic temperature [66]. Similarly, gold NPs were developed and loaded with technetium-99m radiolabelled methotrexate with a potential nano radiopharmaceutical for tumours targeting and further imaging [67]

Iron-oxides NPs

The NPs used for Magnetic resonance imaging (MRI) for the diagnosis of brain tumours are employed with an iron-oxide core made up of polyethylene glycol (PEG). This helps in better diagnosis of brain tumours with detailed information about the extent and location of tumours [68]. A recent study reported whether the usage of NPs might cause reactive oxygen species (ROS) in tumour cells. Consequently, iron oxide antioxidative NPs with caffeic acid for brain tumours theranostic have been developed [69]. Here are a few examples of iron-oxide NPs approved by USFDA for brain tumour imaging: Ferumoxtran, Ferucarbotran, Ferumoxide, Ferumoxytrol. Magnetic particle imaging outperforms MRI in terms of providing 3D information on the distribution of iron-oxide NPs. Although, they do not provide anatomical information related to it. To overcome this problem, researchers have developed a hybrid structure approach such as MPI\MRI, and MRI\CT. Magnetic fluid hyperthermia has been extensively used to kill tumour cells *via* conversion of heat from magnetic NPs. Nanotherm is a marketed formulation of magnetic fluid hyperthermia that has been tested for brain tumour treatment [70].

Silver Nanoparticles

In the field of radiation therapy for brain tumours, silver NPs have become a core technology due to their radiosensitivity effect on tumour cells and increased mean survival time of the patient. Apart from this, they show size-dependent cytotoxicity *i.e.* smaller the size of NPs will show more toxicity to tumour cells [71]. A study reported that polymeric NPs containing the combination of two cytotoxic agents-alisterib and silver NPs help to reduce tumour growth. Jing *et al.* [73], developed unique form of radio-sensitizer silver NPs, to promote the accumulation of aptamer AS1411 and verapamil in tumour cells to improve glioma radiosensitivity. Their research found potential radio-sensitizing characteristics in glioma radiation. Their capacity to penetrate and accumulate in tumour cells, on the other hand, has to be enhanced further [73].

Other metallic Nanoparticles

Among other NPs, zinc oxide NPs, platinum NPs, cerium oxide NPs, manganese oxide NPs shown in Table **1** were used for the brain tumour theranostic. Gao Y *et al.* [74], investigated a study which shows that the use of Platinum NPs decreases the volume and weight of gliomas tumour tissue *via* lethal DNA damage caused by the interaction of Platinum NPs with the DNA phosphate group. Another study demonstrated that the cerium oxide NPs regulate ROS in tumour cells [74].It is a promising tool for some treatment problems associated with brain tumour such as tumour progression due to interaction between tumour cells and the stromal microenvironment [75]. Manganese oxide (MnO) NPs are considered a good contrasting agent in MRI due to their small volume, easy penetration, and low toxicity. Water dispersible MnO nanocrystals have been designed which induce true autophagy that helps MnO nanocrystals to synergize with chemotherapeutic drugs to produce greater lethality against tumour cells and they are independent of P53 activation [76]. Metal NPs have several advantages such as small size, high surface area, easy synthesis, physicochemical properties, and multifunctional theranostic applications due to which recently scientists and researchers have shown great interest in them.

Table 1. List of Nanocarriers, Therapeutics, and diagnostic Agents for Brain Tumour.

Nanocarriers	Drugs	Diagnostic Agents	Cell Lines	Outcomes	Reference
Liposomes	Docetaxel and Quantum dots (QDs)	Arginine-Glycine-Aspatic acid (RGD)	Rat's Brain	Improves imaging and drug target to the brain	[51].
Liposomes	IR780, phospholipid	Near-IR fluorescence	Mouse model	Great potential for clinical imaging and image guided surgery for brain tumour	[40]
Dendrimers	Doxorubicin and dendrimer cationized albumin	-	Rat glioma cell	Improves the drug ability to overcome the BBB	[77]
Liposomes	Apolipoprotein, rabies virus glycoprotein	-	U87 GBM cell line(mouseastrocytomas)	Conjugation of SNA-Liposomes with ApoE or RVG peptides increases the systemic delivery to the brain tumour of syngenic mice	[53]

(Table 1) cont.....

Nanocarriers	Drugs	Diagnostic Agents	Cell Lines	Outcomes	Reference
Liposomes	Paclitaxel, Artemether	-	Glioma cell	Apoptosis induction in brain tumour cells	[54]
Polymeric NPs	Curcumin	-	Rat glioma cell	Inhibits the growth of malignant brain tumour	[60]
Gold NPs	Methotrexate and Doxorubicinorubicin	-	Glioma cell	Cytotoxicity to the tumour cells	[66]
Gold NPs	Technetium-99m radiolabeled methotrexate	Technetium-99m radiolabeled methotrexate	Mice tumour cells	New potential nanoradiopharmaceutical for tumour targeting and further imaging	[67]
Iron oxide NPs	Caffeic acid	Caffeic acid	Tumour cells	Generate ROS in tumour cells	[69]
Silver NPs	Alisterib	-	Brain tumour cell	Reduces the tumour growth	[72]
Cerium oxide NPs	Cerium oxide	-	Anaplastic astrocytoma cell	Regulate ROS in tumour cells	[74]
Manganese oxide nanocrystal	Manganese oxide	Manganese oxide	Tumour cell lines	Produce greater lethality against tumour cells	[76]

Stimuli-Responsive Strategies to Deliver a Drug at Tumour Site

Sometimes control over drug release and that too at the specific site is required for the successful treatment of brain tumour. For this to achieve, a drug delivery responding to endogenous or exogenous stimuli is required. The endogenous stimuli response of drug delivery is beneficial due to the presence of stimuli at the pathological site which increases the targeting of a drug. These triggers can be in the form of pH variation, enzymes, glucose, or redox gradient [56]. The pH-responsive stimuli are very effective in treating the brain tumour as tumour cells are acidic in nature compared to normal cells of the brain which applies the effective use of pH-responsive drug delivery system. The conformation changes or breakage in bonds helps to analyze a change in pH, thus allowing the release of a drug encapsulated inside a dosage form. The redox gradient present inside the cell utilizes the redox responsive stimuli to react for tumorous cells. For example, the presence of glutathione (GSH) at a high concentration regulates the intracellular redox condition that helps in the release of the cargos present in a drug delivery system. The enzyme responsive approach is also very helpful due to the presence of a large number of enzymes in tumours area. The exogenous stimuli in the form of temperature, magnetic field, ultrasound, light, electric pulse, or high radiation are utilized for targeting the tumour cell. The combination of triggers such as pH/temperature, pH/redox, temperature/redox, and temperature/pH/redox, is also possible and tried in recent years [6]. Wang *et al.* [78], formulated a neutrophil exosome system loaded with Doxorubicin having a promising chemotherapeutic approach for the treatment of glioma and brain tumour. *In vivo* zebrafish and C6-Luc, glioma-bearing mice models were used showing that the drug penetrates the brain and reaches the target site. The mouse brain inflammatory study shows that neutrophil exosomes respond to chemotactically inflammatory stimuli and target the inflamed cell of a tumour, thus, showing a stimuli-based response and is clinically used for the treatment of glioma of tumours present in the brain [78]. Naziris *et al.* [79], formulated a functional chimeric nanocarrier that is made up of phospholipid and a deblock copolymer. Antiglioma agent TRAM-34 was incorporated inside the nanocarrier shows the pH-responsive nature and releases its content inside glioblastoma cells. The nanocarrier effectively delivers the anti-glioma agent on pH response with enhanced biocompatibility and cellular internalization [79]. Song *et al.*, (2021) developed a pH/reduction-sensitive carboxymethyl chitosan nanogel (CMCSN). The nanogel was modified by targeting peptide angiopep-2 (ANG) and loaded with Doxorubicin and known to be DOX-ANG-CMCSN. The nanogel (DOX-ANG-CMCSN) possesses good biocompatibility, stability, pH, and reduced sensitivity. The nanogel showed 12.7% drug loading and cumulative release rate up to 24 h to be 82.3% in a stimulated tumour microenvironment. The formulated showed the ability to cross BBB and had targeting capacity towards tumour revealed both *in vivo* and *in vitro* studies with the pH/reduction dual-stimuli response [80].

Non-Invasive Techniques: To Focus Ultrasound-Induced Brain Vascular Permeability Increment

Focused ultrasound (FUS) is a non-invasive method that permits a therapeutic substance to be delivered to a brain tumour. This method uses a combination of ultrasound (FUS) and injectable microbubbles to enhance permeability across the BBB. The FUS is also utilized in conjunction with magnetic resonance imaging (MRI), which aids in the efficient identification of the pharmaceutical target. The BBB is physically modulated by the FUS, which is also known as the cavitation effect, in which circulating microbubbles interact with FUS sonication to produce stable or inertial cavitation (Fig. **3**). The emission of harmonic signals from the bubble causes tight junction modulation in stable cavitation, but inertial cavitation causes vessel rupturing and a degree of bleeding in inertial cavitation. Broadband emissions induce the microbubble to collapse, causing microstreaming and micro-jets to spread across the surrounding region, causing a vascular rupture and irreversible tissue injury. As a result, this method should be utilized with caution to preserve the calibration point for disciplinary microbubble contraction and expansion [81]. Lin *et al.*, (2019) colleagues employed the FUC technique on the gene liposome system to open the BBB and restore motor and neuropathological impairments in pre- to post-symptomatic Huntington's disease transgenic mouse models. To construct a GDNFp-liposome (GDNFp-LPs) complex, liposomes contained GDNF plasmid DNA (GDNFp). The FUS-gene therapy enhanced people's lives [82].

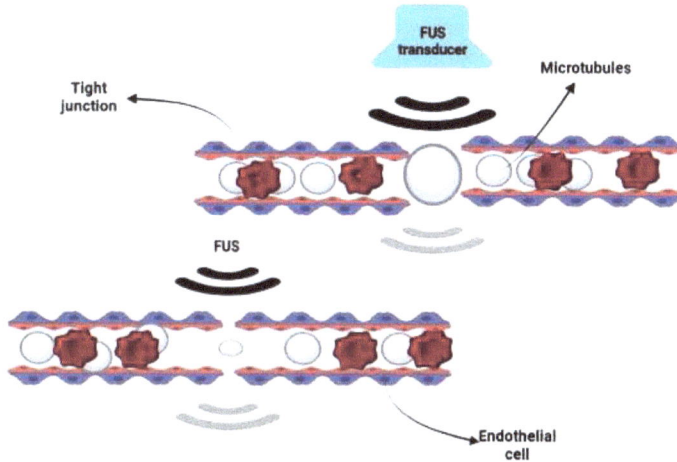

Fig. (3). BBB modulation employing focused ultrasound (FUS) with intravenous injection of microbubbles.

Chen *et al*. [83], showed the administration of local IL-12 into glioblastoma using FUS technology to open the BBB, resulting in enhanced TIL infiltration, anticancer immunological response, and glioma therapeutic effectiveness. The opening of the BBB aids in the delivery of an immune-modulating drug, which improves the anticancer immune response in patients with brain tumours [83]. (Fig. **4**) shows the delivery of IL-12 to the brain tumour by opening BBB using FUS technology.

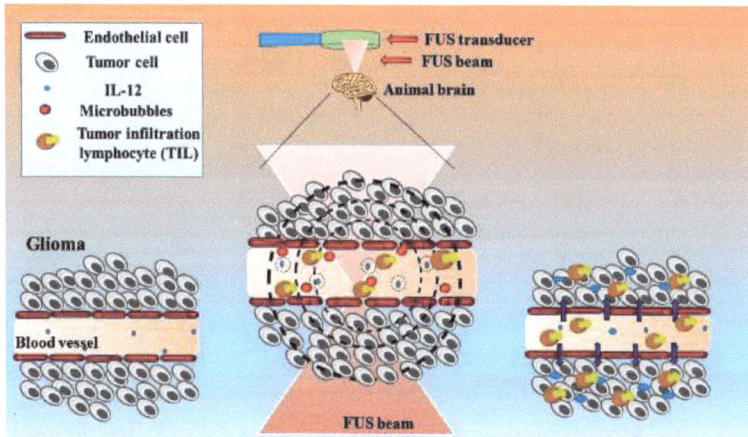

Fig. (4). FUS-induced BBB leaking to enhance IL-12 delivery in brain.

Table 2. Clinical Status of the Nanotheranostics in Brain Tumour.

TITLE	CARRIER SYSTEM		DRUGS	APPLICATION	PATENT NO.	REFERENCE
Gold/lanthanide nanoparticle conjugates and use thereof	Gold nanoparticle	-	Gold,gadolinium, methotrexate, paclitaxel, folic acid	Nanoparticles will allow targeted delivery of imaging agents, and therapeutic compounds to specific cells, tissues, and organs.	US 10, 406, 111 B2	[82]
Encapsulated diagnostics and therapeutics in nanoparticles-conjugated to tropic cells and methods for their use	Micro nanoparticle	-	Biotinylated nanoparticle, Avidin, biotinylated NSC	A therapeutic or diagnostic delivery vehicle comprising a particle conjugated to a tropic cell that targets a brain tumour pathological entity or site	US 2019/0388474 A1	[84]
Selective dendrimer delivery to brain tumour	Dendrimer	-	Poly(amidoamine)hydroxyl	Provides a means for selective delivery through the BBB of chemotherapeutic, immunotherapeutic, and palliative agents	US 10,918,720 B2	[85]
Drug carrier capable of realizing drug delivery specifically targeting tumor and application thereof	Nanoparticles	-	-	Depolymerized full heavy-chain human ferritin combined with the tumor-treating drug again to form nano-particles.	CN104013599A	[86]
Circular coils for deep transcranial magnetic stimulation	-	-	-	Non-invasive technique to apply brief magnetic pulses to the brain	US 9, 808, 642 B2	[87]
Lipid-derived nanoparticles for brain-targeted drug delivery	Nanoparticles	-	-	Facilitate delivery to the brain by crossing blood-brain barrier	US20100076092A1	[43]

CONCLUSION

One of the most lethal diseases, brain tumours have no effective therapy, till today. As primary physiological barriers, the BBB and BBTB, as well as heterogeneity and the invasive character of GB, restrict the entry of diagnostic agents and chemotherapeutics at the tumour site, limiting the efficacies of current therapies. These challenges can impressively be addressed *via* utilizing nanotechnology, which has emerged as a viable option in the diagnosis &

treatment of brain tumours and related ailments. Therapy with nanocarriers has shown promising results in terms of efficacy and safety in mitigating these challenges associated with brain tumour therapy. Nanocarriers are stable in nature and exhibit high drug loading capacity, great tolerability, with resistance to drug degradation. Owing to these attributes, therapies and theranostic drug delivery nanocarrier systems outperform conventional therapy options in different diseases. The topic of "theranostic medicine" has gained a lot of attention in recent years and developing advanced nanocarriers every day for the purpose of diagnosis and treatment in preclinical and clinical subjects. Nanotechnology-based medication delivery system allows the delivery of both therapeutic and diagnostic agents to the targeted location of the body which in turn improves clinical outcomes with lesser adverse effects. However, several other issues *viz.* scale-up issues, drug pharmacokinetics, imaging contrast, high manufacturing costs, *etc.* are yet to be addressed. Thus, there is an urgent need to develop a smart and advanced system(s) for the delivery of TRAM-34 and other therapeutic agents in the diagnosis and treatment of various ailments, especially brain tumours.

ACKNOWLEDGEMENTS

All the authors of this chapter would like to give thanks to Late Prof. Aditya Shastri, Vice-Chancellor of Banasthalli Vidhyapith Rajasthan, India for providing all the necessary facilities for the successful completion of the Chapter.

REFERENCES

[1]   Bhowmik A, Khan R, Ghosh MK. Blood brain barrier: a challenge for effectual therapy of brain tumors. BioMed Res Int 2015; 2015: 1-20.
[http://dx.doi.org/10.1155/2015/320941] [PMID: 25866775]

[2]   d'Angelo M, Castelli V, Benedetti E, *et al.* Theranostic Nanomedicine for Malignant Gliomas. Front Bioeng Biotechnol 2019; 7: 325.
[http://dx.doi.org/10.3389/fbioe.2019.00325] [PMID: 31799246]

[3]   Mendes M, Sousa JJ, Pais A, Vitorino C. Targeted theranostic nanoparticles for brain tumor treatment. Pharmaceutics 2018; 10(4): 181.
[http://dx.doi.org/10.3390/pharmaceutics10040181] [PMID: 30304861]

[4]   Thorat ND, Townely H, Brennan G, *et al.* Progress in remotely triggered hybrid nanostructures for next-generation brain cancer theranostics. ACS Biomater Sci Eng 2019; 5(6): 2669-87.
[http://dx.doi.org/10.1021/acsbiomaterials.8b01173] [PMID: 33405601]

[5]   Wrensch M, Minn Y, Chew T, Bondy M, Berger MS. Epidemiology of primary brain tumors: Current concepts and review of the literature. Neuro-oncol 2002; 4(4): 278-99.
[http://dx.doi.org/10.1093/neuonc/4.4.278] [PMID: 12356358]

[6]   Schiffer D. The origin of gliomas in relation to the histological diagnosis.Brain tumor pathology: Current dagnostic hotspots and ptfalls. 1st ed. Dordrecht: Springer 2006; pp. 3-18.

[7]   Athanasiou E, Gargalionis AN, Boufidou F, Tsakris A. The association of human herpesviruses with malignant brain tumor pathology and therapy: two sides of a coin. Int J Mol Sci 2021; 22(5): 2250.
[http://dx.doi.org/10.3390/ijms22052250] [PMID: 33668202]

[8]   Schwartzbaum JA, Fisher JL, Aldape KD, Wrensch M. Epidemiology and molecular pathology of glioma. Nat Clin Pract Neurol 2006; 2(9): 494-503.
[http://dx.doi.org/10.1038/ncpneuro0289] [PMID: 16932614]

[9]   Tandel GS, Biswas M, Kakde OG, *et al.* A review on a deep learning perspective in brain cancer classification. Cancers (Basel) 2019; 11(1): 111.
[http://dx.doi.org/10.3390/cancers11010111] [PMID: 30669406]

[10]   Chertok B, David AE, Yang VC. Polyethyleneimine-modified iron oxide nanoparticles for brain tumor drug delivery using magnetic targeting and intra-carotid administration. Biomaterials 2010; 31(24): 6317-24.
[http://dx.doi.org/10.1016/j.biomaterials.2010.04.043] [PMID: 20494439]

[11]   Havaei M, Davy A, Warde-Farley D, *et al.* Brain tumor segmentation with deep neural networks. Med Image Anal 2017; 35: 18-31.
[http://dx.doi.org/10.1016/j.media.2016.05.004] [PMID: 27310171]

[12]   Kleihues P, Burger PC, Scheithauer BW. The new WHO classification of brain tumours. Brain Pathol 1993; 3(3): 255-68.
[http://dx.doi.org/10.1111/j.1750-3639.1993.tb00752.x] [PMID: 8293185]

[13]   Ferraris C, Cavalli R, Panciani PP, Battaglia L. Overcoming the blood–brain barrier: successes and challenges in developing nanoparticle-mediated drug delivery systems for the treatment of brain tumours. Int J Nanomedicine 2020; 15: 2999-3022.
[http://dx.doi.org/10.2147/IJN.S231479] [PMID: 32431498]

[14]   Garg T, Bhandari S, Rath G, Goyal AK. Current strategies for targeted delivery of bio-active drug molecules in the treatment of brain tumor. J Drug Target 2015; 23(10): 865-87.
[http://dx.doi.org/10.3109/1061186X.2015.1029930] [PMID: 25835469]

[15]   Chidambaram M, Manavalan R, Kathiresan K. Nanotherapeutics to overcome conventional cancer chemotherapy limitations. J Pharm Pharm Sci 2011; 14(1): 67-77.
[http://dx.doi.org/10.18433/J30C7D] [PMID: 21501554]

[16]   Wei X, Chen X, Ying M, Lu W. Brain tumor-targeted drug delivery strategies. Acta Pharm Sin B 2014; 4(3): 193-201.
[http://dx.doi.org/10.1016/j.apsb.2014.03.001] [PMID: 26579383]

[17]   Liu S, Agalliu D, Yu C, Fisher M. The role of pericytes in blood-brain barrier function and stroke. Curr Pharm Des 2012; 18(25): 3653-62.
[http://dx.doi.org/10.2174/138161212802002706] [PMID: 22574979]

[18]   Keaney J, Campbell M. The dynamic blood-brain barrier. FEBS J 2015; 282(21): 4067-79.
[http://dx.doi.org/10.1111/febs.13412] [PMID: 26277326]

[19]   Xu L, Nirwane A, Yao Y. Basement membrane and blood–brain barrier. Stroke Vasc Neurol 2019; 4(2): 78-82.
[http://dx.doi.org/10.1136/svn-2018-000198] [PMID: 31338215]

[20]   Provenzale JM, Mukundan S, Dewhirst M. The role of blood-brain barrier permeability in brain tumor imaging and therapeutics. AJR Am J Roentgenol 2005; 185(3): 763-7.
[http://dx.doi.org/10.2214/ajr.185.3.01850763] [PMID: 16120931]

[21]   On NH, Mitchell R, Savant SD, Bachmeier CJ, Hatch GM, Miller DW. Examination of blood–brain barrier (BBB) integrity in a mouse brain tumor model. J Neurooncol 2013; 111(2): 133-43.
[http://dx.doi.org/10.1007/s11060-012-1006-1] [PMID: 23184143]

[22]   Khan NU, Miao T, Ju X, *et al.* Carrier-mediated transportation through BBB.Brain Targeted Drug Delivery System. 1st ed. Academic Press 2019; pp. 129-58.
[http://dx.doi.org/10.1016/B978-0-12-814001-7.00006-8]

[23]   Hervé F, Ghinea N, Scherrmann JM. CNS delivery *via* adsorptive transcytosis. AAPS J 2008; 10(3): 455-72.
[http://dx.doi.org/10.1208/s12248-008-9055-2] [PMID: 18726697]

[24]   Pulgar VM. Transcytosis to cross the blood brain barrier, bew advancements and challenges. Front Neurosci 2019; 12: 1019.
[http://dx.doi.org/10.3389/fnins.2018.01019] [PMID: 30686985]

[25]   Zhang Z, Zhan C. Receptor-mediated transportation through BBB. 2019.
[http://dx.doi.org/10.1016/B978-0-12-814001-7.00005-6]

[26]   Guangqing X, Liang Shangm G. Receptor-mediated endocytosis and brain delivery of therapeutic biologics 2013.

[27]   van Tellingen O, Yetkin-Arik B, de Gooijer MC, Wesseling P, Wurdinger T, de Vries HE. Overcoming the blood–brain tumor barrier for effective glioblastoma treatment. Drug Resist Updat 2015; 19: 1-12.
[http://dx.doi.org/10.1016/j.drup.2015.02.002] [PMID: 25791797]

[28]   Belykh E, Shaffer KV, Lin C, Byvaltsev VA, Preul MC, Chen L. Blood-brain barrier, blood-brain tumor Barrier, and fluorescence-guided neurosurgical oncology: Delivering optical labels to brain tumors. Front Oncol 2020; 10: 739.
[http://dx.doi.org/10.3389/fonc.2020.00739] [PMID: 32582530]

[29]   Nag S. Morphology and properties of brain endothelial cells.The blood-brain and other neural barriers Methods in molecular biology. Humana Press 2011; pp. 3-47.
[http://dx.doi.org/10.1007/978-1-60761-938-3_1]

[30]   Vorbrodt AW, Dobrogowska DH. Molecular anatomy of interendothelial junctions in human blood-brain barrier microvessels. Folia Histochem Cytobiol 2004; 42(2): 67-75.
[PMID: 15253128]

[31]   Charles NA, Holland EC, Gilbertson R, Glass R, Kettenmann H. The brain tumor microenvironment. Glia 2011; 59(8): 1169-80.
[http://dx.doi.org/10.1002/glia.21136] [PMID: 21446047]

[32]   Koh I, Kim P. *in vitro* reconstruction of brain tumor microenvironment. Biochip J 2019; 13(1): 1-7.
[http://dx.doi.org/10.1007/s13206-018-3102-6]

[33]   Lorger M. Tumor microenvironment in the brain. Cancers (Basel) 2012; 4(1): 218-43.
[http://dx.doi.org/10.3390/cancers4010218] [PMID: 24213237]

[34]   Chouaib S, Kieda C, Benlalam H, Noman MZ, Mami-Chouaib F, Rüegg C. Endothelial cells as key determinants of the tumor microenvironment: interaction with tumor cells, extracellular matrix and immune killer cells. Crit Rev Immunol 2010; 30(6): 529-45.
[http://dx.doi.org/10.1615/CritRevImmunol.v30.i6.30] [PMID: 21175416]

[35]   Yang D, Guo P, He T, Powell CA. Role of endothelial cells in tumor microenvironment. Clin Transl Med 2021; 11(6)e450
[http://dx.doi.org/10.1002/ctm2.450] [PMID: 34185401]

[36]   Li S, Johnson J, Peck A, Xie Q. Near infrared fluorescent imaging of brain tumor with IR780 dye incorporated phospholipid nanoparticles. J Transl Med 2017; 15(1): 18.
[http://dx.doi.org/10.1186/s12967-016-1115-2] [PMID: 28114956]

[37]   Wang Z, Chen JQ, Liu J, Tian L. Exosomes in tumor microenvironment: novel transporters and biomarkers. J Transl Med 2016; 14(1): 297.
[http://dx.doi.org/10.1186/s12967-016-1056-9] [PMID: 27756426]

[38]   Brassart-Pasco S, Brézillon S, Brassart B, Ramont L, Oudart JB, Monboisse JC. Tumor microenvironment: extracellular matrix alterations influence tumor progression. Front Oncol 2020; 10: 397.

[http://dx.doi.org/10.3389/fonc.2020.00397] [PMID: 32351878]

[39]   Chavanpatil JPD. US20100076092A1 - Lipid-derived nanoparticles for brain-targeted drug delivery - Google Patents. 2010. p. 1–15.

[40]   Krepela E, Vanickova Z, Hrabal P, *et al.* Regulation of fibroblast activation protein by transforming growth factor Beta-1 in glioblastoma microenvironment. Int J Mol Sci 2021; 22(3): 1046.
[http://dx.doi.org/10.3390/ijms22031046] [PMID: 33494271]

[41]   Fitzgerald AA, Weiner LM. The role of fibroblast activation protein in health and malignancy. Cancer Metastasis Rev 2020; 39(3): 783-803.
[http://dx.doi.org/10.1007/s10555-020-09909-3] [PMID: 32601975]

[42]   Mhaidly R, Mechta-Grigoriou F. Fibroblast heterogeneity in tumor micro-environment: Role in immunosuppression and new therapies. Semin Immunol 2020; 48101417
[http://dx.doi.org/10.1016/j.smim.2020.101417] [PMID: 33077325]

[43]   Mohanta BC, Palei NN, Surendran V, *et al.* Lipid based nanoparticles: current strategies for brain tumor targeting. Curr Nanomater 2019; 4(2): 84-100.
[http://dx.doi.org/10.2174/2405461504666190510121911]

[44]   Malam Y, Loizidou M, Seifalian AM. Liposomes and nanoparticles: nanosized vehicles for drug delivery in cancer. Trends Pharmacol Sci 2009; 30(11): 592-9.
[http://dx.doi.org/10.1016/j.tips.2009.08.004] [PMID: 19837467]

[45]   Muthu MS, Feng SS. Theranostic liposomes for cancer diagnosis and treatment: current development and pre-clinical success. Expert Opin Drug Deliv 2013; 10(2): 151-5.
[http://dx.doi.org/10.1517/17425247.2013.729576] [PMID: 23061654]

[46]   Xin H, Jiang J, Wei WXJ. Liposome-based drug delivery for brain tumor theranostics.Nanotechnology-Based Targeted Drug Delivery Systems for Brain Tumors. Academic Press 2018; pp. 245-66.
[http://dx.doi.org/10.1016/B978-0-12-812218-1.00009-9]

[47]   Sonali , Singh RP, Sharma G, *et al.* RGD-TPGS decorated theranostic liposomes for brain targeted delivery. Colloids Surf B Biointerfaces 2016; 147: 129-41.
[http://dx.doi.org/10.1016/j.colsurfb.2016.07.058] [PMID: 27497076]

[48]   Grafals-Ruiz N, Rios-Vicil CI, Lozada-Delgado EL, *et al.* Brain targeted gold liposomes improve RNAi delivery for glioblastoma. Int J Nanomedicine 2020; 15: 2809-28.
[http://dx.doi.org/10.2147/IJN.S241055] [PMID: 32368056]

[49]   Mukhtar M, Bilal M, Rahdar A, *et al.* Nanomaterials for diagnosis and treatment of brain cancer: recent updates. Chemosensors (Basel) 2020; 8(4): 117.
[http://dx.doi.org/10.3390/chemosensors8040117]

[50]   Zhu Q, Ling X, Yang Y, *et al.* Embryonic stem cells-derived exosomes endowed with targeting properties as chemotherapeutics delivery vehicles for glioblastoma therapy. Adv Sci (Weinh) 2019; 6(6)1801899
[http://dx.doi.org/10.1002/advs.201801899] [PMID: 30937268]

[51]   Dong X. Current strategies for brain drug delivery. Theranostics 2018; 8(6): 1481-93.
[http://dx.doi.org/10.7150/thno.21254] [PMID: 29556336]

[52]   Zhu L, Oh JM, Gangadaran P, *et al.* Targeting and therapy of glioblastoma in a mouse model using exosomes derived from natural killer cells. Front Immunol 2018; 9: 824.
[http://dx.doi.org/10.3389/fimmu.2018.00824] [PMID: 29740437]

[53]   Seleci DA, Seleci M, Jonczyk R, *et al.* Niosomes for brain targeting. 2019.
[http://dx.doi.org/10.1201/9780429465079-13]

[54]   De A, Venkatesh N, Senthil M, Sanapalli BKR, Shanmugham R, Karri VVSR. Smart niosomes of temozolomide for enhancement of brain targeting. Nanobiomedicine (Rij) 2018; 5

[http://dx.doi.org/10.1177/1849543518805355] [PMID: 30344765]

[55]   Hu G, Zhang H, Zhang L, Ruan S, He Q, Gao H. Integrin-mediated active tumor targeting and tumor microenvironment response dendrimer-gelatin nanoparticles for drug delivery and tumor treatment. Int J Pharm 2015; 496(2): 1057-68.
[http://dx.doi.org/10.1016/j.ijpharm.2015.11.025] [PMID: 26598487]

[56]   Hu J, Zhang X, Wen Z, *et al.* Asn-Gly-Arg-modified polydopamine-coated nanoparticles for dual-targeting therapy of brain glioma in rats. Oncotarget 2016; 7(45): 73681-96.
[http://dx.doi.org/10.18632/oncotarget.12047] [PMID: 27655664]

[57]   Bhattacharyya S, Kudgus RA, Bhattacharya R, Mukherjee P. Inorganic nanoparticles in cancer therapy. Pharm Res 2011; 28(2): 237-59.
[http://dx.doi.org/10.1007/s11095-010-0318-0] [PMID: 21104301]

[58]   Ghosh P, Han G, De M, Kim C, Rotello V. Gold nanoparticles in delivery applications. Adv Drug Deliv Rev 2008; 60(11): 1307-15.
[http://dx.doi.org/10.1016/j.addr.2008.03.016] [PMID: 18555555]

[59]   Cheng Y, Meyers JD, Agnes RS, *et al.* Addressing brain tumors with targeted gold nanoparticles: a new gold standard for hydrophobic drug delivery? Small 2011; 7(16): 2301-6.
[http://dx.doi.org/10.1002/smll.201100628] [PMID: 21630446]

[60]   Dixit S, Novak T, Miller K, Zhu Y, Kenney ME, Broome AM. Transferrin receptor-targeted theranostic gold nanoparticles for photosensitizer delivery in brain tumors. Nanoscale 2015; 7(5): 1782-90.
[http://dx.doi.org/10.1039/C4NR04853A] [PMID: 25519743]

[61]   Singh P, Pandit S, Mokkapati VRSS, Garg A, Ravikumar V, Mijakovic I. Gold nanoparticles in diagnostics and therapeutics for human cancer. Int J Mol Sci 2018; 19(7): 1979.
[http://dx.doi.org/10.3390/ijms19071979] [PMID: 29986450]

[62]   El-Safoury DM, Ibrahim AB, El-Setouhy DA, Khowessah OM, Motaleb MA, Sakr TM. Amelioration of tumor targeting and *in vivo* biodistribution of 99mTc-methotrexate-gold nanoparticles (99mTc-Mex-AuNPs). J Pharm Sci 2021; 110(8): 2955-65.
[http://dx.doi.org/10.1016/j.xphs.2021.03.021] [PMID: 33812886]

[63]   Orringer DA, Koo YE, Chen T, Kopelman R, Sagher O, Philbert MA. Small solutions for big problems: the application of nanoparticles to brain tumor diagnosis and therapy. Clin Pharmacol Ther 2009; 85(5): 531-4.
[http://dx.doi.org/10.1038/clpt.2008.296] [PMID: 19242401]

[64]   Richard S, Saric A, Boucher M, *et al.* Antioxidative theranostic iron oxide nanoparticles toward brain tumors imaging and ROS production. ACS Chem Biol 2016; 11(10): 2812-9.
[http://dx.doi.org/10.1021/acschembio.6b00558] [PMID: 27513597]

[65]   Dadfar SM, Roemhild K, Drude NI, *et al.* Iron oxide nanoparticles: Diagnostic, therapeutic and theranostic applications. Adv Drug Deliv Rev 2019; 138: 302-25.
[http://dx.doi.org/10.1016/j.addr.2019.01.005] [PMID: 30639256]

[66]   Zhao J, Liu P, Ma J, *et al.* Enhancement of radiosensitization by silver nanoparticles functionalized with polyethylene glycol and aptamer As1411 for glioma irradiation therapy. Int J Nanomedicine 2019; 14: 9483-96.
[http://dx.doi.org/10.2147/IJN.S224160] [PMID: 31819445]

[67]   Zhao J, Li D, Ma J, *et al.* Increasing the accumulation of aptamer AS1411 and verapamil conjugated silver nanoparticles in tumor cells to enhance the radiosensitivity of glioma. Nanotechnology 2021; 32(14)145102
[http://dx.doi.org/10.1088/1361-6528/abd20a] [PMID: 33296880]

[68]   Gao Y, Gao F, Chen K, Ma J. Cerium oxide nanoparticles in cancer. OncoTargets Ther 2014; 7: 835-40.

[http://dx.doi.org/10.2147/OTT.S62057] [PMID: 24920925]

[69]   Sack-Zschauer M, Bader SBP. Cerium oxide nanoparticles as novel tool in glioma treatment: An *in vitro* study. J Nanomed Nanotechnol 2017; 8(6): 1-9.

[70]   Cai X, Zhu Q, Zeng Y, Zeng Q, Chen X, Zhan Y. Manganese oxide nanoparticles as MRI contrast agents In tumor multimodal imaging and therapy. Int J Nanomedicine 2019; 14: 8321-44.
[http://dx.doi.org/10.2147/IJN.S218085] [PMID: 31695370]

[71]   Li, S., Johnson, J., Peck, A. and Xie, Q., 2017. Near infrared fluorescent imaging of brain tumor with IR780 dye incorporated phospholipid nanoparticles. Journal of translational medicine, 15(1), pp. 1-12.

[72]   Locatelli E, Naddaka M, Uboldi C, *et al.* Targeted delivery of silver nanoparticles and alisertib: *in vitro* and *in vivo* synergistic effect against glioblastoma. Nanomedicine (Lond) 2014; 9(6): 839-49.
[http://dx.doi.org/10.2217/nnm.14.1] [PMID: 24433240]

[73]   Wang J, Tang W, Yang M, *et al.* Inflammatory tumor microenvironment responsive neutrophil exosomes-based drug delivery system for targeted glioma therapy. Biomaterials 2021; 273120784
[http://dx.doi.org/10.1016/j.biomaterials.2021.120784] [PMID: 33848731]

[74]   Naziris N, Pippa N, Sereti E, *et al.* Chimeric stimuli-responsive liposomes as nanocarriers for the delivery of the anti-glioma agent TRAM-34. Int J Mol Sci 2021; 22(12): 6271.
[http://dx.doi.org/10.3390/ijms22126271] [PMID: 34200955]

[75]   Song P, Song N, Li L, Wu M, Lu Z, Zhao X. Angiopep-2-Modified carboxymethyl chitosan-based pH/reduction dual-stimuli-responsive nanogels for enhanced targeting glioblastoma. Biomacromolecules 2021; 22(7): 2921-34.
[http://dx.doi.org/10.1021/acs.biomac.1c00314] [PMID: 34180218]

[76]   Chen KT, Wei KC, Liu HL. Theranostic strategy of focused ultrasound induced blood-brain barrier opening for CNS disease treatment. Front Pharmacol 2019; 10(FEB): 86.
[http://dx.doi.org/10.3389/fphar.2019.00086] [PMID: 30792657]

[77]   Lin CY, Tsai CH, Feng LY, *et al.* Focused ultrasound-induced blood brain-barrier opening enhanced vascular permeability for GDNF delivery in Huntington's disease mouse model. Brain Stimul 2019; 12(5): 1143-50.
[http://dx.doi.org/10.1016/j.brs.2019.04.011] [PMID: 31079989]

[78]   Chen PY, Hsieh HY, Huang CY, Lin CY, Wei KC, Liu HL. Focused ultrasound-induced blood–brain barrier opening to enhance interleukin-12 delivery for brain tumor immunotherapy: a preclinical feasibility study. J Transl Med 2015; 13(1): 93.
[http://dx.doi.org/10.1186/s12967-015-0451-y] [PMID: 25784614]

[79]   Georgiou G, Lee CH KT. Engineered antibody fc variants for enhanced serum half life. US 11,059,892 B2, 2021.

[80]   Rangaramanujam, Tyler K, Betty M, *et al.* US20170173172 Selective dendrimer delivery to brain tumors. 2021.

[81]   Xiyun Y, Kelong F, Minmi L, *et al.* CN104013599A - Drug carrier capable of realizing drug delivery specifically targeting tumor and application thereof - Google Patents. CN104013599A, 2014. p. 1–16.

[82]   Yang S, Xu Guizhi, Lei Wang, *et al.* Circular coils for deep transcranial magnetic stimulation. 2016.

[83]   Chen PY, Hsieh HY, Huang CY, Lin CY, Wei KC, Liu HL. Focused ultrasound-induced blood–brain barrier opening to enhance interleukin-12 delivery for brain tumor immunotherapy: a preclinical feasibility study. J Transl Med 2015; 13(1): 93.
[http://dx.doi.org/10.1186/s12967-015-0451-y] [PMID: 25784614]

[84]   Georgiou G, Lee CH, Kang TH. Engineered antibody Fc variants for enhanced serum half life 2021.

[85]   Rangaramanujam K, Tyler BM, Zhang F, Mastorakos P, Mishra MK, Mangraviti A. Selective dendrimer delivery to brain tumors 2021.

[86]   Yan X, Fan K, Liang M. Drug carrier for tumor-specific targeted drug delivery and use thereof 2019.

[87]   Zangen A, Roth Y, Zangen A, Roth Y. Circular Coils For Deep Transcranial Magnetic Stimulation 2016.

CHAPTER 3

Theranostics Polymeric Nanoparticles for Brain Tumor Diagnosis and Treatment

Sivadas Swathi Krishna[1], Ardra Thottarath Prasanthan[1], Nirdesh Salim Kumar[1], Manish Philip[1] and Vidya Viswanad[1,*]

[1] Department of Pharmaceutics, Amrita School of Pharmacy, Amrita Vishwa Vidyapeetham, AIMS Health Science Campus, Kochi, Kerala, India

Abstract: Theranostics, a dual strategy, helps in better tumor imaging, the biodistribution of drugs (the ability to direct therapeutic agents to the tumor site), and understanding the progress and effectiveness of therapy. Theranostics is an emerging technology for the diagnosis and management of brain tumors which differ from peripheral tumors in several ways because of their complexity in the genesis of oncogenes. Several factors must be considered for successful brain tumor-targeted drug delivery. Nanotheranostics for brain cancer therapies have been identified now, and polymeric nanoparticles (PNP) are one of the most efficient and promising nanotechnological platforms. They can be utilized as a new imaging method to optimize chemotherapeutic drug delivery into brain tumors while reducing the drug's dissemination and toxicity in healthy people. Smart carriers and theranostic nanoparticles can diagnose, deliver, and track the therapeutic response synchronized. This chapter gives an insight into superparamagnetic, ultrasound-triggered radionuclide bearing, and fluorescent PNPs as potential theranostic approaches for brain tumor management.

Keywords: Brain tumor targeting, Fluorescent nanoparticles, Polymeric nanoparticles, Superparamagnetic nanoparticles, Theranostics.

INTRODUCTION

Transport of the drug into the brain is a significant defiance owing to the strong brain defense mechanism against foreign molecules. This necessitates the creation of more efficient distribution methods. Targeted drug delivery or targeted nanotechnology implementation is an appealing solution when contemplating all anatomic issues of brain tumors, as it can improve brain drug delivery [1]. A targeted drug delivery system (TDDS) is a technique for delivering therapeutic

* Corresponding Author Vidya Viswanad: Department of Pharmaceutics, Amrita School of Pharmacy, Amrita Vishwa Vidyapeetham, AIMS, Health Science Campus, Kochi, Kerala, India;
E-mails: vidyaviswanad@aims.amrita.edu, vidyanitin26@gmail.com

agents selectively and preferentially to the target site while limiting access to non-target sites. It aims at concentrating the medicament at the target tissue and thereby relatively reducing its concentration in other parts of the body; this increases the effectiveness while lowering the toxicity [2].

Nanoparticles have many benefits over traditional formulations, including the ability for drug conjugation, targeting effects, and improving drug pharmacokinetic characteristics. The half-life of the drugs can be extended using nanoplatforms using molecular probes. This provides various advantages. It provides accurate delivery of the anticancer medicament to the target tissues and releases the drugs with the help of detectors by responding to various stimuli Nanoparticles made of polymeric materials stand out as a powerful tool for increasing drug bioavailability and delivering drugs to their target sites. These are colloidal structures made up of natural or synthetic polymers, and the polymers' flexibility makes them theoretically suitable for meeting the needs of each drug-delivery system [3].

Theranostic nanoparticles appear to be a promising system that offers a novel solution to address present brain tumor management and diagnosis drawbacks. Options such as limiting metabolization of medications, providing simultaneous delivery with combined effects of two or more drugs, and enabling regulated and exact release, reducing adverse effects, are offered by theranostics. This technique aids in tackling the intra- and inter-patient heterogeneity of brain tumors, leading to a potential application of personalized medicine [4]. Nowadays, brain targeted drug delivery has received much interest because of its slow release, controllable and targeted protection.

MECHANISMS OF TARGETED DRUG DELIVERY IN BRAIN TUMOR

Due to the intricacy of brain tumors, several factors should be considered for efficient brain tumor-targeted drug delivery, including the barriers, the microenvironment in the tumor, and tumor cells [5]. Some of the factors which affect brain drug delivery include 1. Drug /polymer concentration gradient. 2. The drug's molecular weight. 3. Cell-to-cell sequestration. 4. Protein affinity for efflux transporters 5. Metabolism by tissues other than the liver. 6. Circulation in the brain. 7. Enzymatic stability throughout the body.8. Drug/polymer clearance rate. 9. The state of the disease. 10. Stability of cellular enzymes. 11. The drug's lipophilicity [6]. To address these problems, various active targeting mechanisms for designing a successful medication delivery system to the brain were used. The blood-brain barrier (BBB) targeting mechanism and the Blood-brain tumor barrier (BBTB) targeting mechanism are the two main types of mechanisms mentioned in Fig. (**1**) [5].

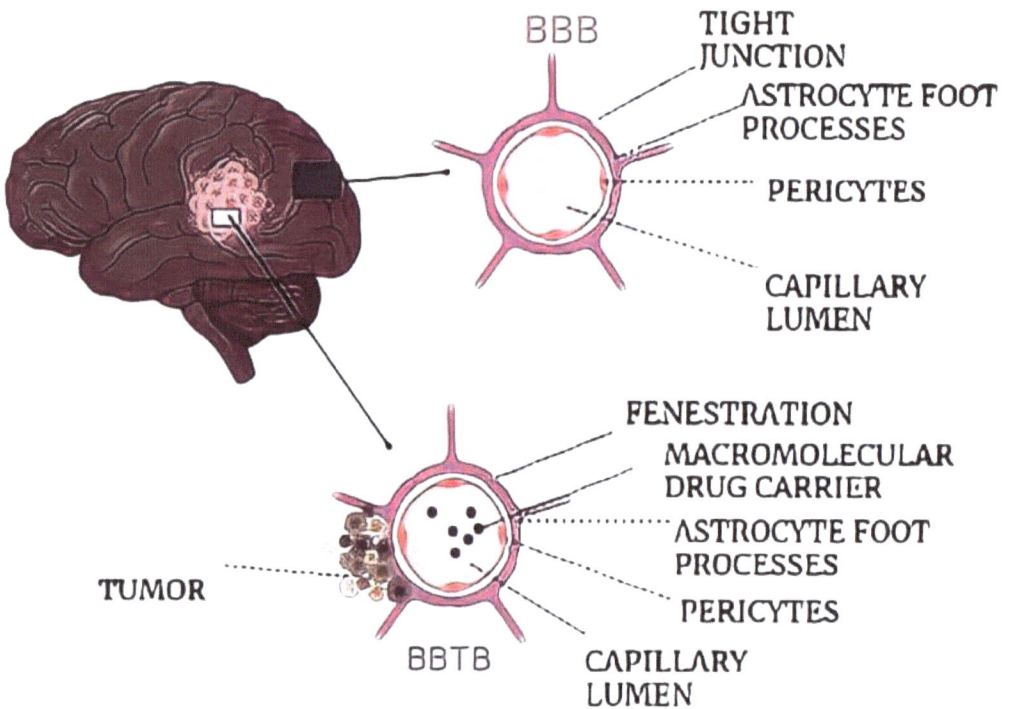

Fig. (1). Argeting mechanisms for brain tumor drug delivery.

The Blood-Brain Barrier Targeting Mechanism

The BBB serves as a physical (tight junctions), metabolic (enzymes), and immunological barrier, limiting drug transport into the brain. The BBB is made up of a variety of cells, including brain capillary endothelial cells (BCECs), pericytes, astrocytes, and neuronal cells, with BCECs being the most abundant. The continuous tight junctions between brain capillary endothelial cells restrict the transport of compounds in a paracellular manner from the blood to the brain and result in exceptionally high trans-endothelial electrical resistance (TEER) between blood and brain, limiting the passive diffusion of compounds. Despite these constraints, the BBB has several overexpressed receptors and carriers that can regulate the movement of various ligands and their drugs. Furthermore, the BBB membrane is negatively charged and has a high affinity for positively charged molecules, which could lead to cell internalization. As a result, these ligands could facilitate NP (nanoparticles) penetration through the BBB through a variety of activities targeting strategies as shown in Fig. (**2**) [7].

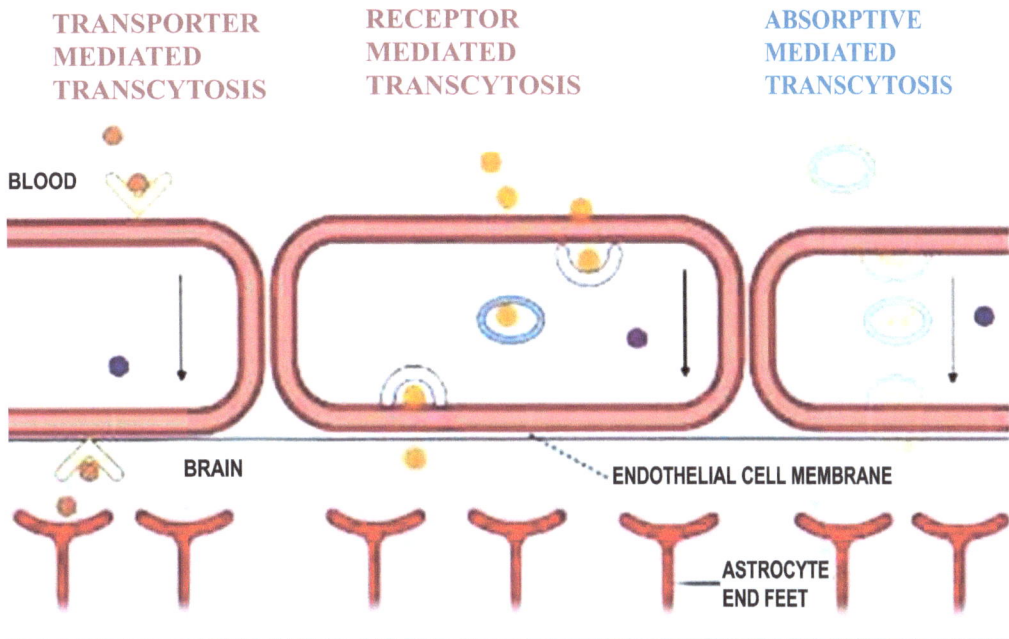

Fig. (2). Active targeting strategies through BBB

Absorptive Mediated Transcytosis

AMT allows cell-penetrating peptides (CPPs) or cationic proteins to transport drugs through the BBB. It is induced by the electrostatic interaction between the protein moieties that have a positive charge and brain endothelial cells that have a negative charge (Fig. **3**) [5]. The BBB's transcytotic pathways and its morphological and enzymatic properties and the high content of mitochondria in cerebral endothelial cells enable molecules to pass through the endothelial cytoplasm. Peptides/proteins, DNA/oligonucleotide, toxins, and nano-drug carriers such as liposomes and micelles have all been delivered using absorptive mediated transcytosis to overcome the lipophilic barrier between the membranes of cells. Since cationic proteins CPPs can bind to any cell membrane that is a negatively charged constituent, the specificity of AMT to the targeted site is reduced. Furthermore, the use of cationic proteins, or CPPs, is restricted due to their possible toxicity and immunogenicity [8].

In a study, aclarubicin (ACL) was integrated into cationic albumin-conjugated pegylated nanoparticle (CBSA-NP-ACL) to assess the potential of its therapy on rats by the intracranial implantation of C6 glioma cells. When labeled with fluorescent probe 6-coumarin, CBSA-NP accumulated much more in tumor mass than ACL-loaded nanoparticles without conjugation of CBSA, indicating its therapeutic potential for glioma treatment [9].

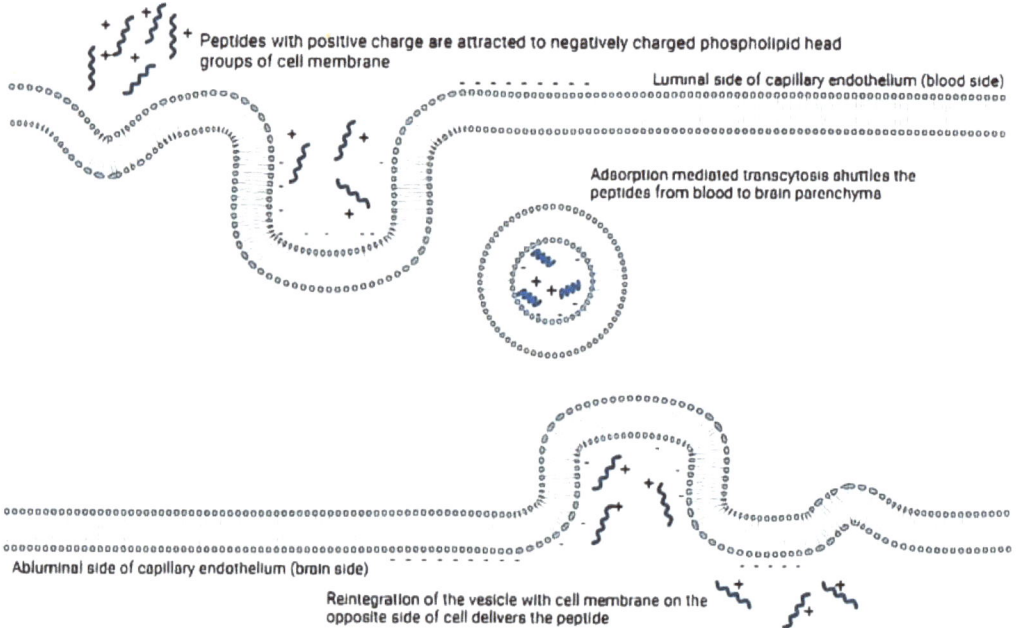

Fig. (3). Mechanism of absorptive mediated transcytosis

In another study, TAT (AYGRKKRRQRRR), a cell-penetrating peptide, was covalently conjugated with cholesterol to prepare doxorubicin-loaded liposomes for brain glioma treatment in which brain capillary endothelial cells (BCECs) and C6 glioma cells were studied for cellular uptake. The survival time of the glioma-bearing rats treated with TAT-modified liposomes was much longer than in other groups [10]. MC-PEI (10 K)/DNA, low molecular weight after being treated with myristic acid and complexed with DNA, nanoparticles were successfully taken up by the mouse brain. The anti-glioblastoma activity of MC-PEI (10 K)/ pORF-hTRAIL was demonstrated using the survival time of intracranial U87 glioblastoma-bearing mice [11].

Transporter Mediated Transcytosis

The cerebral endothelium contains a variety of transport mechanisms for providing the brain with essential nutrients and endogenous substances, TMT exploits these systems as a promising brain targeting strategy. Drugs that have a close resemblance to the substrates present endogenously are allowed for uptake, thereby their transport into the brain occurs. Glucose transporters (GLUT), which aid in glucose transport from the bloodstream to the brain, have a great deal of potential for brain targeting (Fig. **4**) [5].

The cholesterol of glycosyl derivative was formulated to develop novel liposomes to target GLUTs on the BBB and thereby overcome the drawback of poor delivery of the drug to the brain. The cytotoxicity of glucose-mediated brain targeting liposome containing coumarin-6 for brain capillary endothelial cells (BCECs) was lower than that of a traditional liposome [12].

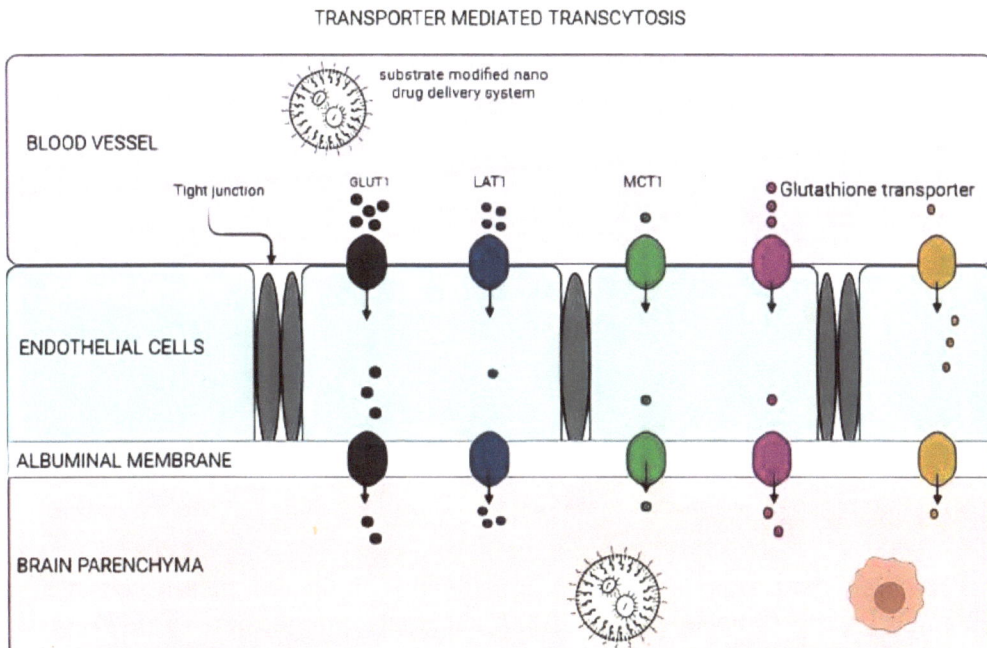

Fig. (4). Mechanism of transporter-mediated transcytosis

Receptor-Mediated Transcytosis

Receptor-mediated transcytosis is one of the most well-established methods for delivering drugs to the brain, with high specificity, selectivity, and affinity. The brain's capillary endothelium expresses various receptors, like the transferrin receptor (TfR), the low-density lipoprotein receptor (LDLR), the insulin receptor, and the nicotinic acetylcholine receptors, which can be targeted by the ligands such as endogenous or exogenous ligands. These receptors and ligands have been taken advantage of to enable receptor-mediated BBB transport and can cause cell internalization due to their ligand specificity [5]. As a result, the appropriate ligands might be functionalized into NPs to help them penetrate the BBB. Targeting efficiency may be lowered because the ligand can influence homeostasis, and also, there may be a chance of competition between natural ligands with therapeutic ligands (Fig. **5**) [7].

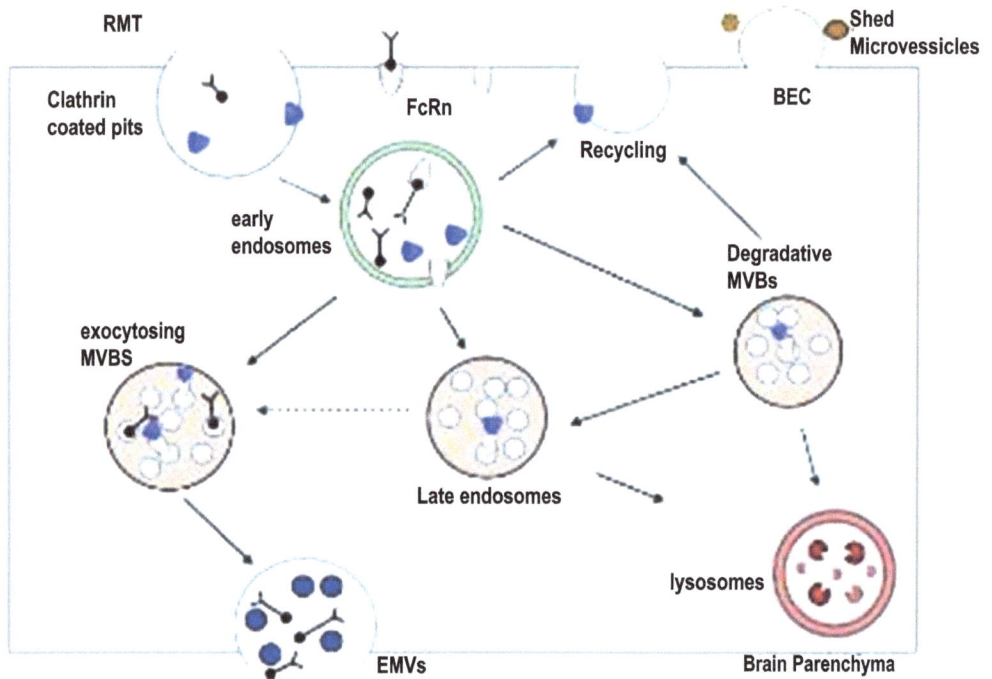

Fig. (5). Mechanism of receptor-mediated transcytosis

The research goal was to develop transferrin-conjugated theranostic d-alph--tocopheryl polyethylene glycol 1000 succinate monoester (TPGS) coated theranostic liposomes carrying docetaxel and quantum dots (QDs) for brain cancer imaging and therapy. *In vivo* data suggested that transferrin receptor-targeted theranostic liposomes could be suitable for brain theranostics, providing better and prolonged brain targeting of docetaxel and quantum dots [13]. The delivery of temozolomide (TMZ), the first-line treatment of Glioblastoma multiforme using poly (lactic-co-glycolic acid) nanoparticles, is established in this study. To assess the drug's *in vitro* cytotoxicity, researchers used glioblastoma tumor cell lines (U215 and U87) targeted with stable nanoparticles functionalized with an OX26 type monoclonal antibody targeting transferrin receptor [14]. Tf-modified paclitaxel-loaded polyphosphoester hybrid micelles (TPM) were produced and examined *in vitro* and *in vivo* for brain-targeting efficacy. TPM showed increased cellular uptake and brain deposition, the maximum anti-glioma activity, and the average survival time of mice with intracranial U-87 MG glioma treated with TPM were considerably longer than that of Taxol®-treated mice [15].

Blood-Brain Tumor Barrier Targeting Mechanism

The blood-brain tumor barrier (BBTB), usually found between tumor tissues in the brain and micro vessels produced by highly sophisticated endothelial cells (ECs), prevents most hydrophilic molecules from reaching tumor tissue *via* paracellular delivery. When the cell clusters of tumors reach a particular size, the BBB gets compromised, and BBTB develops. With the progression of brain tumors, angiogenesis, and progressive BBB damage, BBTB turns the primary impediment to drug delivery nanosystems. Most of the BBTB targeting techniques target high-expression receptors on tumors, including epidermal growth factor receptors and integrins [5].

Antibodies against the epidermal growth factor receptor (EGFR) were coupled to liposomes (immunoliposomes) utilizing the antibody affinity motif of protein A (ZZ) as an adaptor, and sodium borocaptate (BSH) was encased in nickel lipid liposomes. The findings indicate that using immunoliposomes to inject ^{10}B (an isotope of boron) into glioma cells during boron neutron capture therapy (BNCT) is a viable option [16]. In another study, researchers generated a paclitaxel-loaded(RGDyK)-Poly(ethylene glycol)-block-poly(lactic acid) micelle (c(RGDyK)-PEG-PLA-PTX) to take advantage of the strong binding affinity of a cyclic RGD peptide with integrin alpha(v)beta(3)highly-expressed on tumor neovasculature and U87MG glioblastoma. *In vitro* cell toxicity studies demonstrated that the presence of c(RGDyK) increased the anti-glioblastoma cell cytotoxic efficacy by 2.5 folds and the highest tumor growth suppression among the paclitaxel preparations evaluated [17]. To target the EGF-receptor (EGFR), epidermal growth factor (EGF) was used, and a recently synthesized daunorubicin derivative was loaded into the liposome (125) I-Comp1. The effective targeting of the nucleus results in high-ferocity cell killing of cultured U-343MGaCl2:6 cells [18].

Enhanced Permeability And Retention (EPR) Effect-Based Strategies

The enhanced permeability and retention (EPR) effect occurs as the brain tumor grows. The weak microenvironment in the peripheral tumors allows nanosystems with the appropriate particle size to infiltrate the brain tumor through endothelial breaches on microvessels in the brain tumor (Fig. **6**).

Using dtACPP-modified nanoparticles to co-deliver plasmid encoding interfering RNA targeting VEGF (shVEGF) and doxorubicin (dtACPPD/shVEGF-DOX) results in successful blood vessel closure and cell apoptosis inside the tumor itself. dtACPPD/shVEGF-DOX has shown good tumor targetability, excellent antitumor activity, and minimal adverse effects after systemic administration [19].

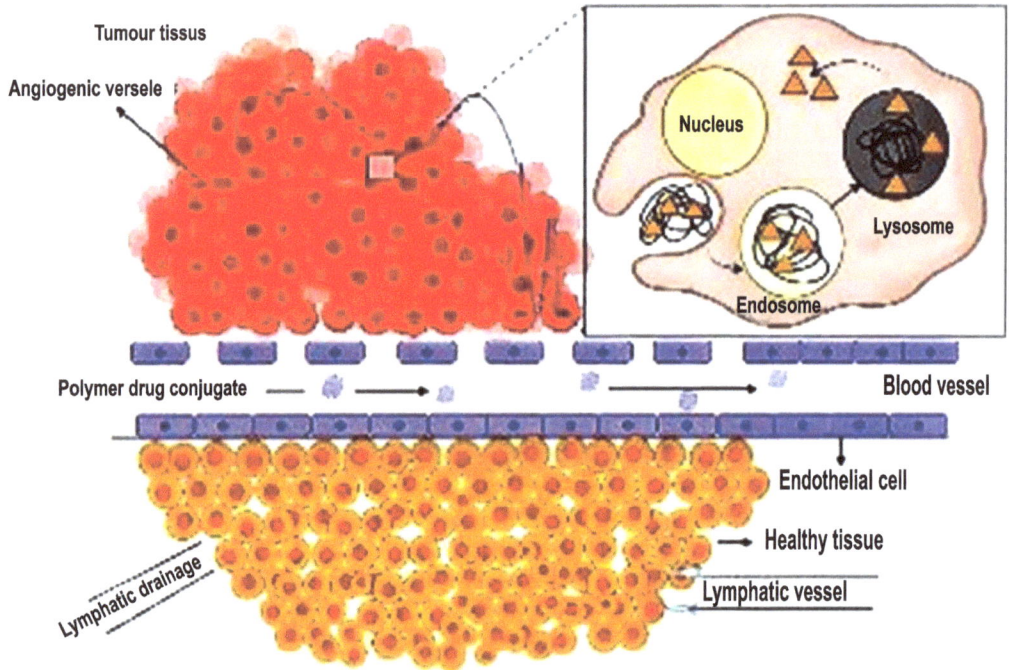

Fig. (6). Mechanism-based on EPR effect

POLYMERIC NANOPARTICLES BASED DIAGNOSIS AND TREATMENT OF BRAIN TUMOR

Polymeric nanoparticles are colloidal systems with a diameter of less than 1000 nm made from various prefabricated synthetic polymers or by polymerization of the monomer. Natural polymers such as albumin, gelatin, chitosan, dextran, dextrin, and hyaluronic acid, as well as pseudo synthetic polymers (different poly(amino) acids), are also used in nanoparticles' development [20, 21]. Furthermore, the surface can be adjusted in various ways to make them suitable for a variety of medical applications. Polysaccharides, proteins, amino acids, polyesters, poly ethyl amines, and other similar materials are widely used to synthesize nanoparticles used in central nervous system applications. Polymeric nanoparticles reach the brain through a variety of pathways:1) Transcytosis by endothelial cells 2) Opening of tight junctions of capillaries in the brain; 3) Attaching to the capillary walls of the brain [20].

TYPES OF POLYMERIC NANOPARTICLES IN DRUG DELIVERY AND TREATMENT

In the case of brain tumor treatment, the ideal drug vehicle should be able to penetrate blood-brain barriers and tumor vasculature. It must be recognized by the target cells specifically and selectively and must retain the specificity of the surface ligands. The drug ligand complex should be stable in plasma, interstitial, and other bio-fluids [21]. The vehicle utilized should be non-toxic, non-immunogenic, and biodegradable. Here we mainly focus on the roles of polymeric nanoparticles such as polymeric micelles and dendrimers in brain tumor management [22].

Polymeric micelles, a type of polymeric nanoparticle, are core-shell nanospheres made up of self-assembling amphiphilic block copolymers [23]. They are difficult to detect and extract due to their nano-dimensions. The phagocytic mechanism enhances the permeability and retention of their hydrophilic shells [24]. Its small size also provides a high structural solubility for administering hydrophobic medications to malignant brain tumors [23].

In a study, Aptamer-functionalized poly (ethylene glycol)-poly (D, L lactic-c--glycolic acid) PEG-PLGA nanoparticles were developed for anti-glioma delivery of paclitaxel. A pre-clinical study demonstrated extended circulation and intensified drug accumulation of Ap-PTX-NP (PEG-PLGA nanoparticles for anti-glioma delivery of paclitaxel), showing that these polymeric nanoparticles act through aptamer-nucleolin interaction, which results in increased nanoparticle penetration into C6 glioma cells, consequently resulting in increased cytotoxicity to tumor cells [23].

The docetaxel-loaded bio-adhesive micelles for brain tumor therapy act by enhanced transport of the docetaxel-encapsulated micelles system into C6 glioma cells. It shows that targeted and non-targeted nano-micelles had 4.08- and 2.89-times higher bioavailability, respectively compared to pristine Dorcel after 48 hr treatment [24]. Polymeric biodegradable nanoparticles comprising nanosphere and nanocapsule topologies are also promising for BBB-impenetrable therapeutic delivery. These devices can also regulate medication payload release and safeguard drugs from environmental contamination.

A preclinical study showed inhibition of glioma cell proliferation and extension of survival time in a rat tumor model when polysorbate-80 coated PBCA nanoparticles were administered with nucleoside reductase inhibitor in c6 glioma cells [23].

Dendrimers are highly branched, a well-ordered nano-scale structure with multivalent functional groups that allow therapeutic agents to get easily incorporated into their structure. These hyper branched polymers are thought to be promising drug carriers because of their well-engineered three-dimensional framework and broad surface functionalities. Drug molecules may be entrapped within the dendrimer's internal vacuum or bound to the surface groups. A range of functional groups on the dendrimer surface has led to the generation of a variety of therapeutic molecules and compounds. They have innumerable advantages over other nanosystems, including nano-scale size, size consistency, large functional classes, quick cell entry, adjustable size, reduced macrophage absorption, targeted delivery, and widespread transcytosis *via* biological membranes [24]. Distinct kinds of stimulus-sensitive groups can be used to induce controlled drug release from dendrimers. Several investigations have shown that they can cross the BBB and improve the build-up of the drug at the brain tumor site [23]. To achieve targeted and selective brain delivery, dendrimers' surfaces can be coated with targeting ligands that aid in the reconstitution of cancer cells without affecting normal cell viability [24].

A study shows that researchers created a pH-responsive dual-targeting dendrimer for the treatment of brain gliomas coupled with transferrin and tamoxifen. Doxorubicin, an anticancer medication, was covalently bonded to the dendrimer poly(amidoamine) (PAMAM) through a pH-sensitive hydrazone bond. At a pH of 7.4, only 6% of the drug was released, while at a pH of 4.5, 32% release was detected. In an *in vitro* BBB model, these dendrimers outperformed non-targeted and transferrin-targeted dendrimers in transport efficiency [23]. Dendritic polymers, such as the poly (amidoamine) (PAMAM) dendrimer, have risen to prominence as reliable polymeric nanostructures for delivering targeted genes and drugs in cancer care. As a result, several PAMAM dendrimer-driven nano-theragnostic drug delivery systems have been developed to take advantage of their potential for brain targeting.

Another study shows that BBB-penetrating nanocarrier device by integrating angiopep-2 peptide, conjugated to epidermal growth factor receptor (EGFR) enhances the glioma-targeting effect after using the fourth-generation PAMAM dendrimer after BBB penetration [24].

POLYMERIC NANOPARTICLES IN BRAIN TUMOR DIAGNOSIS

High-resolution imaging is crucial before surgery, especially for an extremely invasive brain tumor. Because of the invasiveness, determining a definite tumor boundary is challenging preoperatively and postoperatively. Accurate imaging of a tumor is crucial for determining tumor distribution and responsiveness to a treatment program [23]. Optical imaging, computed tomography, photo acoustic imaging, positron emission tomography, and fluorescence imaging techniques are already accessible tools for visualizing and diagnosing brain tumors and cancer [24]. Contrast-enhanced T1-weighted MRI is by far the most popular approach for imaging brain malignancies [23] to overcome these limitations, a system as a part of nanotechnology called polymeric NPs has been developed as it has the potential to improve not only drug delivery to diseases but also accurate imaging of cancerous tissues in the brain. Surface chemistry, topology, shape, solubility, stability, and other physical features of NPs have made them a good choice for usage as image contrast agents. If biocompatible nanomaterials are used, their nano-dimension extends the circulation time and enhances the safety profile. As a response to phagocytosis by cells in the brain, nano diagnostics reduces the frequency of signaling in brain malignancies and tumors. Because NPs have improved penetration and retention in tumor-associated cells and macrophages, they can be used to image malignant tissues and distinguish them from normal cells [24]. It also provides better information about the extent of the tumor [25]. Modulating the tropism of nanostructures with specific peptide, bio-conjugate, and nucleotide coatings is one such technique for high-precision malignancies [24]. Magnetic resonance imaging is one of the most advanced applications of nanotechnology in diagnosing brain cancers. Many nanoparticles have been designed as MRI contrast agents [25]. The polymeric nanoparticles with a dextran and iron oxide core were first utilized *in vivo* in people for diagnostic reasons, exploiting their superparamagnetic effect [22].

Researchers used polymer-coated nanoparticles to deliver the anti-cancer medication epirubicin and other molecules infusing brain tissue with an MRI contrast agent. The researchers used ultrasound to create microbubbles that changed the permeability of the BBB, allowing the magnetic nanoparticles to pass through. They also confirmed under the direction of MRI, synergistic targeting and image monitoring are effective approaches for delivering macromolecular chemotherapeutic drugs into the CNS [26].

Another study using Photofrin® and iron oxide coupled with F3 in a polymeric nanoparticle formulation for MRI and PDT exemplifies theranostic systems. Under light exposure, Photofrin® was able to produce singlet oxygen and instigate cytotoxicity. Due to the magnetic characteristics of iron oxide, the pharmacokinetics of the nanoparticles might be assessed using MRI. The F3 modified nanoparticles had a 2-fold increase in contrast enhancement and longer retention in the brain tumor site compared to untargeted nanoparticles. A study also conveyed that targeted theranostic nanoparticles considerably enhanced survival rates in test objects with a brain tumor after PDT-mediated laser irradiation compared to non-targeted theranostic nanoparticles or Photofrin® alone. After the trial, 40% of the tested object in the targeted theranostic nanoparticle treatment group was tumor-free [23].

Another study formulated and analyzed a nontoxic dye–loaded polyacrylamide nanoparticle that has the potential to distinguish neoplastic tissue under normal lighting settings. 9L gliosarcoma cells have been demonstrated to stain with Coomassie-blue-loaded nanoparticles, and *in vivo* data is now being collected [25].

Other than drug targeting, dendrimers are useful in diagnosis of brain tumors because of their high-density surface groups. A study shows that fluorescein isothiocyanate, an imaging dye, folic acid, the targeting molecule, and paclitaxel (anti-cancer agent) were incorporated with PAMAM dendrimer [27]. A group of researchers demonstrated that 5-aminolaevulinic acid using dendrimer technology was used for glioblastoma imaging to circumscribe tumor margins for surgery. Dendrimers targeting this acid specifically could improve the precision of this approach. Over the last two decades, gadolinium (Gd) paramagnetic contrast agents have been fused with dendrimer molecules to create imaging complexes for MRI. It increases clearance properties, improves contrast, and the possibility of being targeted [20].

In an *in vivo* investigation with fluorescent polysorbate 80 overlaid with PBCA nanoparticles, there was direct evidence of nanoparticles entering the brain. The nanoparticles were tagged *in situ* with a fluorescent dye and coated with polysorbate 80 after being synthesized using a mini emulsion method. The BBB was studied *in vitro* using human brain microvascular endothelial cells (BMECs). The cells demonstrated substantial growth in the *in vitro* model (transwell system), and the transcytosis was absent [22]. Reported data of theranostic nanoparticle is given in Table **1** below.

Table 1. Reported data of Theranostics Polymeric Nanoparticles.

CARRIERS / TRANSPORRTERS	FORMULATIONS	DRUG / MOLECULES
MICELLES	LIGAND MOLECULES WITH CYCLIC ARG-GLY-ASP	PLATINUM
	PLURONIC P-105	DOXORUBICIN
	TRANSFERRIN CONJUGATED WITH PCL-PEEP	PACLITAXEL
	CHITOSAN FUSED WITH STEARIC ACID	DOXORUBICIN
	POLYMERIC MICELLES TREATED WITH P-HA	DOCETAXEL

(Table 1) cont.....

CARRIERS / TRANSPORRTERS	FORMULATIONS	DRUG / MOLECULES
DENDRIMERS	DENDRIMER BIOCONJUGATES OF CETUXIMAB (IMC-C225)	DOXORUBICIN
	POLYAMIDOAMINE DENDRIMERS	DOXORUBICIN
	TRANSFERRIN (TF) AND WHEAT GERM AGGLUTININ PEGYLATED FOURTH-GENERATION PAMAM DENDRIMER (WGA)	DOXORUBICIN
NANOEMULSION	PINE NUT OIL	PACLITAXEL
LIPOSOMES	GLUTATHIONE PEGYLATED LIPOSOME	DOXORUBICIN
	LACTOFERRIN CONJUGATED WITH PEGYLATED LIPOSOME	RADIO-ISOTOPE COMPLEX, 99MTC - BMEDA
	PEGYLATED LIPOSOME	DOXORUBICIN
	AB-CONJUGATED WITH LIPOSOME (IMMUNOLIPOSOME)	DAUNOMYCIN
	LIPOSOME WHICH IS THERMOSENSITIVE	CIS-DIAMINE-DICHLORO-PLATINUM (CDDP)
	LIPOSOME CONJUGATED WITH INTERLEUKIN-13	DOXORUBICIN
	D-A-TOCOPHERYL PEG 1000 SUCCINATE MONO-ESTER	DOCETAXEL
	LIPOSOMES CONJUGATED WITH ATHEROSCLEROTIC PLAQUE-SPECIFIC PEPTIDE-1 (AP-1)	DOXORUBICIN

[28 - 43]

THERANOSTICS

Theranostics, which focuses on patient-centered treatment, is emerging as a precise, effective, and efficient therapy that integrates diagnosis and treatment. It works as a gateway between traditional medicine and personalized medicine. It deals with a personalized care plan based on each person's specific characteristics, resulting in the right prescription for the right patient at the right time [44]. The goal is to detect and cure illnesses as early as possible when they are most likely curable [45]. It acquires diagnosis and delivers a treatment dose of radiation to the patient using various biological pathways in the human body [46]. It also offers a cost-efficient, highly effective treatment regimen and focuses mainly on pharmacogenetic, proteomics, and biomarker profiling (Fig. **7**) [45]. Among theranostics, nano theranostics or theranostic nanomedicine is most commonly used for medical purposes (Fig. **8**) [46]. These therapeutic and diagnostic agents are combined into a single theranostic arena in nanomedicine, which can be integrated into biological ligands for targeted delivery. It can attain systemic circulation, evade host immunity, and deliver drugs and diagnostic agents to the targeted site, accounting for cellular and molecular diagnosis and treatment [45]. This new technological phenomenon combines inorganic and organic nanoparticles to achieve combined properties in a nanoparticle, using organic NPS for drug delivery and inorganic NPS for imaging [1, 46]. This advanced technology offers several benefits over traditional drug products in precise targeting the ability to boost pharmacokinetics and biodistribution of established therapeutic agents to target tissues, increased stability, and site-specific delivery inside solid tumors *via* leaky vasculature. As a result, theranostics is a comprehensive shift from trial-and-error medicine to prognostic, prophylactic, and customized medicine, resulting in better pharmacotherapy treatment [44].

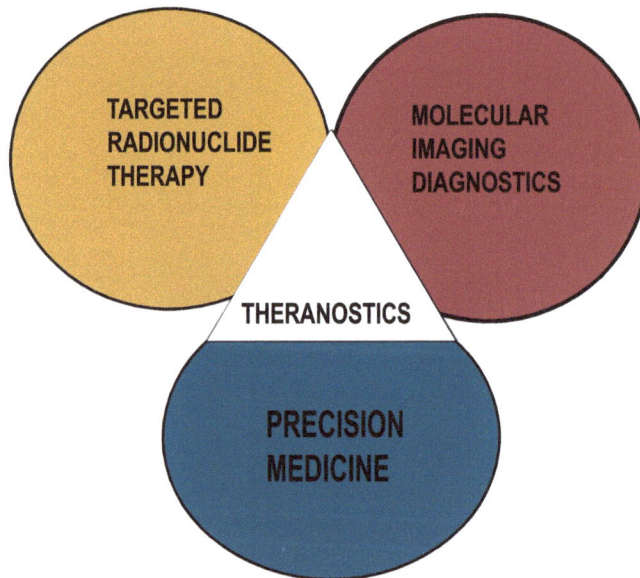

Fig. (7). Pictorial representation of the application of theranostics

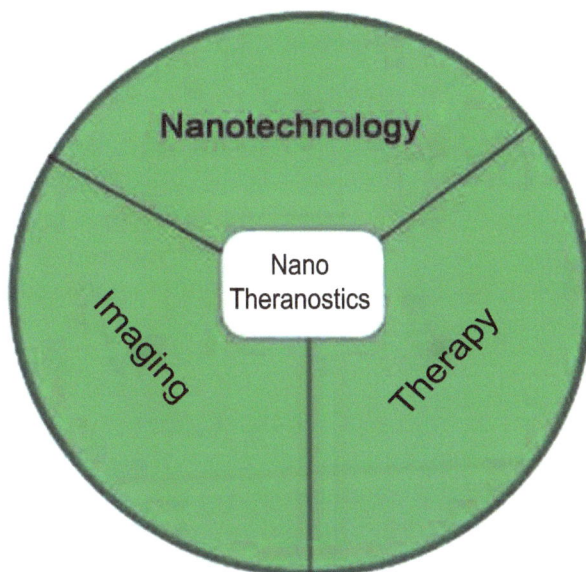

Fig. (8). Diagram representing nano theranostics

THERANOSTICS IN BRAIN TUMOR MANAGEMENT

Detecting and treating brain cancer in its early stages is difficult because of extracellular fluid accumulation surrounding the tumor area. Traditional diagnostic and therapeutic agents had poor biodistribution and pharmacokinetics, resulting in inadequate tumor dissemination. They're also non-specific, which can build up in healthy organs, resulting in high toxicity. In three dimensions, new vistas in cancer treatment are being opened – theranostics is a technique for diagnosing, treating, and monitoring a patient's response, particularly with the help of nanotechnology [44]. Several successful nano theranostics therapies for brain cancers have been identified, but further research is needed. Nanoparticle-augmented imaging of the CNS at the subcellular level pinpoints the intracranial neoplasms region with greater precision. Furthermore, nanoparticle-enhanced neuroimaging is extremely helpful in understanding physiological processes such as apoptosis, ischemia, inflammation, cell differentiation, and mitosis, and serves as the primary method for future study; if a diagnostic molecule is attached, the extent of curative effect inside the brain tumor may be sensed [46].

An *in vitro* model has been developed based on differentiated cells or brain endothelial cell culture and shows how nanoparticles aid in the transfer of drugs into the targeted sites in the brain. For *e.g* a group of researchers in a study tested the impacts of chitosyme nanoparticles on BBB integrity, tight junction proteins (ZO-1, occludin), and extracellular matrix impacts. Paclitaxel (PTX) was also created with a cyclic Arg-Gly-Asp (RGD) peptide as a targeting ligand to pass through the BBB using a targeting technique in other experiments. The nanocarriers were examined on a 3D glioma spheroid of glioma cells cultured on agarose. They demonstrated selective accumulation into tumor spheroids and outstanding infiltration relative to traditional nanocarriers, implying that they could be used in the future for therapy. Theranostic nanosystems in conjunction with a targeting agent recognize specific targets in brain cancer cells. They bind and permeate into the tumor through a specific mechanism. Gold Nanoparticles (AuNPs) and Quantum Dots (QDs) are two nanomaterials with inherent diagnostic and therapeutic properties, which are mentioned in the coming sections [2].

Glioblastoma, an invasive brain tumor, is difficult to diagnose and treat. According to current advances in GB therapy and diagnosis, there has been no substantial decrease in the number of people dying from GB. Treatment inefficiency can be attributed to various factors, including tumor heterogeneity, imprecise drug delivery, and failure in initial stage diagnosis. Theranostic approaches allow for the diagnosis of GB, the understanding of its location and stage of disease, and the perception of the progression of the tumor. These approaches aid in addressing intra- and interpatient diversification in GB, pointing to a future application in personalized medicine [1]. Numerous NPSs (lipidic, magnetic, liposomal, fluorescent, and polymeric) have been created to cross the BBB for the treatment of GB, with active, passive, and stimuli-targeting approaches taken into account. It also helps to reduce toxicity caused by a high and invasive dose, resulting in better patient outcomes [2]. It uses organic and inorganic NPs to obtain several properties in a single NP, taking advantage of organic NPs for drug delivery and inorganic NPs for imaging.

A study showed that micro-RNA (miRNAs) are used as theranostics for a brain tumor. They proposed miRNAs as an ideal diagnosis marker and a prognosis marker. MiRNAs are an effective therapy for an exceedingly diverse tumor type due to their broad mechanism of action. It has been found that it is a good source for glioblastoma treatment. Data from *in vivo* treatment revealed that miRNAs could revitalize the immune system and reduce drug resistance, two of the existing therapies' limitations. The movement of RNA drugs into the Central Nervous System through the blood-brain barrier is one of the most significant limitations of this unmet medical need. Novel carriers have been developed and synthesized in recent years to address this constraint, and miRNAs are optimal for loading these delivery mechanisms due to their structure and small-scale molecular weight [47]. Some of the examples of polymeric nanoparticle-coated drugs for glioma which are under clinical trials are given in Table **2** below [48].

Table 2. Examples of polymeric nanoparticle-coated drugs for glioma.

DRUGS	TYPE OF TUMORS	PHASES OF CLINICAL TRIAL
NAB-RAPAMYCIN	HIGH-GRADE GLIOMA RECURRENCE, NEWLY DIAGNOSED GLIOBLASTOMA	II
NANOLIPOSOMAL CPT-11	HIGH-GRADE GLIOMA RECURRENCE	COMPLETED I PHASE
FERUMOXYTOL	HIGH-GRADE GLIOMA RECURRENCE	I
9-ING-41	GLIOBLASTOMA	II
PEGYLATED LIPOSOMAL DOXORUBICINE+ TEMOZOLOMIDE	GLIOBLASTOMA	COMPLETED II PHASE

APPLICATION OF VARIOUS POLYMERIC NANOPARTICLES AS THERANOSTICS IN BRAIN TUMOR

Gold Nanoparticles

Gold Nanoparticles with gold centers are a novel system for theranostic applications. They're biocompatible and come in various shapes and sizes, including spheres, wire, rods, cubes, and cages. AuNPs, like other inorganic nanoparticles, cause oxidative stress, which leads to cytotoxicity. The ultraviolet (UV) absorption of spheroidal AuNPs is at 520 nm, while the absorption of gold nanorods is in the infrared range (690–900 nm). AuNPs can be used as a variety of theranostic medicines in clinical settings due to their intrinsic optical properties. AuNPs exhibited diagnostic properties, adaptable core size, minimal toxicity, surface plasmon absorption, ease of production, and light scattering properties [49]. Gold-based nanoshells having optical and magnetic properties coupled with a targeted moiety and explored as a treatment for head and neck cancer and have been demonstrated to benefit the treatment of gliomas; for example, combining AuNPs with irradiation improved survival relative to radiation therapy alone [50]. Furthermore, AuNPs are a promising possibility for tumor margin identification, which could help in brain cancer surgery resection [51].

E.g: the radio-sensitizing efficacy of gold theranostic micelles integrated with polyethylene glycol-polycaprolactone (PEG-PCL) for GBM (glioblastoma management)treatment was demonstrated. It can be employed as an innovative agent of contrast for both MRI and CT examinations [51].

Magnetic Nanoparticle

Magnetic nanoparticles (MNPs) have been proposed as viable nanocarriers for tumor-targeted medication administration, with the bonus of MRI traceability. Magnetically targeted delivery is improved by the magnetic response (iron oxide core). In a preclinical study, it has been demonstrated that intravenous delivery of these moieties can reach the tumor site and also act as a promising tool for increased accretion of MNPs in brain tumors and conducting non-invasive MRI screening [2].

Quantum Dots

Quantum dots (QDs) are nanocrystals of inorganic semiconductors with a nanoscale (10 nm) that could be used for theranostic purposes. Because of their structure, composition, and size, they emit light with a wavelength that can be modified. Cadmium selenide/zinc sulfide-based QDs are the most commonly used nanomaterials for diagnostic purposes. They consists of a CdSe (silica-coated cadmium selenide) core covered in ZnS lamina. Furthermore, the surface of the QDs can be covalently or non-covalently coupled with targeting probes such as antibodies, peptides, nucleic acids, folate aptamers, and other small molecules to obtain affinity and target the cancer location. One of the most effective ways to conjugate targeted compounds is avidin-biotin cross-linking. HER2, which is significantly expressed in glioblastoma, CD44, proteins, antibodies, folic acid, and other cancer cell-specific ligands, can be attached to QDs. Remarkably, QDs can be coupled with RGD peptides in paramagnetic liposomal compositions and used as an investigative tool in tumor angiogenesis utilizing MRI. Because of their possible toxicity in humans, QDs in theranostic have a potential clinical limit. To solve this issue, more research is needed to develop biocompatible, excretable, surface-modified QDs [2]. Essential requirements for the clinical application of nano theranostics are the capacity to execute various roles in biological systems and toxicity and biodistribution [1].

BRAIN TUMOR TREATMENT AND DIAGNOSIS- SOLUTIONS THROUGH NANO THERANOSTICS

Table **3** demonstrates the various types of treatment used to overcome the barriers issues.

Table 3. Different types of therapies to overcome the barriers.

STRATEGIES FOR THERAPY	BARRIERS TO CONVENTIONAL THERAPY	SOLUTION THROUGH NANOTECHNOLOGY
SURGERY	DIFFICULTY IN IDENTIFYING TUMOR BOUNDARIES	NANOPARTICLE-BASED IMAGING PROBES FOR INTRAOPERATIVE IMAGING GUIDANCE TO DISTINGUISH DISSEMINATED TUMOR MARGINS FROM HEALTHY BRAIN TISSUE WITH HIGH SPECIFICITY, SENSITIVITY, AND RESOLUTION.
RADIATION THERAPY	RADIO-RESISTANCE	1. DELIVER A HIGH-Z ELEMENT RADIOSENSITIZER BASED ON NANOPARTICLES. 2. TO TREAT TUMOR HYPOXIA. 3. NANOPLATFORMS ARE USED TO DELIVER GASOTRANSMITTERS LIKE NO AND H_2S
CHEMOTHERAPY	• BBB • DRUG RESISTANCE • WHEN DRUG ACCUMULATION IN TUMORS IS MINIMAL.	4. ENCAPSULATION OF NANO-DRUG WITH TARGETING LIGANDS. 5. DEVELOP A "ALL-IN-ONE" MEDICATION COCKTAIL BASED ON NANOPARTICLES FOR USE IN COMBINATION THERAPY. 6. ENCAPSULATE THERAPEUTIC PHARMACEUTICALS IN NANOCARRIERS FOR LONGER HALF-LIVES IN CIRCULATION AND ON-DEMAND DRUG RELEASE.

NANOPLATFORMS FOR BRAIN TUMOR IMAGING

Table **4** illustrates the different nanoplatforms in diagnosing diseases

Table 4. Various nanoplatforms in diagnosing diseases.

TYPES	CHARACTERISTICS	EXAMPLES
MRI (MAGNETIC RESONANCE IMAGING)	• EXCEPTIONAL SPATIAL RESOLUTION • UNRESTRICTED PENETRATION • SENSITIVITY ISSUES • ACQUISITION TIME IS HIGH.	SPION, GD-DTPA DENDRIMER NP

(Table 4) cont.....

TYPES	CHARACTERISTICS	EXAMPLES
FL IMAGING (FLUORESCENCE IMAGING)	• EXCEPTIONAL SENSITIVITY • NON-INTRUSIVENESS • PENETRATION IS RESTRICTED. • INSUFFICIENT SPATIAL RESOLUTION	SEMI-CONDUCTING QDS, CARBON DOTS, CARBON NANOTUBES, RARE-EARTH DOPED NPS, ORGANIC DYE-BASED NPS
ULTRASOUND	• CAN GENERATE SOUND WAVES THAT ARE GREATER THAN 20KHZ • ITS HEATING EFFECT HELPS IN THE RELEASE OF THERAPEUTIC AGENTS. • HELPS IN REVERSIBLE OPENING OF BBB.	TANNIC ACID AND POLY(*N*-VINYLPYRROLIDONE) COATED DOXORUBICIN
SUPERPARAMAGNETIC	• HIGH DRUG LOADING AND ENCAPSULATION EFFICIENCY • SPECIFICALLY, IN THE IDENTIFICATION OF TUMOUR LOCATION	P80-TMZ/SPIO-NPS, DSPE-PEG 2000
RADIONUCLIDE	• EARLY DIAGNOSIS • SENSITIVITY AND SPECIFICITY IN THE DETECTION OF SMALL PRIMARY TUMORS OR METASTASES	[8]GA-DOTATATE AND [177]LU-DOTATATE

PERSONALIZED MEDICINE: A POSSIBLE SCENARIO IN THERANOSTICS

Personalized medicine views pharmacogenomics, pharmacoproteomic, and pharmacogenetics data as critical for prescribing therapeutics tailored to - individual patients. Because of a greater comprehension of the condition at a molecular level, personalized medicine in oncology appears to be a promising strategy. With the introduction of a high-quality personalized medicine program, individualized medicine can be effective in managing cancers with precision and specificity. Personalized medicine helps to customize the design of nanoparticles by using pharmacogenetic, pharmacogenomic, and pharmacoproteomic methods and the comprehensive genetic and molecular profile of the patient. Specific molecular biomarkers may interact with targeted nanoparticles, which decides how the disease progresses and how well it responds to treatments. Nanoparticles used in customized medicine are tailored to each patient's needs, considering their unique characteristics. However, crucial steps in developing personalized cancer therapy, such as a thorough evaluation of biological characteristics of tumors from each client and validated methods to classify groups or subgroups of patients that may benefit more from therapy, are required. A clear example of a treatment using personalized medicine is the one applied to cancer based on the genotype of each person [1]. As mentioned above, glioma, an invasive tumor is very difficult to treat and diagnose. Hence, researchers recommend that personalized medicine with the comprehension of cancer (glioblastoma) microenvironment with the use of TNPs will improve its therapeutic and diagnostic potency.

POLYMER-BASED SUPERPARAMAGNETIC NANOPARTICLES AS THERANOSTICS FOR BRAIN TUMOR

Drug delivery systems have progressed to the point that they can combine the capabilities of various imaging techniques with an externally applied field or the action of a drug in a therapeutic manner. The development of these efficacious nanoplatforms, which combine magnetic nanoparticles and polymer, is advantageous because the latter can serve as a reservoir of drugs and a tool for extra functioning (for cell targeting or imaging). In contrast, magnetic NPs enable MRI, MPI, and hyperthermia—a cancer treatment that can be combined with the effect of medication [52]. In this regard, the iron structure is noteworthy, partly because iron is abundant and is used in a multitude of sectors. Furthermore, Ferro-and ferrimagnetic materials are gaining popularity, particularly in magnetic imaging and targeting. Magnetically sensitive magnetite (Fe_3O_4) and maghemite (γFe_2O_3)-based crystalline particles are easily manufactured as nanoscale (3.0100.0 nm) formulations. These formulations are accessible to surface manipulation and functionalization because they include atom vacancies and surface defects and polar amphoteric OH arrangement. These NPs are superparamagnetic, which shows that their magnetism appears to be zero on average at certain temperatures without applying a magnetic field externally. Due to their relatively high magnetic susceptibility in this state, the magnetization of nanoparticles can be done with the help of a magnetic field applied externally, giving them a suitable platform for magnetic targeting, magnetism-based hyperthermia, and imaging techniques such as MRI or magnetic particle imaging (MPI) [53]. Furthermore, iron oxides combined with transition metal ions such as copper, cobalt, nickel, and manganese were found to have superparamagnetic characteristics and hence fall into the SPION group (Fig. **9**) [54].

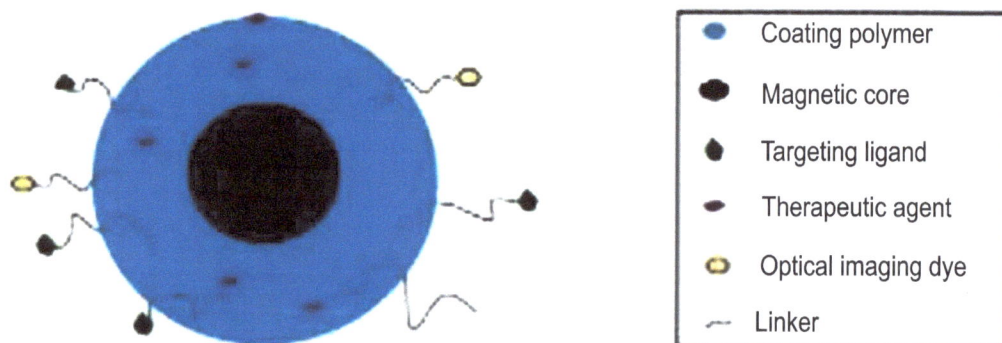

●	Coating polymer
◆	Magnetic core
◗	Targeting ligand
►	Therapeutic agent
◯	Optical imaging dye
～	Linker

Fig. (9). Diagram representing the active targeting of drug-using SPION core

The SPION core is typically made of magnetite (Fe_3O_4) or maghemite (γ-Fe_2O_3), which varies from 10 nm to 100 nm in diameter. The surface of the superparamagnetic core is coated with a compatible coating such as dextran, polyethylene glycol (PEG), poly-L-Lysine, D-mannose, or other polymers to avert agglomeration and improve biocompatibility. Here, active molecules can be coated with it, which allows the nanoparticle to be tailored for specific applications like active targeting (Fig. **8**). SPIONs are synthesized using various processes, including the sol-gel process, hydrothermal method, thermal decomposition, microemulsion system, high-energy ball mining technique, and microwave-assisted synthesis, the most common of which is co-precipitation. SPIONs are a promising tool for MRI of brain tumors because of their negative function, improving image contrast by suppressing the T2 MRI signal. Its relaxivity can be improved by tuning the core size and coating. Also, different ligands and bioactive compounds that can detect target receptors present in cancer cells can be implanted on the SPION surface to improve tumor imaging selectivity. Several tumor ligands are frequently used as potential options for active tumor targeting, including lactoferrin, neuropilin-1, and epidermal growth factor receptor (EGFR) deletion-mutant (EGFRvIII). Chitosan surface modification boosted the surface charge of dextran-coated SPIONs, resulting in improved internalization in GB cells. Furthermore, hybrid chitosan-dextran SPIONs can exhibit strong MRI contrast-enhancing properties for characterizing a brain tumor [55].

SPIONs not only improve contrast for MRI diagnosis, but they may also aid in the direct release of chemotherapeutic drugs at the tumor site. SPION nanoshells with hollow structures were employed as carriers for hydrophobic anticancer medicines delivered intracellularly. SPION Targeting strategies can be grouped into passive targeting, active targeting, and magnetic focusing. Passive targeting takes advantage of the nanoparticles' characteristic size, tumor microenvironment, and distinctive properties. Nanoparticles penetrate cancerous cells through these pores and are retained for longer periods than normal cells due to malignant tissue's inadequate lymphatic drainage system, a phenomenon known as the increased penetration and retention effect. Targeting ligands that are anchored to the surface of magnetic nanoparticles interact with receptors that are overexpressed in their target areas' active targeting. In magnetic focusing, external magnets provide an appropriate magnetic field gradient over the targeted area, ensuring considerable loading of drug-loaded SPIONs. The intensity of the applied magnetic field can be adjusted to modify drug release in the desired manner, resulting in the best therapeutic benefit [54].

P80-TMZ/SPIO-NPs, polysorbate 80 coated temozolomide-loaded PLGA-based superparamagnetic nanoparticles, were developed efficiently and identified as drug transporter and diagnostic agents for malignant glioma P80-TMZ/SPIO-NPs had shown high drug loading and entrapment efficiency and 15-day, sustained drug release performance [56]. Hydrophobic superparamagnetic iron oxide nanoparticles (SPIO NPs) were created using thermal decomposition approaches. They were coated with 1,2-stearoyl-sn-glycero-3-phosphoethanolamine-*N*-[methoxy (polyethylene glycol)-2000] (DSPE-PEG 2000) and Doxorubicin (DOX) employing a thin-film hydration technique followed by loading of indocyanine green (ICG) into the phospholipid layer. The multifunctional NPs generated were able to offer a sustained release of DOX with enhanced cellular uptake of DOX compared with that of free DOX. *In vivo* fluorescence and MRI indicated that NPs not only cross these dynamic barriers but are also stacked specifically at the tumor location [57] intravenously administered IL-1Ra or SPION-IL-1Ra at various concentrations to rats with intracranial C6 glioma. The conjugates of synthesized SPION-IL-1Ra have the characteristics of a negative contrast agent with high relaxation efficiency factors. SPION-IL-1Ra nanoparticles showed high intracellular incorporation and had no toxic effect on C6 cells or lymphocyte viability and proliferation *in vitro*, suggesting that SPION-IL-1Ra could be a candidate for theranostic approaches in neuro-oncology for both brain tumor diagnosis and management of peritumoral edema [58].

One of the significant disadvantages of delivering drugs *via* coating the surface of SPIONs is the low entrapment effectiveness of drug molecules, as only a minimal dose of medication can be conjugated. Another challenge is the formation of extremely reliable links as a response to covalent interaction between drugs and the surface of SPIONs, which results in the drug molecule failing to be released at the targeted location. When a promoter, such as a catalyst, like copper, is utilized in the covalent binding of medication to the SPION surface, it can produce *in vivo* toxicity if it is not adequately refined [54].

ULTRASOUND-TRIGGERED POLYMERIC NANOPARTICLES AS THERANOSTICS FOR BRAIN TUMOR

Ultrasound is a powerful method that can be used to enhance biological changes in the human body in a broad-spectrum manner with the help of acoustic variability in intensity, exposure, and length. For imaging such as obstetrics, low-intensity ultrasound helps obtain diagnostic information without inducing cellular damage. At high intensities, instantaneous tissue necrosis is produced, and this method is widely used in medical oncology [59].

The piezoelectric transducer is an Ultrasound generating modality that can generate sound waves greater than 20 kHz. In a non-invasive manner, this generated ultrasound causes the heating of localized tissues by the thermal and mechanical energy deposited in the body. This localized heating can cause radiation and cavitation acoustically. This, in turn, causes localized drug release from the nanocarriers, thereby producing a localized therapeutic effect [60].

With the help of ultrasound, polymeric microbubbles can be expanded and contracted with the help of variable intensity, which induces microstreaming. This microstreaming causes variations in cell permeability by ion channel/ receptor modulation. This causes a reversible opening of the dynamic barrier by disrupting the tight junctions [61].

Polyethylene oxide (PEO) can be used for the encapsulation of anti-cancer drugs. PEO is a thermo- responsive polymer that has shown potential in a controlled release of drugs by activating thermal energy produced by ultrasound [60]. Polypyrrole hollow microspheres, microbubbles, hollow microspheres, temperature-sensitive liposomes, biodegradable poly-based microcapsules, *etc.*, can be used for cancer therapy using ultrasound [62].

A polymeric microbubble is typically a gaseous core present inside a shell of lipids or proteins. With the help of highly intense ultrasound, it can be used to enhance drug delivery in Enhanced Permeation and Retention mediated therapy. The drugs present in microbubbles are resistant to intracellular reactions. High-Frequency Focused Ultrasound of the drug doxorubicin can be employed using lipid microbubbles [63].

Ultrasound-targeted microbubble destruction causes the reversible opening of the Blood-Brain Barrier with the help of circulating microbubbles. Two ultrasound radiations are involved. In the first radiation, the lipid-based nanodroplets temporarily overcome the tumor barriers. By destroying lipid microbubbles by ultrasound, the polylactic co-glycolic acid-based nanodroplets accumulate in the intra- tumor region. This process helps in the entry of therapeutic agents (doxorubicin) directly into the tumors by generating pores. In the second radiation, more efficient delivery of medicaments into the tumor tissue occurs [64].

The release of drugs and the bioeffects are the two ways to enhance permeability and retention of the acoustic waves created by ultrasound to treat and diagnose tumors. By controlling the various ultrasound parameters like frequency, power density, and pulse duration, it is possible to determine the rate of release of a drug from its carrier. High-frequency ultrasound is used to treat superficial tumors with the help of targeted drugs. Whereas low-frequency ultrasound, due to its high permeability, has been used to treat large and deeply located tumors [63].

POLYMERIC NANOPARTICLES BEARING RADIONUCLIDE AS THERANOSTICS FOR BRAIN TUMOR [6]

A radionuclide is an unstable nucleus that emits radioactive rays and can be used as a detector in medical imaging modalities such as PET and SPECT and therapeutic applications. Polymer nanoparticles should be excellent DDS (drug delivery system) carriers of radionuclides in the nucleus because they can contain most diagnostic and therapeutic substances. They have a correct design of polymers with a hydrophilic and hydrophobic nature [65]. Rather than focusing on physical changes in tissues, as MRI does, radionuclide imaging is used in medicine to determine how an illness has progressed based on cellular metabolism and physiology within the body [66]. Nanomaterials can be developed to include multivalent cancer-targeting molecules and have a high loading capacity for therapeutic radioisotopes. These functional carriers have greater therapeutic benefits and can influence the pharmacokinetics of radionuclides. The nonspecific radiation emitted by unbonded radioisotopes in normal tissues is one of the most serious problems connected with radionuclide treatment [1]. Despite significant advances in radiation technology, one difficult challenge that remains unsolved is how to increase dose deposition in brain cancer-affected tissues while avoiding harming the remainder of the body's critical organs. Two considerations determine the best radionuclide (radioactive species) for treatment. (Fig. **10**).

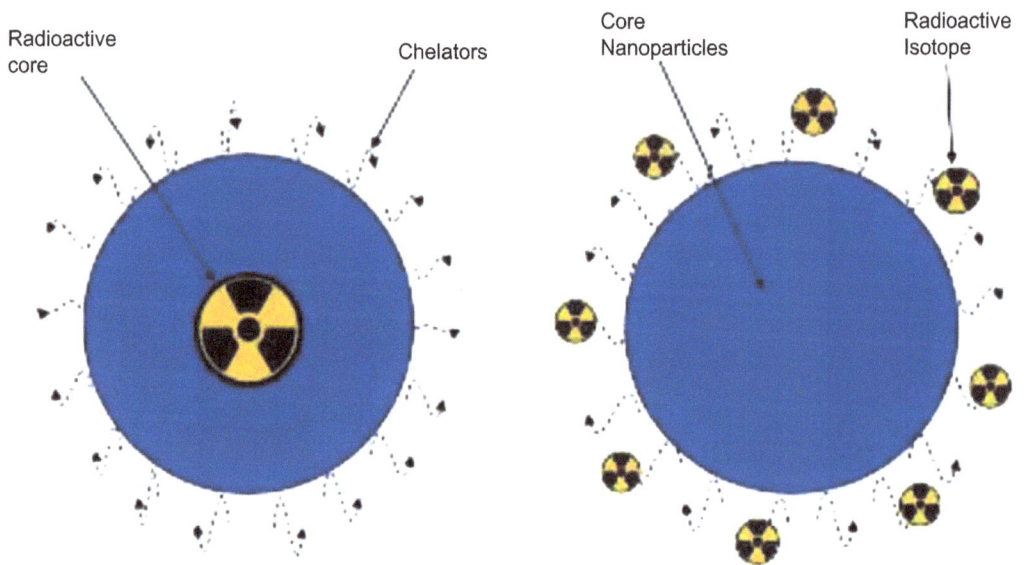

Fig. (10). Diagram representing two methods to create radioactive polymeric nanoparticles

1-Physical parameters such as the type of emission, energy radiation, daughter product, mode of generation, purity of radionuclide, and effective half-life are included in the first.

2- The second category comprises biological aspects such as tissue targeting, tumor retention, stability, and toxicity. Two approaches can be used to create radioactive polymeric NPs for imaging purposes.

In the first procedure, a radioactive element is incorporated into nano-sized clumps. The second method is to attach radioactive to a nanoparticle. (Fig. **9**) Polymeric nanoparticles of various sorts are designed for medicinal and diagnostic purposes. These include;

- A nanosphere containing radioactive material is loaded in a polymeric matrix.
- A nanocapsule with a polymeric shell that contains radioactive material.
- Dendrimers with radioactive material linked to polymeric nanoparticles.
- Surface modification *via* direct labeling with radioactive material linked to polymeric NP5- surface modification by indirect labeling using radioactive material linked to polymeric nanoparticles [67].

By copolymerization accompanied by radiolabeling, polymeric vesicles can be produced to carry radionuclide ligands. Researchers have designed and generated two newer forms of theranostic agents for tumor-targeting using radionuclides. Anticancer medication taxoid (SB-T-1214), tumor-targeting moiety biotin, and two arms carrying 64Cu for PET and 99mTc for single-photon emission tomography make up theranostic agents (SPECT) [60].

For brain cancer therapy, several radiolabeled nanomaterials are being studied. As a result, stable integration of α-/βemitters in nanostructures and precise delivery to specific tumor locations is required for successful cancer treatment and toxicity reduction. Furthermore, radionuclides that radiate energetic α- or β-particles are most usually employed to treat massive tumors; otherwise, tiny clusters of tumors are treated with radionuclides that release energetic α- or βparticles. Äuger electrons emitting radionuclides are favored due to their strong cytotoxic effect and short biological efficacy [60]. α-, β, and Auger electron-emitting radionuclides are the three types of radionuclides investigated to treat glioblastoma, a type of brain tumor [68]. PNPs (Polymeric Nanoparticles) have been radio-labeled using a cross-linking agent. Secondary γ -radiation decay may be seen in several-emitting radionuclides. When radioisotopes are combined with NPS as imaging agents, it is possible to evaluate their *in vivo* disposition using PET, Cerenkov luminescence (CL), positron, or single-photon emission computed tomography (SPECT) [60].

For the treatment of glioblastoma, lutetium-177, iodine-131, rhenium-186, rhenium-188, or yttrium-90 are usually used. However, astatine-211, actinium-225, or bismuth-213 in targeted-particle therapy (TAT) is gaining traction. One of the most important factors in TRT is to match the radionuclide to the tumor features (size, radiosensitivity, and amount of heterogeneity), which includes the decay pathway, effective tissue range, linear energy transfer (LET), and relative biological effectiveness (RBE).

Alpha-particles have unique radiobiological properties, such as a short tissue range (40–100 m) and a high LET, which results in a high tumor cell-killing efficiency and RBE. According to calculations, only five high LET-particle passing through the nucleus can kill a cell, but 10,000–20,000 low LET-particle traversals are required to achieve the same death. TAT has also been proposed as a facilitator for overcoming tumoral resistance to chemotherapy. Among all the known -particle-emitting radionuclides, three have attracted the greatest interest for TAT and RIT: actinium-225, astatine-211, and bismuth-213. These may be able to eliminate micro metastasis in the brain and recurring GB lesions in GB tumors.

β-emitting radionuclides, such as iodine-131 and yttrium-90, are employed in roughly 90 percent of current clinical TRT applications. Their cross-fire effect

(100–300 cell diameters) and relatively extended range (0.2–12 mm) make them especially effective for treating common bulky, heterogeneous primary (not requiring homogeneous distribution), and recurrent GB with an average size of >0.5 mm. For example, yttrium-90 (maximum range 12 mm) might treat medium-large GB tumors, while lutetium-177 (maximum range 2 mm) might be used to treat smaller GB tumors. However, because of their lower LETs (0.2–2 keV/m) and RBEs, these -emitters are only effective when tumor oxygenation and proliferation are adequate, making them less suited for the treatment of radioresistant and hypoxic tumors [68 - 71].

Auger electrons (AE) emitters have a shorter wavelength range (less than 100 nm) and a high LET and RBE. Importantly, because AE emitters are less dependent on the oxygenation condition of the tumor environment, these high LET emitters may be able to withstand hypoxia and necrosis. Because target-negative GB cells may evade the fatal effects of AE-mediated therapy, homogeneous antigen expression inside the GB tumor is required. This is particularly difficult for various types of GBs [69, 72]. When AE-emitting radionuclides are integrated into DNA, they are most effective. They cause direct DNA double-strand breaks when they are shuttled into the region of the cell nucleus (DSB). As a result, while evaluating the radionuclide properties, internalization into the GB cells and nucleus is an important design consideration in conjunction with the appropriate medications. As a result, when evaluating the features of the radionuclide in combination with appropriate medicines, internalization into the GB cells and nucleus is a significant design component [73, 74]. One of the examples for AE is based on its MA properties. It directly impacts the amount of energy given to independent cancer cells per receptor-recognition event, and it may result in the loss of critical crossfire effects. Although AE-emitters have shown significant therapeutic efficacy in preclinical studies, clinical efficacy has been reported in a small number of human studies, except for some positive results with [125I] iodo-deoxyuridine ([125I] iodo-UdR) and [111In] In DTPA-octreotide. Using an [125I] iodomAb 425/TMZ combination to treat GB patients resulted in improved survival with minimal normal tissue harm, leading to the registration of a Phase III clinical trial [75 - 77].

One of the most significant advantages of radioactive polymeric nanoparticles is better targeting for a specific location, which may result in a lower radioactive dose in the final drug while still generating the desired effect. Furthermore, increased targeting could imply an early diagnosis, providing clinicians more time to treat individuals who are at risk. Finally, polymeric nanoparticles, which are radioactive show an evolution [78].

FLUORESCENT POLYMERIC NANOPARTICLES AS THERANOSTICS FOR BRAIN TUMOR

Fluorescence imaging is one of the common detection techniques in nanomedicine because of its high sensitivity, less toxicity, and simplicity in use [79]. In biological imaging, fluorescence microscopy techniques play a critical role. It has been used *in vitro* and *in vivo* to perform real-time diagnostics. Most of the existing optical theranostic approaches use emitted photons as the signal readout, which suffers from an autofluorescence backdrop in the tissue and lower light penetration efficiency, impacting diagnostic accuracy [80]. NIR fluorescence dyes have been coupled with therapeutic drugs in a polymer-based theranostic system. NIR nanoprobes, such as QDs, rare-earth-doped NPs, carbon nanotubes, and organic dye-based NPs, have addressed these issues [48]. For polymeric nanoparticles, fluorophores such as fluorescein isothiocyanate (FITC), rhodamine, cyanines (Cy3 and Cy5), and coumarin are widely utilized as imaging labels [79]. Several innovative CPs and relevant imaging techniques have been used to fulfill the requirements of *in vivo* applications. Conjugated polymers (CPs) are a type of macromolecule with a significant number of π-conjugated backbones. Because of its great light-absorbing efficiency, numerous emissive wavelengths, the flexibility of customization, and unique ability to capture and expel light energy can be efficiently converted into fluorescence. CPNs also have good photostability and low cytotoxicity and have recently gotten a lot of attention in the biological world for imaging and sensing with fluorescence. Agents that have the potential to be theranostic because of their high quality CPNs feature light-harvesting and light-amplifying capabilities [80]. Fluorescence is also a part of photodynamic therapy (PDT), which uses a different mechanism other than medication or gene delivery to produce its therapeutic impact. Nanotheranostic particles utilized in PDT directly destroy their targets, rather than administering cancer-fighting medication or protein or altering gene expression. PDT is a minimally invasive approach for killing tumor cells in the presence of oxygen by releasing ROS when a photoreceptor is activated by light. Fluorescence and PDT combinations are effective in colorectal tumors as per preclinical studies. So, it is expected to be useful in brain tumor if it crosses the dynamic barrier with further modifications in the polymeric particles that are permeable to BBB [66]. Also, self-fluorescent polymer nanogels are used for simultaneous imaging and medication delivery in a novel technique recently published. This method enables imaging to be done more efficiently and completed without externally hired personnel fluorescent probes, which opens a new field of research for direct cell imaging and treatment [81].

It has been found that quantum dots (QDs) are an appealing tool for imaging malignancies due to their adjustable features and flexibility to be employed with fluorescent properties such as significant Stokes shifts and narrow emission bands for high-resolution images. They can also be utilized as dual-modality during surgery to map abnormalities in the brain. (Fig. **11**), below, shows the interaction of the mechanism of generation of fluorescence imaging of cells.

The commonly used major semiconducting QDs is NIR fluorophore because of its controlled size, configurable surface, high photoluminescence quantum yield, high photostability, and tunable emission wavelength. *In vivo* brain malignancies have been detected using a self-assembled matrix metalloproteinase (MMP)-2 activated QD. Here the CdTe QDs are coated with fluorescent units of low-molecular-weight heparin (LMWH) and quencher MMP-2 substrate cleavable low-molecular-weight protamine. Then it is supplied with fluorescence and thereby creates fluorophore prodrug drug. This prodrug is then integrated with the T7 peptide. It helps in detecting brain tumors and is hence concluded as a good brain tumor diagnosis tool. Also, a study shows that photoluminescent carbon dots play a role in non-invasive glioma diagnosis. A self-targeting carbon dot (CD-ASP) exhibited a continuous full-color photoluminescence emission, and CD-Asp easily entered the BBB within 5 min and showed a significant contrast in 15 min and helped to measure the tumor size [4]. Another study shows that PEG-coated QDs according to CdSe/ZnS were investigated as potential glioma nanoprobes. These QDs contain asparagines-glycine-arginine peptides (NGR) that target the CD13 glycoprotein on tumor cells. In an *in vivo* examination, these NGR-PE--QDs were able to target CD13 on glioma tissues and their input to fluorescence, which could aid in glioma surgical resection. It has been found that fluorescence-based surgery is an emerging technology, and a preclinical study shows that A QD-labeled aptamer (QD-Apt) was devised to bind precisely to the tumor surface based on this notion. The A32 aptamer was used because of its capability to bind the epidermal growth factor receptor variation III (EGFRvIII), which is present on the surface of glioma cells. The QD-Apt nanoprobes were less toxic and crossed the BBB to photograph tumor tissues with EGFRvIII. The researchers created new green fluorescent polysaccharide QDs nano-bioconjugates. L-cysteine and poly-L-arginine were used to functionalize carboxymethylcellulose nanostructures. The cellular uptake of the nanohybrids was investigated using confocal microscopy. These non-toxic nanoconjugates held a lot of promise for brain cancer bioimaging [24].

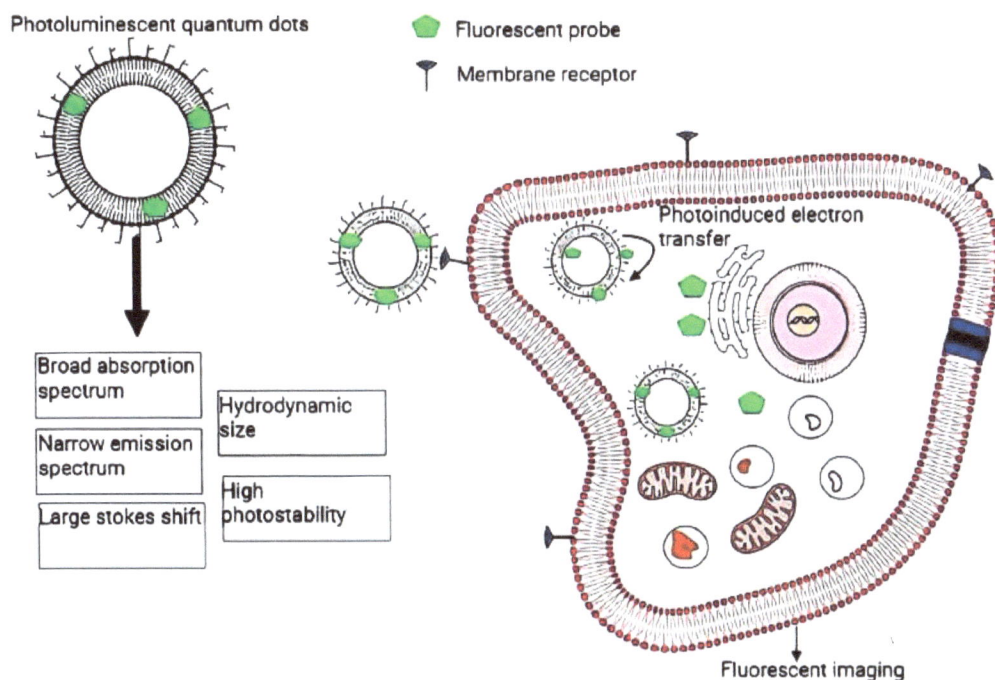

Photoluminescent quantum dots

Fluorescent probe

Membrane receptor

Photoinduced electron transfer

Broad absorption spectrum

Narrow emission spectrum

Large stokes shift

Hydrodynamic size

High photostability

Fluorescent imaging

Fig. (11). Mechanism of generation of fluorescence imaging of cells

CHALLENGES AND FUTURE DIRECTIONS

The future of targeted theranostic nanoparticles for brain tumor treatment is likely to be part of simultaneous drug administration and enhanced use of targeting agents and imaging agents. Because different medications can be delivered simultaneously, treatment can be personalized to the patient, making targeted nanoparticles essential delivery vehicles for medication mixtures. Increased usage of targeted drugs will improve therapeutic efficacy by increasing accretion in brain tumors while decreasing accumulation in non-cancerous brain tissue. Improved use of imaging agents will aid in the diagnosis of cancer at an earlier stage, allowing for the best chance of survival and the monitoring of brain tumors through the course of treatment.

The design of complex systems necessitates a grasp of numerous elements that comprise the delivery vehicle in its entirety. Therefore the future remains tough. Future theranostics targeted nano particle delivery systems that can use simultaneous drug delivery, targeting specific brain tumor surface indicators, and concurrent drug delivery imaging will require a deep understanding of how each cofactor works. Moreover, success with one core material may not necessarily translate to success with another, and long-term research is important.

Implications of these fundamental elements on human health and their biodistribution features are presently under investigation.

In treating brain tumors, positive outcomes have been found with nanotechnology-based techniques such as polymeric, lipid-based, and hybrid nanoparticles. Prospects in brain tumor therapy also include biotechnological breakthroughs such as carrier peptides and gene therapy. As a result, these customized delivery systems for brain tumor treatment will be advantageous in clinical practice.

CONCLUSION

Brain tumors are the most dismal diseases involving various intricate molecular pathways, gene mutations, and tumor microenvironments. Despite numerous studies, there is still an unmet medical urge to treat invasive brain tumors. Nanotechnology-based methods, such as nanoparticles that can be tailored to optimize transport and allow the targeting of multiple pathways inside the tumor microenvironment, are now being researched extensively.

The cargo release precisely at the desired site occurs through the brain cells overexpressed with proteins, receptors, and the EPR effect. A nonspecific process is AMT in which macromolecules are conveyed within membrane-bound vesicles and it is made possible by the ample supply of polyanions enveloping BBB endothelial cells that can interact electrostatically with circulating cationic molecules. Nutrients, hormones, and carrier systems at the BBB level have been utilized to deliver medications closely resembling endogenous carrier substrates to the brain using TMT. RMT occurs when the ligand binds to a transmembrane receptor-like TfR, LDLR, and insulin receptor, which is present on the apical plasma membrane of the endothelial cell.

Because of their biodegradable and biocompatible behavior inside the human body and the limitless forms and attributes they may be modified into, polymeric NPs are garnering increased interest in the treatment of brain tumors. Polymeric micelles have recently drawn much interest due to their improved permeability, retention of their hydrophilic shells, and small size, which allow for high structural solubility when administering hydrophobic drugs. Vehicles like Biodegradable polymeric nanoparticles modulate medication payload release and prevent drugs from environmental contamination. Nanoscale size, size homogeneity, vast functional classes, rapid cell entry, tunable size, reduced macrophage absorption, targeted distribution, and extensive transcytosis over biological membranes are advantages of dendrimers over conventional drug delivery technologies.

With the potential to combine treatment and imaging in a single NP, the use of NPs may result in a milestone in brain cancer care. Theranostic NPs can diagnose, deliver, and track the therapeutic response in sync as smart carriers. This chapter has discussed superparamagnetic, ultrasound triggered, radionuclide bearing, and fluorescent PNPs as potential theranostic approaches for brain tumor management.

SPIONs function as a negative contrast agent, improving image contrast by suppressing the T2 MRI signal. SPIO nanoshells aid in the direct release of hydrophobic anticancer medicines at the tumor site. Focused ultrasound (FUS) with microbubbles can safely and reversibly open the BBB employing two radiations, the first temporarily overcoming tumor barriers and the second more efficiently delivering therapeutic chemicals into tumor tissue. PNPs are radiolabeled by copolymerization or conjugation in radionuclide PNPs. Radionuclides that emit energetic α- or β-particles, Äuger electrons, and Secondary γ -radiation decay are most usually employed to treat dense and massive tumors. In a fluorescence-based theranostic system, NIR fluorescence dyes like fluorescein isothiocyanate (FITC), rhodamine, cyanines (Cy3 and Cy5), and coumarin have been coupled with therapeutic drugs.

Knowing the concentrations of chemotherapeutic agents and safer pharmacokinetic profiles, as well as legit surveillance of biodistribution and specific site accretion, visualization of target receptor density, and evaluation of therapeutic efficacy, may be advantageous in therapy selection and planning, which can be accomplished using novel theranostic techniques, thereby extending the patient's survival as well as life-quality.

RECOMMENDATIONS

Further study is required to investigate the current clinical platform of NPs in conjunction with new diagnostic NPs to build diverse and intelligent theranostic applications.

The utilization of the body's cells (Immune cells and stem cells) as a medication delivery platform is a revolutionary method of targeted drug delivery. They can penetrate the intact BBB, possibly allowing therapeutic compounds and nanocarriers to be transported.

The potential harm of nanomedicines to individuals and the environment necessitates long-term research. As a result, a thorough assessment of novel nanomaterials' probable acute and chronic toxicity effects on humans and the environment is required. Biodegradable material with no immunogenicity or biotoxicity that can be retrieved from the brain should be used in NDDS from a biosafety standpoint. Therefore, novel natural biomaterials have remained in high demand because they are biodegradable, biocompatible, readily available, regenerative, and low in toxicity. Despite recognizing natural biopolymers like polysaccharides and proteins, research into making them more durable in production environments and biological matrixes through methodologies like crosslinking is currently one of the most advanced study areas.

Even though numerous theranostic NPs are in development, most of them lack proof of concept due to a lack of concordance between *in vitro* and *in vivo* findings. With our deep understanding of diseases at the molecular level, nano theranostics will become the more extensively adopted treatment strategy.

REFERENCES

[1]   Mendes M, Sousa JJ, Pais A, Vitorino C. Targeted theranostic nanoparticles for brain tumor treatment. Pharmaceutics 2018; 10(4): 181.
[http://dx.doi.org/10.3390/pharmaceutics10040181] [PMID: 30304861]

[2]   Choudhary S, Waghmare S, Kamble H. A review: targeted drug delivery system.

[3]   Begines B, Ortiz T, Pérez-Aranda M, *et al.* Polymeric nanoparticles for drug delivery: Recent developments and future prospects. Nanomaterials (Basel) 2020; 10(7): 1403.
[http://dx.doi.org/10.3390/nano10071403] [PMID: 32707641]

[4]   d'Angelo M, Castelli V, Benedetti E, *et al.* Theranostic nanomedicine for malignant gliomas. Front Bioeng Biotechnol 2019; 7: 325.
[http://dx.doi.org/10.3389/fbioe.2019.00325] [PMID: 31799246]

[5]   Wei X, Chen X, Ying M, Lu W. Brain tumor-targeted drug delivery strategies. Acta Pharm Sin B 2014; 4(3): 193-201.
[http://dx.doi.org/10.1016/j.apsb.2014.03.001] [PMID: 26579383]

[6]   Iu P, Jiang C. Brain-targeting drug delivery systems. Wiley Interdiscip Rev Nanomed Nanobiotechnol. 2022 Sep; 14(5): e1818. Epub 2022 May 20.
[http://dx.doi.org/10.1002/wnan.1818] [PMID: 35596258]

[7]   Gao H. Progress and perspectives on targeting nanoparticles for brain drug delivery. Acta Pharm Sin B 2016; 6(4): 268-86.
[http://dx.doi.org/10.1016/j.apsb.2016.05.013] [PMID: 27471668]

[8]   Hervé F, Ghinea N, Scherrmann JM. CNS delivery *via* adsorptive transcytosis. AAPS J 2008; 10(3): 455-72.
[http://dx.doi.org/10.1208/s12248-008-9055-2] [PMID: 18726697]

[9]   Lu W, Wan J, Zhang Q, She Z, Jiang X. Aclarubicin-loaded cationic albumin-conjugated pegylated nanoparticle for glioma chemotherapy in rats. Int J Cancer 2007; 120(2): 420-31.
[http://dx.doi.org/10.1002/ijc.22296] [PMID: 17066446]

[10]   Qin Y, Chen H, Zhang Q, *et al.* Liposome formulated with TAT-modified cholesterol for improving brain delivery and therapeutic efficacy on brain glioma in animals. Int J Pharm 2011; 420(2): 304-12.
[http://dx.doi.org/10.1016/j.ijpharm.2011.09.008] [PMID: 21945185]

[11]   Li J, Gu B, Meng Q, *et al.* The use of myristic acid as a ligand of polyethylenimine/DNA nanoparticles for targeted gene therapy of glioblastoma. Nanotechnology 2011; 22(43)435101
[http://dx.doi.org/10.1088/0957-4484/22/43/435101] [PMID: 21955528]

[12]   Qin Y, Fan W, Chen H, *et al. In vitro* and *in vivo* investigation of glucose-mediated brain-targeting liposomes. J Drug Target 2010; 18(7): 536-49.

[http://dx.doi.org/10.3109/10611861003587235] [PMID: 20132091]

[13] Sonali, Singh RP, Singh N, Sharma G, Vijayakumar MR, Koch B, et al. Transferrin liposomes of docetaxel for brain-targeted cancer applications: formulation and brain theranostics. Drug Delivery. 2016; 23(4): 1261–71.

[14] Ramalho MJ, Sevin E, Gosselet F, *et al.* Receptor-mediated PLGA nanoparticles for glioblastoma multiforme treatment. Int J Pharm 2018; 545(1-2): 84-92.
[http://dx.doi.org/10.1016/j.ijpharm.2018.04.062] [PMID: 29715532]

[15] Zhang P, Hu L, Yin Q, Zhang Z, Feng L, Li Y. Transferrin-conjugated polyphosphoester hybrid micelle loading paclitaxel for brain-targeting delivery: Synthesis, preparation and *in vivo* evaluation. J Control Release 2012; 159(3): 429-34.
[http://dx.doi.org/10.1016/j.jconrel.2012.01.031] [PMID: 22306333]

[16] Feng B, Tomizawa K, Michiue H, *et al.* Delivery of sodium borocaptate to glioma cells using immunoliposome conjugated with anti-EGFR antibodies by ZZ-His. Biomaterials 2009; 30(9): 1746-55.
[http://dx.doi.org/10.1016/j.biomaterials.2008.12.010] [PMID: 19121537]

[17] Zhan C, Gu B, Xie C, Li J, Liu Y, Lu W. Cyclic RGD conjugated poly(ethylene glycol)-co-poly(lactic acid) micelle enhances paclitaxel anti-glioblastoma effect. J Control Release 2010; 143(1): 136-42.
[http://dx.doi.org/10.1016/j.jconrel.2009.12.020] [PMID: 20056123]

[18] Fondell A, Edwards K, Ickenstein LM, Sjöberg S, Carlsson J, Gedda L. Nuclisome: a novel concept for radionuclide therapy using targeting liposomes. Eur J Nucl Med Mol Imaging 2010; 37(1): 114-23.
[http://dx.doi.org/10.1007/s00259-009-1225-7] [PMID: 19662408]

[19] Huang S, Shao K, Liu Y, *et al.* Tumor-targeting and microenvironment-responsive smart nanoparticles for combination therapy of antiangiogenesis and apoptosis. ACS Nano 2013; 7(3): 2860-71.
[http://dx.doi.org/10.1021/nn400548g] [PMID: 23451830]

[20] Krůpa P, Řehák S, Diaz-Garcia D, Filip S. Nanotechnology - new trends in the treatment of brain tumours. Acta Med (Hradec Kralove) 2014; 57(4): 142-50.
[http://dx.doi.org/10.14712/18059694.2015.79] [PMID: 25938897]

[21] Moein Moghimi S. Recent developments in polymeric nanoparticle engineering and their applications in experimental and clinical oncology. Anticancer Agents Med Chem 2006; 6(6): 553-61.
[http://dx.doi.org/10.2174/187152006778699130] [PMID: 17100563]

[22] Mailänder V, Landfester K. Interaction of nanoparticles with cells. Biomacromolecules 2009; 10(9): 2379-400.
[http://dx.doi.org/10.1021/bm900266r] [PMID: 19637907]

[23] Cheng Y, Morshed RA, Auffinger B, Tobias AL, Lesniak MS. Multifunctional nanoparticles for brain tumor imaging and therapy. Adv Drug Deliv Rev 2014; 66: 42-57.
[http://dx.doi.org/10.1016/j.addr.2013.09.006] [PMID: 24060923]

[24] Mukhtar M, Bilal M, Rahdar A, *et al.* Nanomaterials for diagnosis and treatment of brain cancer: Recent updates. Chemosensors (Basel) 2020; 8(4): 117.
[http://dx.doi.org/10.3390/chemosensors8040117]

[25] Orringer DA, Koo YEL, Chen T, *et al. In vitro* characterization of a targeted, dye-loaded nanodevice for intraoperative tumor delineation. Neurosurgery 2009; 64(5): 965-72.
[http://dx.doi.org/10.1227/01.NEU.0000344150.81021.AA] [PMID: 19404156]

[26] Meyers JD, Doane T, Burda C, Basilion JP. Nanoparticles for imaging and treating brain cancer. Nanomedicine (Lond) 2013; 8(1): 123-43.
[http://dx.doi.org/10.2217/nnm.12.185] [PMID: 23256496]

[27] Pridgen EM, Langer R, Farokhzad OC. Biodegradable, polymeric nanoparticle delivery systems for cancer therapy. Nanomedicine (Lond) 2007; 2(5): 669-80.
[http://dx.doi.org/10.2217/17435889.2.5.669] [PMID: 17976029]

[28]   Niu J, Wang A, Ke Z, Zheng Z. Glucose transporter and folic acidreceptor-mediated Pluronic P105 polymeric micelles loaded withdoxorubicin for brain tumor treating 2014.

[29]   Syu WJ, Yu HP, Hsu CY, *et al.* Improved photodynamic cancer treatment by folate-conjugated polymeric micelles in a KB xenografted animal model. Small 2012; 8(13): 2060-9.
[http://dx.doi.org/10.1002/smll.201102695] [PMID: 22508664]

[30]   Xie YT, Du YZ, Yuan H, Hu FQ. Brain-targeting study of stearic acid-grafted chitosan micelle drug-delivery system. Int J Nanomedicine 2012; 7: 3235-44.
[PMID: 22802685]

[31]   XiaoLi W, XiaoYu Z, WeiYue L. p-Hydroxybenzoicacid (p-HA) modified polymeric micelles for brain-targeted docetaxeldelivery. Special Issue: Nano-Biomedical OptoelectronicMaterials and Devices 2013; 58(21): 2651-6.

[32]   Gaillard PJ, Appeldoorn CCM, Dorland R, *et al.* Maussang,Tellingen O. Pharmacokinetics, Brain Delivery, and Efficacy inBrain Tumor-Bearing Mice of Glutathione Pegylated LiposomalDoxorubicin (2B3-101). PLoS One 2014; 9(1): 1-10.
[http://dx.doi.org/10.1371/journal.pone.0082331] [PMID: 24416140]

[33]   Hau P, Fabel K, Baumgart U, *et al.* Pegylated liposomal doxorubicin-efficacy in patients with recurrent high-grade glioma. Cancer 2004; 100(6): 1199-207.
[http://dx.doi.org/10.1002/cncr.20073] [PMID: 15022287]

[34]   Huang FY, Chen WJ, Lee WY, Lo ST, Lee TW, Lo JM. *In vitro* and *in vivo* evaluation of lactoferrin-conjugated liposomes as a novel carrier to improve the brain delivery. Int J Mol Sci 2013; 14(2): 2862-74.
[http://dx.doi.org/10.3390/ijms14022862] [PMID: 23434652]

[35]   Huwyler J, Wu D, Pardridge WM. Brain drug delivery of small molecules using immunoliposomes. Proc Natl Acad Sci USA 1996; 93(24): 14164-9.
[http://dx.doi.org/10.1073/pnas.93.24.14164] [PMID: 8943078]

[36]   Kakinuma K, Tanaka R, Takahashi H, Watanabe M, Nakagawa T, Kuroki M. Targeting chemotherapy for malignant brain tumor using thermosensitive liposome and localized hyperthermia. J Neurosurg 1996; 84(2): 180-4.
[http://dx.doi.org/10.3171/jns.1996.84.2.0180] [PMID: 8592219]

[37]   Madhankumar AB, Slagle-Webb B, Wang X, *et al.* Efficacy of interleukin-13 receptor–targeted liposomal doxorubicin in the intracranial brain tumor model. Mol Cancer Ther 2009; 8(3): 648-54.
[http://dx.doi.org/10.1158/1535-7163.MCT-08-0853] [PMID: 19276162]

[38]   Muthu MS, Kulkarni SA, Raju A, Feng SS. Theranostic liposomes of TPGS coating for targeted co-delivery of docetaxel and quantum dots. Biomaterials 2012; 33(12): 3494-501.
[http://dx.doi.org/10.1016/j.biomaterials.2012.01.036] [PMID: 22306020]

[39]   Yang FY, Yang F-Y, Wang , *et al.* Treating glioblastoma multiforme with selective high-dose liposomal doxorubicin chemotherapy induced by repeated focused ultrasound. Int J Nanomedicine 2012; 7: 965-74.
[http://dx.doi.org/10.2147/IJN.S29229] [PMID: 22393293]

[40]   Desai A, Vyas T, Amiji M. Cytotoxicity and apoptosis enhancement in brain tumor cells upon coadminstration of paclitaxel and ceramide in nanoemulsion formulations. J Pharm Sci 2008; 97(7): 2745-56.
[http://dx.doi.org/10.1002/jps.21182] [PMID: 17854074]

[41]   Cui D, Xu Q, Gu S, Shi J. CheHe X. P AMAM-drug complex fordelivering anticancer drug across blood-brain barrier *in vitro* and *in vivo* Afr J Pharm Pharmacol 2009; 3(5): 227-33.

[42]   He H, Li Y, Jia XR, *et al.* PEGylated Poly(amidoamine) dendrimer-based dual-targeting carrier for treating brain tumors. Biomaterials 2011; 32(2): 478-87.
[http://dx.doi.org/10.1016/j.biomaterials.2010.09.002] [PMID: 20934215]

[43]   Wu G, Barth RF, Yang W, Kawabata S, Zhang L, Green-Church K. Targeted delivery of methotrexate to epidermal growth factor receptor–positive brain tumors by means of cetuximab (IMC-C225) dendrimer bioconjugates. Mol Cancer Ther 2006; 5(1): 52-9.
[http://dx.doi.org/10.1158/1535-7163.MCT-05-0325] [PMID: 16432162]

[44]   Jeelani S, Jagat Reddy RC, Maheswaran T, Asokan GS, Dany A, Anand B. Theranostics: A treasured tailor for tomorrow. J Pharm Bioallied Sci 2014; 6(5) (Suppl. 1): 6.
[http://dx.doi.org/10.4103/0975-7406.137249] [PMID: 25210387]

[45]   Muthu MS, Leong DT, Mei L, Feng SS. Nanotheranostics- application and further development of nanomedicine strategies for advanced theranostics. Theranostics. 2014; 4(6): 660.

[46]   Shrivastava S, Jain S, Kumar D, Soni SL, Sharma M. A review on theranostics: an approach to targeted diagnosis and therapy. Asian Journal of Pharmaceutical Research and Development. 2019 Apr 14; 7(2): 63-9.

[47]   Petrescu GED, Sabo AA, Torsin LI, Calin GA, Dragomir MP. MicroRNA based theranostics for brain cancer: basic principles. J Exp Clin Cancer Res 2019; 38(1): 231.
[http://dx.doi.org/10.1186/s13046-019-1180-5] [PMID: 31142339]

[48]   Tang W, Fan W, Lau J, Deng L, Shen Z, Chen X. Emerging blood–brain-barrier-crossing nanotechnology for brain cancer theranostics. Chem Soc Rev 2019; 48(11): 2967-3014.
[http://dx.doi.org/10.1039/C8CS00805A] [PMID: 31089607]

[49]   Xie J, Lee S, Chen X. Nanoparticle-based theranostic agents. Adv Drug Deliv Rev 2010; 62(11): 1064-79.
[http://dx.doi.org/10.1016/j.addr.2010.07.009] [PMID: 20691229]

[50]   Hainfeld JF, Smilowitz HM, O'Connor MJ, Dilmanian FA, Slatkin DN. Gold nanoparticle imaging and radiotherapy of brain tumors in mice. Nanomedicine (Lond) 2013; 8(10): 1601-9.
[http://dx.doi.org/10.2217/nnm.12.165] [PMID: 23265347]

[51]   Sun L, Joh DY, Al-Zaki A, *et al.* Theranostic application of mixed gold and superparamagnetic iron oxide nanoparticle micelles in glioblastoma multiforme. J Biomed Nanotechnol 2016; 12(2): 347-56.
[http://dx.doi.org/10.1166/jbn.2016.2173] [PMID: 27305768]

[52]   Gauger AJ, Hershberger KK, Bronstein LM. Theranostics based on magnetic nanoparticles and polymers: Intelligent design for efficient diagnostics and therapy. Front Chem 2020; 8: 561.
[http://dx.doi.org/10.3389/fchem.2020.00561] [PMID: 32733850]

[53]   Israel LL, Galstyan A, Holler E, Ljubimova JY. Magnetic iron oxide nanoparticles for imaging, targeting and treatment of primary and metastatic tumors of the brain. J Control Release 2020; 320: 45-62.
[http://dx.doi.org/10.1016/j.jconrel.2020.01.009] [PMID: 31923537]

[54]   Wahajuddin AS, Arora S. Superparamagnetic iron oxide nanoparticles: magnetic nanoplatforms as drug carriers. Int J Nanomedicine 2012; 7: 3445-71.
[http://dx.doi.org/10.2147/IJN.S30320] [PMID: 22848170]

[55]   Marekova D, Turnovcova K, Sursal TH, Gandhi CD, Jendelova P, Jhanwar-Uniyal M. Potential for treatment of glioblastoma: New aspects of superparamagnetic iron oxide nanoparticles. Anticancer Res 2020; 40(11): 5989-94.
[http://dx.doi.org/10.21873/anticanres.14619] [PMID: 33109536]

[56]   Ling Y, Wei K, Zou F, Zhong S. Temozolomide loaded PLGA-based superparamagnetic nanoparticles for magnetic resonance imaging and treatment of malignant glioma. Int J Pharm 2012; 430(1-2): 266-75.
[http://dx.doi.org/10.1016/j.ijpharm.2012.03.047] [PMID: 22486964]

[57]   Shen C, Wang X, Zheng Z, *et al.* Doxorubicin and indocyanine green loaded superparamagnetic iron oxide nanoparticles with PEGylated phospholipid coating for magnetic resonance with fluorescence imaging and chemotherapy of glioma. Int J Nanomedicine 2018; 14: 101-17.

[http://dx.doi.org/10.2147/IJN.S173954] [PMID: 30587988]

[58]   Shevtsov MA, Nikolaev BP, Yakovleva LY, *et al*. Recombinant interleukin-1 receptor antagonist conjugated to superparamagnetic iron oxide nanoparticles for theranostic targeting of experimental glioblastoma. Neoplasia 2015; 17(1): 32-42.
[http://dx.doi.org/10.1016/j.neo.2014.11.001] [PMID: 25622897]

[59]   ter Haar G. Therapeutic applications of ultrasound. Prog Biophys Mol Biol 2007; 93(1-3): 111-29.
[http://dx.doi.org/10.1016/j.pbiomolbio.2006.07.005] [PMID: 16930682]

[60]   Indoria S, Singh V, Hsieh MF. Recent advances in theranostic polymeric nanoparticles for cancer treatment: A review. Int J Pharm 2020; 582(119314)119314
[http://dx.doi.org/10.1016/j.ijpharm.2020.119314] [PMID: 32283197]

[61]   Liu HL, Fan CH, Ting CY, Yeh CK. Combining microbubbles and ultrasound for drug delivery to brain tumors: current progress and overview. Theranostics 2014; 4(4): 432-44.
[http://dx.doi.org/10.7150/thno.8074] [PMID: 24578726]

[62]   Sneider A, VanDyke D, Paliwal S, Rai P. Remotely triggered nano-theranostics for cancer applications. Nanotheranostics 2017; 1(1): 1-22.
[http://dx.doi.org/10.7150/ntno.17109] [PMID: 28191450]

[63]   Cao Y, Chen Y, Yu T, *et al*. Drug release from phase-changeable nanodroplets triggered by low-intensity focused ultrasound. Theranostics 2018; 8(5): 1327-39.
[http://dx.doi.org/10.7150/thno.21492] [PMID: 29507623]

[64]   Duan L, Yang L, Jin J, *et al*. Micro/nano-bubble-assisted ultrasound to enhance the EPR effect and potential theranostic applications. Theranostics 2020; 10(2): 462-83.
[http://dx.doi.org/10.7150/thno.37593] [PMID: 31903132]

[65]   Makino A, Kimura S. Solid tumor-targeting theranostic polymer nanoparticle in nuclear medicinal fields. ScientificWorldJournal 2014; 2014: 1-12.
[http://dx.doi.org/10.1155/2014/424513] [PMID: 25379530]

[66]   Luk BT, Zhang L. Current advances in polymer-based nanotheranostics for cancer treatment and diagnosis. ACS Appl Mater Interfaces 2014; 6(24): 21859-73.
[http://dx.doi.org/10.1021/am5036225] [PMID: 25014486]

[67]   Wu S, Helal-Neto E, Matos APS, *et al*. Radioactive polymeric nanoparticles for biomedical application. Drug Deliv 2020; 27(1): 1544-61.
[http://dx.doi.org/10.1080/10717544.2020.1837296] [PMID: 33118416]

[68]   Ersahin D, Doddamane I, Cheng D. Targeted radionuclide therapy. Cancers (Basel) 2011; 3(4): 3838-55.
[http://dx.doi.org/10.3390/cancers3043838] [PMID: 24213114]

[69]   Ku A, Facca VJ, Cai Z, Reilly RM. Auger electrons for cancer therapy – a review. EJNMMI Radiopharm Chem 2019; 4(1): 27.
[http://dx.doi.org/10.1186/s41181-019-0075-2] [PMID: 31659527]

[70]   Gudkov S, Shilyagina N, Vodeneev V, Zvyagin A. Targeted radionuclide therapy of human tumors. Int J Mol Sci 2015; 17(1): 33.
[http://dx.doi.org/10.3390/ijms17010033] [PMID: 26729091]

[71]   Karagiannis TC. Comparison of different classes of radionuclides for potential use in radioimmunotherapy. Hell J Nucl Med 2007; 10(2): 82-8.
[PMID: 17684582]

[72]   Cornelissen B, A Vallis K. Targeting the nucleus: an overview of Auger-electron radionuclide therapy. Curr Drug Discov Technol 2010; 7(4): 263-79.
[http://dx.doi.org/10.2174/157016310793360657] [PMID: 21034408]

[73]   Sgouros G, Bodei L, McDevitt MR, Nedrow JR. Radiopharmaceutical therapy in cancer: clinical advances and challenges. Nat Rev Drug Discov 2020; 19(9): 589-608.
[http://dx.doi.org/10.1038/s41573-020-0073-9] [PMID: 32728208]

[74]   Wygoda Z, Kula D, Bierzyńska-Macyszynz G, *et al.* Use of monoclonal anti-EGFR antibody in the radioimmunotherapy of malignant gliomas in the context of EGFR expression in grade III and IV tumors. Hybridoma (Larchmt) 2006; 25(3): 125-32.
[http://dx.doi.org/10.1089/hyb.2006.25.125] [PMID: 16796458]

[75]   Rebischung C, Hoffmann D, Stéfani L, *et al.* First human treatment of resistant neoplastic meningitis by intrathecal administration of MTX Plus [125] IUdR. Int J Radiat Biol 2008; 84(12): 1123-9.
[http://dx.doi.org/10.1080/09553000802395535] [PMID: 19061137]

[76]   Emrich JG, Brady LW, Quang TS, *et al.* Radioiodinated (I-125) monoclonal antibody 425 in the treatment of high grade glioma patients: ten-year synopsis of a novel treatment. Am J Clin Oncol 2002; 25(6): 541-6.
[http://dx.doi.org/10.1097/01.COC.0000041009.06780.E5] [PMID: 12477994]

[77]   Quang TS, Brady LW. Radioimmunotherapy as a novel treatment regimen: 125I-labeled monoclonal antibody 425 in the treatment of high-grade brain gliomas. Int J Radiat Oncol Biol Phys 2004; 58(3): 972-5.
[http://dx.doi.org/10.1016/j.ijrobp.2003.09.096] [PMID: 14967458]

[78]   Jeon J. Review of therapeutic applications of radiolabeled functional nanomaterials. Int J Mol Sci 2019; 20(9): 2323.
[http://dx.doi.org/10.3390/ijms20092323] [PMID: 31083402]

[79]   Zhang W, Mehta A, Tong Z, Esser L, Voelcker NH. Development of polymeric nanoparticles for blood–brain barrier transfer—strategies and challenges. Adv Sci (Weinh) 2021; 8(10)2003937
[http://dx.doi.org/10.1002/advs.202003937] [PMID: 34026447]

[80]   Qian C, Chen Y, Feng P, *et al.* Conjugated polymer nanomaterials for theranostics. Acta Pharmacol Sin 2017; 38(6): 764-81.
[http://dx.doi.org/10.1038/aps.2017.42] [PMID: 28552910]

[81]   Krasia-Christoforou T, Georgiou TK. Polymeric theranostics: using polymer-based systems for simultaneous imaging and therapy. J Mater Chem B Mater Biol Med 2013; 1(24): 3002-25.
[http://dx.doi.org/10.1039/c3tb20191k] [PMID: 32261003]

CHAPTER 4

Theranostic Liposome for Brain Tumor Diagnosis and Treatment

Payal Kesharwani[1,2], **Shiv Kumar Prajapati**[3], **Devesh Kapoor**[4], **Smita Jain**[1] and **Swapnil Sharma**[1,*]

[1] *Department of Pharmacy, Banasthali Vidyapith, Banasthali, Rajasthan, India*

[2] *Rameesh Institute of Vocational and Technical Education, Greater Noida, India*

[3] *Institute of Pharmaceutical Research, GLA University, Mathura, Uttar Pradesh, India*

[4] *Dr. Dayaram Patel Pharmacy College, Bardoli, Surat, Gujarat, India*

Abstract: The treatment of brain tumours is often a challenging task due to the low permeability of drugs through the blood-brain barrier and their poor penetration into the tumour tissues. Liposomes enhance the delivery of chemotherapeutics to the brain without using any invasive approach. Liposomes are biomimetic nanocarriers that exhibit good biocompatibility, high loading capacity, and the ability to reduce the amount of encapsulated drugs. It is a promising candidate performing a dual function of both drug delivery and diagnosis. This approach helps to locate the tumour tissue with appropriate biodistribution of liposomes. The theranostic liposomes provide a platform for imaging tumour cells for early diagnosis and simultaneously, delivery to the brain enhances the targeting delivery. Fluorescent dyes, magnetic resonance imaging, and nuclear imaging are the few approaches used in the diagnosis of tumour cells. A new approach involving semi-conductor-based quantum dots has emerged as an imaging reagent for brain tissues. The theranostic application of liposomes provides the real-time monitoring of the administered drug, reducing the risk of under-or over-dosing and allowing for more customized therapy regimens. This chapter highlights the techniques for directing liposomes to solid tumours in-depth, potential targets in cancer cells, such as extracellular and intracellular targets, and targets in the tumour microenvironment or vasculature. Additionally, this chapter also concludes recent efforts for improving anticancer drug delivery at the tumour site using surface functionalization techniques, and the different contrast agents which help in diagnosis are discussed.

Keywords: Liposomes, MRI, Nuclear Imaging, Surface Modification, Theranostics.

---

* **Corresponding author Swapnil Sharma:** Department of Pharmacy, Banasthali Vidyapith, Banasthali, P.O. Rajasthan-304022-India; E-mail: skspharmacology@gmail.com

INTRODUCTION

Liposomes structurally can be defined as spherical vesicular moiety with lipid base having 100- 200 nm diameter. Soon after their development in the early 1960s, the potential utility of these vesicles as a carrier system for therapeutically active chemicals was realized [1, 2]. It is composed of a phospholipid which forms a lipid bilayer enclosing the aqueous core. The aqueous core helps in the encapsulation of hydrophilic drugs or small molecules [3]. Liposomes have been studied in recent yearsas carriers of therapeutic drugs, imaging agents, and for the delivery of genes, with a focus on neurological diseases, their therapy, and/or diagnostics [4]. Scientists are more focused on the development of active targeting of liposomes to a specific cell type which can be achieved by conjugation or surface modification with ligands such as monoclonal antibodies, antibody fragments, proteins, peptides, carbohydrates, glycoproteins, aptamers, and small molecules [5]. These substances can be attached to the surface of the liposomes making them targeted to a specified surface receptor [6]. Such strategies are very effective while targeting the brain tumour. The brain is the most complicated part of the body and it is very difficult to deliver the therapeutic entity to the targeted area in the brain due to the presence of BBB [7]. Therefore, it becomes challenging to diagnose and treat the tumour at the primary stage. The conventional treatment of brain tumour includes surgery and chemotherapy or radiotherapy which usually produces side effects on the human body [8]. Liposomes are the emerging strategy that acts as a drug carrier to deliver drug[s] at the targeted site without any systemic toxicity. It allows the active targeting of cell receptors with a surface-attached ligand which delivers a drug to a tumour-associated stromal cells [6].

Theranostic medicines are playing an important role to improvise both diagnosis and therapeutics [9]. The liposomes are also successfully emerged to be utilized in the theranostic nanoplatform encapsulating the contrast agent which successfully helps in MR microangiography of the neurovascular as well as monitoring CED of drugs to brain tumours [10]. Liposomes allow achieving desirable properties in accordance with pharmacokinetics, target specificity, therapy monitoring, and signal amplification in contrast agent MR imaging-based liposomal contrast agents [11]. It increases the specific behavior and efficacy of the anticancer drugs [12]. The theranostic liposomes provide various advantages such as high biosafety, prolonged half-life in the circulatory system, concomitant loading of therapeutic and contrast agents, small size, high surface functionalization, and the ability to perform concomitantly diagnosis/monitoring and therapeutic approaches in real-time [13]. This strategy is very helpful in diagnostics and to obtain therapeutic efficacy in brain tumour. The theranostic nanosystem is developed to such an extent that it provides the encapsulation of magnetic nanoparticles inside the liposome core and acts as a responsive drug delivery system [13]. There are many key challenges that are faced during the development of surface-modified liposomes when established to scale up production. It becomes very difficult to characterize the ligand-functionalized liposome formulations, as well as the inadequate recapitulation of *in vivo* tumours in the preclinical models currently used to evaluate their performance [6]. This chapter explains the advantage of using liposomes for brain tumour imaging along with various contrast agents used in diagnosis. It also depicts in detail various strategies used for targeting tumour in brain cancer. Techniques such as dual-targeted liposomes, gene therapy-based targeting liposome, proteins as targets, small molecules as targets, are discussed.

MECHANISM OF LIPOSOMES TARGETING BBB AND BBTB

The human brain is a very complex organ of the body that governs and coordinates several important functions at the same time and makes a balance [14]. Successful drug delivery to a brain tumour is restricted because of the barrier possessed by the brain to reach the targeted area after systemic circulation [15]. Tight junctions, transporters, receptors, enzymes, and the ATP-dependent 170-kDa efflux pump P-glycoprotein all contribute to the BBB's physical barrier, which is made up of vascular endothelial cells [16]. The BBB restricts the passage of compounds with amolecular weight of more than 500 Da, as well as some of the small molecules (Fig. **1**) [17]. ATP-binding P-gp also serves as an efflux pump for xenobiotics, and their high expression prevents substrates from passing across the BBB. Because the bulk of chemotherapeutics are hydrophobic and have a greater molecular size, they are unable to cross the BBB on their own [18]. Chemotherapeutics are also substrates for multidrug-resistant drug efflux pumps, which are found in tumour vascular cells as well as the BBB [19]. Liposomes have the unique property to incorporate hydrophilic, lipophilic, and hydrophobic therapeutic agents because of their unique physicochemical characteristics [20]. Furthermore, cationic lipids enable the adsorption of polyanions, like DNA and RNA [21]. They also exhibit high biocompatibility and biodegradability, as well as minimal toxicity, drug-targeted delivery, and controlled drug release in order to enhance blood circulation and supply to the brain [22]. Included macromolecules such as polymers, polysaccharides, peptides, antibodies, or aptamers can further modify the liposome surface [23].

Drug-loaded liposomes must easily penetrate the highly electrostatic BBB for more effective therapeutic effects. The surface charge of the liposomes is one of the criteria for improved brain permeability (positive, negative, and neutral) [3]. Cationic liposomes are mostly used due to their effectiveness in carrying a drug molecule and genes. The most convenient reason for this conclusion is the electrostatic interaction between the cationic liposomes and the negatively charged cell membranes, which promote the nanoparticle uptake by adsorptive-mediated endocytosis, that has been reported in several studies [18]. Thus, making the cationic nanocarriers more efficient vehicle for drug delivery to the brain than conventional, neutral, or anionic liposomes [23]. The drawback of using cationic liposomes for brain delivery is the large quantities required to achieve therapeutic efficacy due to nonspecific absorption by peripheral tissues and their binding to serum proteins, which attenuates their surface charge, and those carriers are potentially lethal [24]. Liposomes may also be transported to the brain using glucose, which is the brain's primary source of energy. By modifying the surface of drug-loaded liposomes with glycosylate, which interacts with GLUT transporters and helps the liposomes cross the BBB, this method improves their permeability to the brain. N-acetylglucosamine [NAG] and Arginine-Glycin--Aspartic[RGD] have been shown to improve brain delivery [25]. The functionalization of physiologically active agents such as peptides, antibodies, aptamers, viral vectors (marked by high gene transfection efficiency) and others promote liposome transportation across the BBB (Fig. **2**) [13].

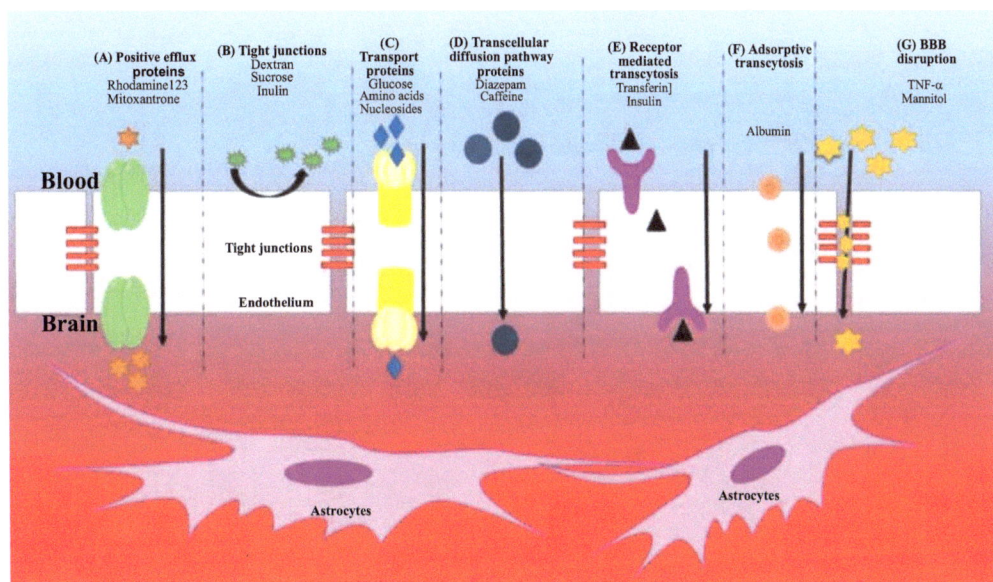

Fig. (1). Transport of drugs across BBB

STRATEGIES TO TARGET BRAIN TUMOUR USING LIPOSOMES

Conventional liposomes are made of phospholipids [**A**]; PEGylated/stealth liposomes contain a layer of polyethylene glycol [PEG] at the surface of liposomes [**B**]; targeted liposomes contain a specific targeting ligand to target a cancer site [**C**]; and multifunctional such as theranostic liposomes, which can be used for diagnosis and treatment of solid tumors [**D**] Multifunctional liposome [**E**] Receptors, ligands and proteins for drug binding.

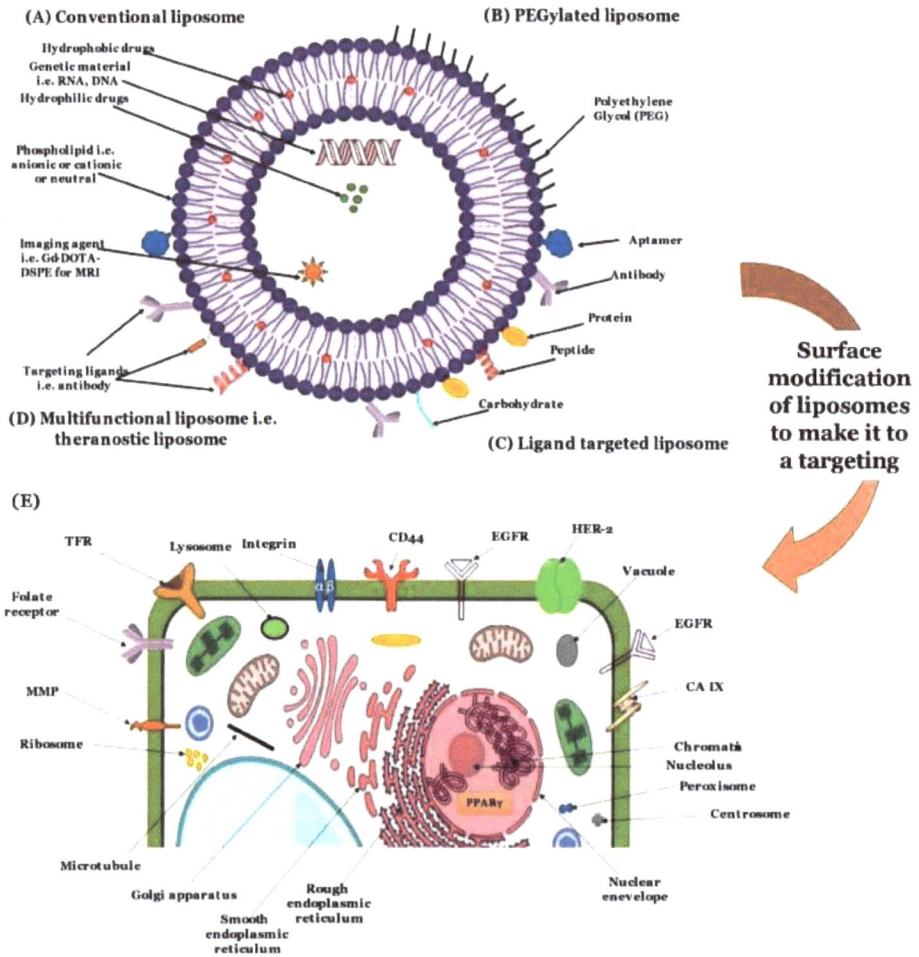

Fig. (2). Surface modification of liposomes

Protein Targets

Scientist have engineered an encouraging technique against tumour which involves the alteration of liposomes with small peptides, antibodies, *etc* [20]. The epidermal growth factor receptor [EGFR] is selected for targeting therapy in most of the cases like biomedical tools in diagnostic and therapeutic areas. Such ligand-attached liposomes are used for EGFR- and human epidermal growth factor receptor 2 [HER2]-positive malignancies, neurodegenerative diseases, autoimmune and infectious diseases, cardiovascular and inflammatory disorders [26]. This strategy is successfully used for efficient delivery of Doxorubicin against tumour cells confirmed by working animal xenograft models [5].

For the drug delivery to the brain, modified proteins or antibodies are used which have the ability to undergo absorptive-mediated or receptor-mediated transcytosis through BBB [27]. The brain consists of several receptors which are expressed on the surface of brain endothelial cells that help in the transportation of amino acid, glucose, or nucleic acid across BBB. This is a non-invasive approach of delivering drugs to the brain that provides active targeting through receptor-mediated transcytosis [28]. The vectors used for brain targeting include cationized albumin, the OX26 monoclonal antibody to the rat transferrin receptor, or monoclonal antibodies to the insulin receptor [27]. Transferrin is one such receptor present on both tumour cells and brain endothelial helping in targeting tumours [28]. The proteins can be effectively attached to liposomes through amino-reactive homo-bifunctional cross-linkers, water-soluble carbodiimide linkage, disulfide bonds, thioester linkages, *etc*. Disulfide and thioester linkages are used and reported widely in literature [29]. The only drawback of using liposomes and proteins together is that the PRG chain shows a strong shielding effect which prevents the meeting of bound receptor ligands and its receptor [27].

Lakkadwala *et al.* [28] formulated a liposome having dual function by modifying the surface of BBB with transferrin [Tf] and a cell-penetrating peptide [CPP] for receptor and adsorptive mediated transcytosis, respectively. The influence of insertion of CPP on Tf-liposomes helps to improve biocompatibility, cellular uptake, and transport across the BBB both *in vitro* and *in vivo* studied. The mice brain model was examined for the biodistribution of Doxorubicin and erlotinib. The distribution was found to be significant when delivered through liposomes [28]. Mahmud *et al.* [30] designed M-CTX-Fc conjugated liposomes encapsulating Doxorubicin. The U251MG-P1 cells [xenograft model of human glioblastoma cells] were used as the target model in this study. The liposome surface was modified with M-CTX-Fc having a diameter of 100–150 nm with high encapsulation efficiency and loading capacity. The *in vitro* and *in vivo* studies showed the high uptake capacity of the tumour cells with promising ability to suppress the tumour cells [30].

Small Molecules as Targets

Small molecules such as folate, antibody, carbohydrate, and others are utilized astargeting ligands attached on the surface of liposome for the targeting approach to brain tumours [29]. The small hydrophilic anticancer agent has a fast clearance, an irregular distribution, and poor intracellular absorption with toxicity. Surface-modified liposomes encapsulating small compounds can overcome these constraints [31]. Immunoliposomes based drug delivery systems are used for targeting such molecules which are used in micromolar concentrations in a target tissue to have a pharmacological effect [25].

Dual Targeting Approach

Dual-ligand liposomes are a new approach used for targeting two tumour cell receptors thus, overcoming the heterogeneity of targeting multiple cell types. Such a strategy helps to overcome the therapeutic limitation of current therapies and increases the possibility of liposomes binding to different cancer cells [6]. There are many reported studies defining the modified liposomes with two surface bound ligands that have the ability to bind to the specific receptor on the tumour cell. They also facilitate the transport of drug across the BBB for the successful delivery of drugs. Dual targeting daunorubicin liposomes were prepared with the help of p-aminophenyl-α-D-manno-pyranoside [MAN] and transferrin [TF] from crossing BBB and Brain tumour barrier. The *in vitro* models include C6 glioma cells *in vitro*, avascular C6 glioma tumour spheroids *in vitro*, and C6 glioma-bearing rats *in vivo*, respectively. The transport ratio across the BBB was increased by 24.9%, and uptake by C6 glioma cells was verified using flow cytometry and a confocal lens microscopy. The inhibitory rate against C6 glioma cells was also enhanced by 64.0%. *In vitro* and *in vivo* studies, the dual-targeting daunorubicin liposomes can increase the efficacy of treatment in brain glioma [32]. In another study, a dual targeting functionalized drug delivery was developed by modifying the liposome's surface with transferrin [Tf] for receptor-mediated transcytosis and a cell-penetrating peptide-penetrating [Pen] for enhanced cell penetration. Doxorubicin and erlotinib were encapsulated inside liposomes to transport them across the BBB to reach the brain tumour. The excellent biocompatibility study was demonstrated by *In vitro* cytotoxicity and hemocompatibility studies during *In vivo* administration. The dual targeting liposome increased the accumulation of Doxorubicin and erlotinib to ~12 and 3.3-fold respectively. It increased the regressing up to ~90% of tumour in mice brains in 36 days with no toxic effect. Thus, it turned out to be very effective in treating brain tumour [28]. A dual-functionalized thermosensitive liposomal system [DOX@P1NS/TNC-FeLPs] was developed by Shi *et al*. [33] to offer a targeted delivery, the GBM-specific cell-penetrating peptide [P1NS] and an anti-GBM antibody were coupled into a liposome. Doxorubicin and super paramagnetic iron oxide nanoparticles [SPIONs], were enclosed in a liposome allowing for thermo-triggered drug administration to the target location. The results of the *in vitro* BBB model showed that this approach was effective in assisting transport *via* the BBB. DOX@P1NS/TNC-FeLPs selectively penetrated U-87 human GBM cells and reduced tumour cell growth without affecting healthy brain cell function, according to results from immunofluorescent [IF] labeling and RT-qPCR. As a result, this method showed potential in terms of drug delivery across the BBB [33]. Sun *et al.* [34] designed a dual modified cationic liposome [DP-CLPs] with surviving siRNA and paclitaxel [DP-CLPs–PTX–siRNA] that has a dual-targeting character (Fig **3**). This helps in the diagnosis and treatment of glioma cells [CD133+ glioma stem cells] as well as brain microvascular endothelial cells. With increased selective death of CD133+ glioma stem cells and its differentiation, the method demonstrated very little cytotoxicity. It also suppressed carcinogenesis, promoted CD133+ glioma cell death, and enhanced survival rates in cerebral glioma tumour-bearing nude mice. As a result, it demonstrated a long-term capacity to attach glioma cells and brain microvascular endothelial cells [34].

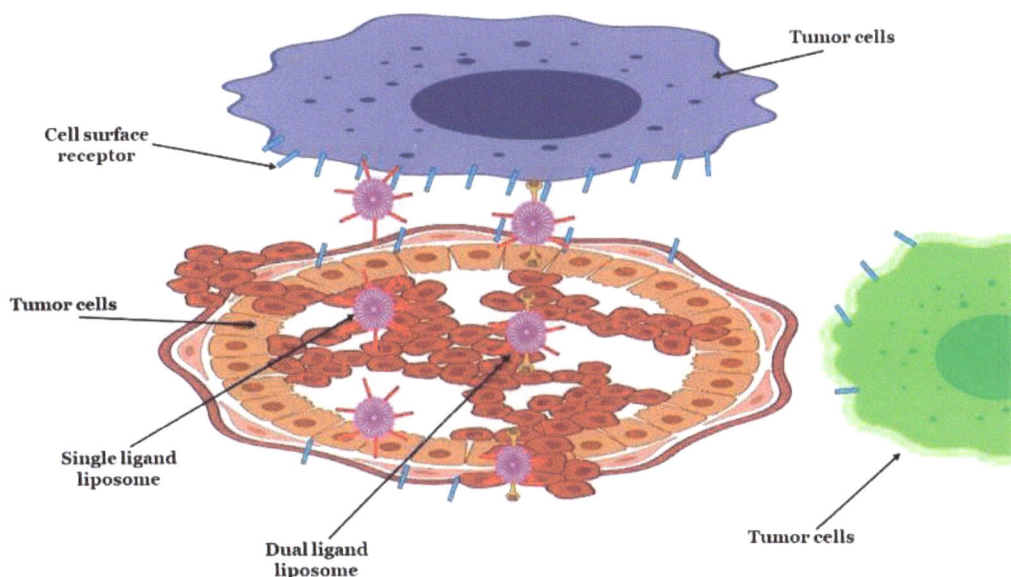

Fig. (3). Dual targeted liposomes as a strategy to cross BBB

Gene Therapy-Based Targeting Liposome

The modified genetic material can be delivered into the cell through nucleic acid which is known as a gene vector that helps in correcting the inaccurate genes present in the cell by the production of the therapeutic protein. But such vectors cannot be easily transported through the membrane present in the cell and genetic material easily gets degraded when administered externally into the body. Therefore, liposomes are used as a carrier that encapsulates, protects, and transports the genetic material inside the cell [35]. Till now, no gene therapy for a brain tumour has been approved in the US or Europe, but there are a total of 77 clinical trials going which are listed on US government website as of 2018. Gene therapy is very effective for treating brain tumour when detected at the early stage which can be corrected with invasive gene therapy procedures [36]. Because gliomas are caused by the progressive accumulation of genetic changes, gene therapy looks to be a viable therapeutic option for brain tumours. Direct intracerebral implantation of genes with viral vectors like adenovirus or herpes simplex virus, on the other hand, induces inflammation and demyelination. The Immunoliposome method, which incorporates DNA in the inner portion, aids in the inhibition of immunological responses. It is possible to create a neutral liposome with a targeted vector/DNA combination that encapsulates DNA and helps in delivery to a specific region of the brain [37]. Liposome-templated hydrogel nanoparticles [LHNPs] being used as a versatile system that uses CRISPR/Cas9-delivery tool for the detailed study of tumours and for translating the cancer gene therapy. [CRISPR]–CRISPR-associated protein 9 [CRISPR/Cas9] is the widely used genome editing technology for the tumour [38]. The liposome-based delivery of a vector is designed to effectively deliver the gene to a target-specific cell using a targeting molecule [39].

LIPOSOMES AS A CARRIER FOR IMAGING AGENT

Liposomes are a very useful tool for MR imaging-based nanoparticle contrast agents which is successfully demonstrated in animal models. The liposomes provide encapsulation of contrast agents, surface modification, and dual-action [40]. Imaging techniques such as fluorescence imaging, MRI, ultrasonography, and nuclear imaging are used [41]. Some theranostic applications of liposomes are discussed in Table **1**.

Fluorescence Imaging

Fluorescence imaging is one of the promising approaches for the diagnosis of living cells or tissues to understand in detail their biological function with the visualization of biomolecule or imaging probe location, gene expression, and enzyme activity found inside the cell [42]. It is nowadays commonly used for preclinical tumour detection and clinical image-guided oncological surgery. The commonly used dyes for the fluorescent effect in the brain are cyanine dye IR780 [43], fluoro-3,6-dioxatetracosane [44], Evans's blue, and carbocyanine dyes. But due to its inability to cross the BBB, a carrier is needed. Liposomes are used as a carrier for the diagnostic contrast agent with improved pharmacokinetic properties that helps in the transport of fluorescence imaging agents to the target area [3, 45]. The nanosized liposomes encapsulated with a positron emitter and labeled with fluoro-3,6-dioxatetracosane is used for the imaging of a tumour by positron emission tomography (PET). It showed a promising result for the diagnosis of brain tumour by targeting the cancerous cell without harming the normal cells of the brain [44]. Self-assembled IR780-liposomes were prepared for the identification of glioma cells using confocal lens microscopy. U87MG glioma ectopic and orthotopic xenograft models, as well as a spontaneous glioma mouse model caused by RAS/RTK activation, were used to test the *in vivo* brain tumour targeting and near-infrared fluorescence NIRF imaging capability of IR780-nanoparticles. Thus, the outcomes of study showed a potential for clinical imaging and image-guided surgery of brain tumours [43].

Magnetic Resonance Imaging [MRI]

Since 1973, MRI has been a vital tool in clinical and scientific contexts. This method, which is based on nuclear magnetic resonance [NMR] fundamental theories, allows for real-time monitoring of the dynamics of medicinal therapies [46]. It shows a good anatomic resolution of cells and tissues and excellent soft-tissue contrast imaging capabilities. The MRI contrast agent helps in improving the image contrast by producing a good image that differentiates between a diseased and healthy tissue enhancing the MRI sensitivity and accuracy [47]. Some of the commonly used contrast agents for MRI are gadolinium [Gd] chelates, iron oxide nanoparticles, *etc*. Liposomes may carry a wide range of MRI contrast agents, enabling efficient administration and controlled release of these probes for better imaging. The aqueous core of liposomes [known as H-MLs] decreases particle aggregation in physiological circumstances, increases tissue accumulation, and boosts imaging capabilities [48]. Furthermore, covering the liposome surface with PEG polymer prevents the intake of the contrast agent by local phagocytic cells at the injection site [49]. A stealth-type liposome was formulated encapsulating Doxorubicin for targeting brain tumour. A dynamic contrast-enhanced (DCE-MRI) was utilized to enhance the heterogenicity in tumour vasculature. The normal and tumour space were determined by voxel-wise analysis using a general tracer kinetic model [GTKM] to obtain a DCE-MRI image. The present model showed a better result compared with conventional liposomes for delivery to the brain in case of tumour [50].

Ultrasound Imaging

Medical ultrasonography is another extensively used non-invasive diagnostic imaging technology that offers unique and crucial potential to improve molecular imaging and medication administration [51]. Sound waves interact with stabilized gas bubbles to produce echoes, which are then used to generate visuals. To improve transmembrane and extravascular drug transport, sound waves can also free encapsulated pharmaceuticals from microbubbles and liposomes [52].

Liposomes having the characteristic of echogenicity or ultrasound responsiveness reflected by a microbubble are the dynamic feature for ultrasound imaging [51]. Acoustic liposomes with a diameter of 100-200 nm can also be utilized as a drug delivery device that uses the EPR effect to passively localize to tumour tissue. Acoustic liposomes can be utilized to test both drug transport efficiency and antitumor effects when combined with high-frequency ultrasound [HF-US] [53]. In a study, Zhan [54], used a combination therapy of drug delivery using liposomes along with FUS-MB-induced disruption of BBB. Thus, the strategy helps to successfully cross the BBB in case of a brain tumour [54]. In another study, FUS (focused ultrasound) in combination with DNA-loaded MBs can cause a non-invasive, reversible, local breach of the BBB that allows for targeted exogenous gene transfer into the central nervous system. Glioma enlargement was delayed by the development of phospholipid complex with adequate gene loading and peptide-mediated targeting. MBs were bound to shBirc5-lipo-NGR, which served as both a tumour cell target and an efficient gene loader. An apoptotic assay, real-time PCR, western blotting [WB], and a volume measurement survival analysis *in vivo* were used to assess the silencing impact of shBirc5. The experimental group showed a substantial therapeutic effect, but the FUS-only, MB-shBirc5-lipo-NGR-only, and FUS-aided MB-shControl-lipo-NGR groups showed no difference in tumour enlargement or survival time [P.01] [55]. Aryal *et al.* [56] conducted a similar investigation in which liposomes encapsulating Doxorubicin were coupled with ultrasound-induced breakdown of the blood–tumor and BBB. The efficacy of the formulation was determined using a 9L rat glioma model, which revealed that median survival time was much longer in the FUS-MB formulation than in the basic Doxorubicin formulation. In this rat glioma model, the FUS-MB method to improve liposomal Doxorubicin administration had a significant therapeutic impact [56].

LIPOSOMES AS NANOCARRIERS FOR DIAGNOSTIC APPLICATIONS

Earlier, the detection and diagnosis of brain tumour were very difficult at the primary stages due to the accumulation of extracellular fluid which surrounds the tumour. So, the primary modality to handle the brain tumour was surgical resection and/or chemotherapy [57]. The conventional strategies used for diagnostic purposes show uneven biodistribution and pharmacokinetics of an agent which causes the propagation of tumour in a body [22]. Introduction to nano theranostics approach has helped to overcome the concern related to diagnosis and treatment of brain tumour. Many nano theranostics brain cancer therapies have been identified which are under investigation for better and more efficient results [58]. The liposome-based neuroimaging is an emerging field which helps to understand the physiological processes such as apoptosis, ischemia, inflammation, cell differentiation, and mitosis, in detail which act as the main tool in the diagnosis of a brain tumour [23]. The contrast agents delivered using liposomes have allowed for cellular and molecular imaging, monitoring of drug delivery to tumours, and efficient surgical removal of solid tumours. Liposomes are also very helpful in preclinical studies for brain tumour models which allows the molecular targeting of tumour cells with cytotoxic agents. The diagnostic imaging takes place due to the sufficient intensity of the signal obtained from tumour cells which distinguishes it from the healthy cells [51]

The various contrast agents such as Gadolinium [Gd]-based compounds, like Gd–diethylenetriaminepentaacetic acid, gadodiamide, and gadoteridol are used for scanning MRI images [59]. The Gd-based compounds used with liposomes help to conveniently locate the tumour site using the EPR effect [enhanced permeability and retention]. Further, pH-responsive Gd liposomes have also been developed which release the imaging agent at 0.2 pH precision *i.e.* acid tumour microenvironment [60]. The optical imaging of glioma is based on the process known as fluorescence. The commonly used dye for producing fluorescence in lipid binding is carbocyanine dyes DiD [4,4′-diisothiocyanatostilbene-2,-′-disulfonic acid, disodium salt], DiO [3,3′-dioctadecyloxacarbocyanine perchlorate], and DiI [1,1′-dioctadecyl-3,3,3,′3,′-tetramethylinocarbocyanine perchlorate] used for imaging studies [61]. These dyes are not able to cross the BBB, therefore encapsulated inside the liposomes. One of the studies suggested that Evans blue dye encapsulated inside the liposomes circumscribes visually the invasive gliomas [62].

Kostevšek *et al.* [40], formulated a liposome encapsulating IO-based T2 contrast agent. The study was conducted to analyze the influence of different phospholipids on the relaxivity [r^2] values of magneto-liposomes showing a deep relation between bilayer fluidity and r^2. For the improvement of relaxivity 5-nm, IO NPs were embedded into the lipid bilayer. *In vitro*, MRI measurements revealed that selective contrast agents were preferentially taken up by cancerous T24 cells. This approach efficiently helped in identifying the cancerous cell from healthy cells [40]. Magnevist [Gd/DTPA] is a very effective MRI contrast agent used to detect the tumour at its early stages. But the only limitation is that it cannot cross the BBB. Therefore, it needs to be encapsulated in a liposome to cross BBB. Xiaoli *et al.* [63] designed a liposome conjugated with IL-13 encapsulating a Magnevist [Gd-DTPA] as a MRI contrast agent. Intracranial glioma mouse model was validated histologically to evaluate the MR image intensity. The MRI signal intensity was increased after the 15% injection of IL-13-liposome-Gd-DTPA into the normal brain tissue. MRI detected small tumour masses in the brain area. Thus, this approach helped in the early detection of a brain tumour [63]. Xiaoli *et al.* [64], also formulated IL-13-liposome encapsulating Gd-DTPA and DOX. For the detection of tumour glioma U251 and glioma stem cells T3691 and athymic nude mice with intracranial glioma were selected. The formulation confirmed the detection of tumour in the model [64].

Table 1. Theranostic applications of some brain targeted liposome formulation

Liposome Type	Drug	Theranostic Agent	Remark	Reference
TPGS liposomes	Docetaxel	QDs	Sustained drug release for more than 72 hr. The *in vivo* study confirmed the brain targeted theranostic potential of transferrin receptor-targeted liposomes.	[65]
TPGS liposomes	Docetaxel	QDs	RGD-TPGS decorated theranostic liposomes have reduced ROS generation effectively and did not show any signs of brain damage or edema in brain histopathology.	[66]
MRI-detectable liposomal hydrogel	Gemcitabine	barbituric acid	The imaging tactic preferred allowed simultaneous and independent monitoring of both the drug and the liposome carrier in the hydrogel matrix.	[67]
Liposomes	-	Gadolinium	Real-time MRI monitoring of liposomes containing gadolinium allowed direct visualization of a robust distribution. MRI of liposomal gadolinium was highly accurate at determining tissue distribution, as confirmed by comparison with histological results from concomitant administration of fluorescent liposomes.	[68]
Liposomes	-	Gadoteridol/rhodamine	Gadoteridol/rhodamine-loaded liposomes were distributed in the putamen, corona radiata and brain stem of non-human primates. Distribution was monitored by real-time MRI throughout infusion procedures and allowed accurate calculation of the volume of distribution within anatomical structures.	[69]

(Table 1) cont.....

Liposome Type	Drug	Theranostic Agent	Remark	Reference
Multifunctional liposomes	Apomorphine	QDs	The results showed that QD-loaded liposomes, but not free, QDs were transported across the BBB. Liposomes were observed to have been efficiently endocytosed into bEND3 cells.	[51]
TPGS liposomes	-	Fluorescein isothiocyanate	The TPGS enhanced blood circulation. The developed liposomes showed the distribution of liposomes in the cytoplasm confirmed by green fluorescence.	[70]
TPGS Liposomes	Docetaxel	Gold	The *in vivo* results demonstrated that targeted gold liposomes were able to significantly deliver DCX into the brain than the Docel™	[71]
Multifunctional liposomes	Cisplatin	QDs	The cellular uptake of quantum dot liposomes [QDLs] confirmed effective internalization and significant fluorescence in melanoma cells. The ex vivo studies revealed significant fluorescent intensity and accumulation of cisplatin in the brain and skin.	[72]
QDs and superparamagnetic iron oxide [SPIO] liposomes [QSC-Lip]	-	QDs and SPIO	*In vivo*, MRI and fluorescence imaging revealed that QSC-Lip not only enhanced the negative contrast of gliomas on MRI but also caused the tumour to radiate fluorescence on magnetic targeting.	[73]

MAJOR CHALLENGES FACED DURING THE DEVELOPMENT OF LIGAND-GATED LIPOSOMES

The quality consistency ofliposomes is a key problem in their production. Temperature, cholesterol content, pH, and surface charge potential impact the long-term stability of liposomes, keeping the production process's dependability and repeatability at risk. To minimize the steps of production and the usage of organic solvents, the processing method needs to be optimized. Furthermore, while liposome surface coating improves the transportation of substances through BBB efficiently, it complicates the system and may pose problems for large-scale good manufacturing [cGMP] production. For the clinical translation of surface-modified liposomes, a cost-benefit analysis is required [74]. As a result, specialists should communicate and collaborate at all phases of the process, including manufacturing, laboratory research, and clinical evaluation. Despite promising preclinical research in the field of ligand-directed liposomes for the treatment of solid tumours and other illnesses, tailored liposome formulations are delayed to reach clinical trials. There are various important parameters that need to be considered in the development of targeted liposomes for preclinical studies. These include large-scale development of ligand-gated liposomes, their characterization, models that accurately reflect tumour heterogeneity, accounting for the enhanced permeability and retention effect in the preclinical setting [6].

CONCLUSION AND FUTURE PROSPECTIVE

Drug targeting against cancer tissue has been greatly aided by liposomes. Free drugs were unable to produce targeting to the tumour site due to the reticuloendothelial system. When compared to free medicines, drug distribution using ligand-targeted liposomes has enhanced therapy. The *in vitro* and *in vivo* studies have clearly suggested that the toxicity, biodistribution, and pharmacokinetics of the liposomes show safety and effective results in clinical trial studies. Theranostic application along with liposomes uses a combined approach of both diagnosis and therapeutics which helps in the early detection of brain tumour. Theranostic liposomes help the drug particle be released in the affected area thus targeting the over-expressed proteins and receptors that are present on brain cancerous cells. Surface-modified liposomes are a new class of pharmacological tools that will be studied further in the future to provide better and more precise targeting of brain tumours. The low drug loading capacity needs to be studied in detail in order to successfully deliver the potent drug to the targeted area. In addition, nano theranostics will become more prevalent in brain cancer detection techniques. In the future, liposomes will play a vital role in personalized medicine for individual patients by reducing the cost and duration of therapy. Multifunctional liposomes having certain features, *e.g.*, sustained release, targeted delivery, triggered release, and synergistic functionalities using a variety of surface functionalization and modification approaches, will play a vital role in tumour therapy.

LIST OF ABBREVIATION

ATP	Adenosine triphosphate
BBB	Blood brain barrier
CPP	Cell penetrating peptide
DNA	Deoxyribonucleic acid
DOX=	Doxorubicin

EGFR	Epidermal growth factor receptor
FUS	Focused ultrasound
Gd	Gadolinium
GLUT	Glucose transporter
HER2	Human epidermal growth factor receptor 2
HF-US	high-frequency ultrasound
LHNPs	superparamagnetic iron oxide nanoparticles
MAN	p-aminophenyl-α-D-manno-pyranoside
MB	Microbubbles
MR	Magnetic Resonance
MRI	Magnetic Resonance Imaging
NAG	N-acetylglucosamine
NMR	nuclear magnetic resonance
PCR	Polymerase chain reaction
P-gp	P-glycoprotein
RNA	Ribonucleic acid
SPIONs	Superparamagnetic iron oxide nanoparticles
Tf	Transferrin
U251MG-P1cells	Xenograft model of human glioblastoma cells
WB	Western blotting

ACKNOWLEDGEMENT

All the Authors of this chapter would like to thank Late Prof. Aditya Shastri, Vice-Chancellor of Banasthalli Vidhyapith Rajasthan, India for providing all the necessary facilities for the successful completion of the Chapter.

REFERENCES

[1]   Patra JK, Das G, Fraceto LF, *et al.* Nano based drug delivery systems: recent developments and future prospects. J Nanobiotechnology 2018; 16(1): 71.
[http://dx.doi.org/10.1186/s12951-018-0392-8] [PMID: 30231877]

[2]   Jain S, Prajapati SK, Jain S, Jain S, Jain A. Propylene glycol-liposome for anticoagulant drug delivery through skin. Journal of Bionanoscience 2018; 12(5): 721-7.
[http://dx.doi.org/10.1166/jbns.2018.1586]

[3]   Bozzuto G, Molinari A. Liposomes as nanomedical devices. Int J Nanomedicine 2015; 10: 975-99.
[http://dx.doi.org/10.2147/IJN.S68861] [PMID: 25678787]

[4]   Lamichhane N, Udayakumar T, D'Souza W, *et al.* Liposomes: Clinical Applications and Potential for Image-Guided Drug Delivery. Molecules 2018; 23(2): 288.
[http://dx.doi.org/10.3390/molecules23020288] [PMID: 29385755]

[5]   Eloy JO, Petrilli R, Trevizan LNF, Chorilli M. Immunoliposomes: A review on functionalization strategies and targets for drug delivery. Colloids Surf B Biointerfaces 2017; 159: 454-67.
        [http://dx.doi.org/10.1016/j.colsurfb.2017.07.085] [PMID: 28837895]

[6]   Belfiore L, Saunders DN, Ranson M, Thurecht KJ, Storm G, Vine KL. Towards clinical translation of ligand-functionalized liposomes in targeted cancer therapy: Challenges and opportunities. J Control Release 2018; 277: 1-13.
        [http://dx.doi.org/10.1016/j.jconrel.2018.02.040] [PMID: 29501721]

[7]   He Q, Chen J, Yan J, *et al.* Tumor microenvironment responsive drug delivery systems. Asian Journal of Pharmaceutical Sciences 2020; 15(4): 416-48.
        [http://dx.doi.org/10.1016/j.ajps.2019.08.003] [PMID: 32952667]

[8]   Wang X, Xuan Z, Zhu X, Sun H, Li J, Xie Z. Near-infrared photoresponsive drug delivery nanosystems for cancer photo-chemotherapy. J Nanobiotechnology 2020; 18(1): 108.
        [http://dx.doi.org/10.1186/s12951-020-00668-5] [PMID: 32746846]

[9]   Prajapati SK, Malaiya A, Kesharwani P, Soni D, Jain A. Biomedical applications and toxicities of carbon nanotubes. Drug Chem Toxicol 2022; 45(1): 435-50.
        [http://dx.doi.org/10.1080/01480545.2019.1709492] [PMID: 31908176]

[10]   Al-Jamal WT, Kostarelos K. Liposomes: from a clinically established drug delivery system to a nanoparticle platform for theranostic nanomedicine. Acc Chem Res 2011; 44(10): 1094-104.
        [http://dx.doi.org/10.1021/ar200105p] [PMID: 21812415]

[11]   Ren L, Chen S, Li H, *et al.* MRI-guided liposomes for targeted tandem chemotherapy and therapeutic response prediction. Acta Biomater 2016; 35: 260-8.
        [http://dx.doi.org/10.1016/j.actbio.2016.02.011] [PMID: 26873364]

[12]   Hare JI, Lammers T, Ashford MB, Puri S, Storm G, Barry ST. Challenges and strategies in anti-cancer nanomedicine development: An industry perspective. Adv Drug Deliv Rev 2017; 108: 25-38.
        [http://dx.doi.org/10.1016/j.addr.2016.04.025] [PMID: 27137110]

[13]   d'Angelo M, Castelli V, Benedetti E, *et al.* Theranostic nanomedicine for malignant gliomas. Front Bioeng Biotechnol 2019; 7: 325.
        [http://dx.doi.org/10.3389/fbioe.2019.00325] [PMID: 31799246]

[14]   Sporns O. Structure and function of complex brain networks. Dialogues Clin Neurosci 2013; 15(3): 247-62.
        [http://dx.doi.org/10.31887/DCNS.2013.15.3/osporns] [PMID: 24174898]

[15]   Jain KK. A Critical overview of targeted therapies for glioblastoma. Front Oncol 2018; 8: 419.
        [http://dx.doi.org/10.3389/fonc.2018.00419] [PMID: 30374421]

[16]   Sanchez-Covarrubias L, Slosky L, Thompson B, Davis T, Ronaldson P. Transporters at CNS barrier sites: obstacles or opportunities for drug delivery? Curr Pharm Des 2014; 20(10): 1422-49.
        [http://dx.doi.org/10.2174/13816128113199990463] [PMID: 23789948]

[17]   Banks WA, Greig NH. Small molecules as central nervous system therapeutics: old challenges, new directions, and a philosophic divide. Future Med Chem 2019; 11(6): 489-93.
        [http://dx.doi.org/10.4155/fmc-2018-0436] [PMID: 30912980]

[18]   Liu C, Zhang L, Zhu W, *et al.* Barriers and strategies of cationic liposomes for cancer gene therapy. Mol Ther Methods Clin Dev 2020; 18: 751-64.
        [http://dx.doi.org/10.1016/j.omtm.2020.07.015] [PMID: 32913882]

[19]   Li YS, Sahi J. The role of drug transporters at the blood brain barrier. Eur Pharm Rev 2016; 21(1): 15-9.

[20]   Daraee H, Etemadi A, Kouhi M, Alimirzalu S, Akbarzadeh A. Application of liposomes in medicine and drug delivery. Artif Cells Nanomed Biotechnol 2016; 44(1): 381-91.
        [http://dx.doi.org/10.3109/21691401.2014.953633] [PMID: 25222036]

[21]   Guevara ML, Persano F, Persano S. Advances in lipid nanoparticles for mRNA-based cancer immunotherapy. Front Chem 2020; 8589959
[http://dx.doi.org/10.3389/fchem.2020.589959] [PMID: 33195094]

[22]   Din F, Aman W, Ullah I, *et al.* Effective use of nanocarriers as drug delivery systems for the treatment of selected tumors. Int J Nanomedicine 2017; 12: 7291-309.
[http://dx.doi.org/10.2147/IJN.S146315] [PMID: 29042776]

[23]   Vieira D, Gamarra L. Getting into the brain: liposome-based strategies for effective drug delivery across the blood–brain barrier. Int J Nanomedicine 2016; 11: 5381-414.
[http://dx.doi.org/10.2147/IJN.S117210] [PMID: 27799765]

[24]   Upadhyay RK. Drug delivery systems, CNS protection, and the blood brain barrier. Biomed Res Int. 2014;2014.

[25]   Wang ZY, Sreenivasmurthy SG, Song JX, Liu JY, Li M. Strategies for brain-targeting liposomal delivery of small hydrophobic molecules in the treatment of neurodegenerative diseases. Drug Discov Today 2019; 24(2): 595-605.
[http://dx.doi.org/10.1016/j.drudis.2018.11.001] [PMID: 30414950]

[26]   Taneja P, Sharma S, Sinha VB, Yadav AK. Advancement of nanoscience in development of conjugated drugs for enhanced disease prevention. Life Sci 2021; 268118859
[http://dx.doi.org/10.1016/j.lfs.2020.118859] [PMID: 33358907]

[27]   Schnyder A, Huwyler J. Drug transport to brain with targeted liposomes. NeuroRx 2005; 2(1): 99-107.
[http://dx.doi.org/10.1602/neurorx.2.1.99] [PMID: 15717061]

[28]   Lakkadwala S, dos Santos Rodrigues B, Sun C, Singh J. Biodistribution of TAT or QLPVM coupled to receptor targeted liposomes for delivery of anticancer therapeutics to brain *in vitro* and *in vivo*. Nanomedicine 2020; 23: 102112-2.
[http://dx.doi.org/10.1016/j.nano.2019.102112] [PMID: 31669083]

[29]   Riaz M, Riaz M, Zhang X, *et al.* Surface functionalization and targeting ltrategies of Liposomes in solid tumor therapy: A review. Int J Mol Sci 2018; 19(1): 195.
[http://dx.doi.org/10.3390/ijms19010195] [PMID: 29315231]

[30]   Mahmud H, Kasai T, Khayrani AC, *et al.* Targeting glioblastoma cells expressing CD44 with liposomes encapsulating doxorubicin and displaying chlorotoxin-IgG Fc fusion protein. Int J Mol Sci 2018; 19(3): 659.
[http://dx.doi.org/10.3390/ijms19030659] [PMID: 29495404]

[31]   Eloy JO, Claro de Souza M, Petrilli R, Barcellos JPA, Lee RJ, Marchetti JM. Liposomes as carriers of hydrophilic small molecule drugs: Strategies to enhance encapsulation and delivery. Colloids Surf B Biointerfaces 2014; 123: 345-63.
[http://dx.doi.org/10.1016/j.colsurfb.2014.09.029] [PMID: 25280609]

[32]   Ying X, Wen H, Lu WL, *et al.* Dual-targeting daunorubicin liposomes improve the therapeutic efficacy of brain glioma in animals. J Control Release 2010; 141(2): 183-92.
[http://dx.doi.org/10.1016/j.jconrel.2009.09.020] [PMID: 19799948]

[33]   Shi D, Mi G, Shen Y, Webster TJ. Glioma-targeted dual functionalized thermosensitive Ferri-liposomes for drug delivery through an *in vitro* blood–brain barrier. Nanoscale 2019; 11(32): 15057-71.
[http://dx.doi.org/10.1039/C9NR03931G] [PMID: 31369016]

[34]   Sun X, Chen Y, Zhao H, *et al.* Dual-modified cationic liposomes loaded with paclitaxel and survivin siRNA for targeted imaging and therapy of cancer stem cells in brain glioma. Drug Deliv 2018; 25(1): 1718-27.
[http://dx.doi.org/10.1080/10717544.2018.1494225] [PMID: 30269613]

[35]   Duan L, Xu L, Xu X, *et al.* Exosome-mediated delivery of gene vectors for gene therapy. Nanoscale 2021; 13(3): 1387-97.

[http://dx.doi.org/10.1039/D0NR07622H] [PMID: 33350419]

[36] Chen X, Gole J, Gore A, *et al*. Non-invasive early detection of cancer four years before conventional diagnosis using a blood test 2020.
[http://dx.doi.org/10.1038/s41467-020-17316-z]

[37] Banerjee K, Núñez FJ, Haase S, *et al*. Current Approaches for Glioma Gene Therapy and Virotherapy. Front Mol Neurosci 2021; 14621831
[http://dx.doi.org/10.3389/fnmol.2021.621831] [PMID: 33790740]

[38] Chen Z, Liu F, Chen Y, *et al*. Targeted Delivery of CRISPR/Cas9-Mediated Cancer Gene Therapy *via* Liposome-Templated Hydrogel Nanoparticles. Adv Funct Mater 2017; 27(46)1703036
[http://dx.doi.org/10.1002/adfm.201703036] [PMID: 29755309]

[39] Zylberberg C, Gaskill K, Pasley S, Matosevic S. Engineering liposomal nanoparticles for targeted gene therapy. Gene Ther 2017; 24(8): 441-52.
[http://dx.doi.org/10.1038/gt.2017.41] [PMID: 28504657]

[40] Kostevšek N, Cheung CCL, Serša I, *et al*. Magneto-liposomes as MRI contrast agents: A systematic study of different liposomal formulations. Nanomaterials (Basel) 2020; 10(5): 889.
[http://dx.doi.org/10.3390/nano10050889] [PMID: 32384645]

[41] Xin H, Jiang Y, Lv W, *et al*. Liposome-Based Drug Delivery for Brain Tumor Theranostics.Nanotechnology-Based Targeted Drug Delivery Systems for Brain Tumors. Academic Press 2018; pp. 245-66.
[http://dx.doi.org/10.1016/B978-0-12-812218-1.00009-9]

[42] Keller DS, Ishizawa T, Cohen R, Chand M. Indocyanine green fluorescence imaging in colorectal surgery: overview, applications, and future directions. Lancet Gastroenterol Hepatol 2017; 2(10): 757-66.
[http://dx.doi.org/10.1016/S2468-1253(17)30216-9] [PMID: 28895551]

[43] Li S, Johnson J, Peck A, Xie Q. Near infrared fluorescent imaging of brain tumor with IR780 dye incorporated phospholipid nanoparticles. J Transl Med 2017; 15(1): 18.
[http://dx.doi.org/10.1186/s12967-016-1115-2] [PMID: 28114956]

[44] Oku N, Yamashita M, Katayama Y, *et al*. PET imaging of brain cancer with positron emitter-labeled liposomes. Int J Pharm 2011; 403(1-2): 170-7.
[http://dx.doi.org/10.1016/j.ijpharm.2010.10.001] [PMID: 20934495]

[45] Bhaskar S, Tian F, Stoeger T, *et al*. Multifunctional Nanocarriers for diagnostics, drug delivery and targeted treatment across blood-brain barrier: perspectives on tracking and neuroimaging. Part Fibre Toxicol 2010; 7(1): 3.
[http://dx.doi.org/10.1186/1743-8977-7-3] [PMID: 20199661]

[46] Grover VPB, Tognarelli JM, Crossey MME, Cox IJ, Taylor-Robinson SD, McPhail MJW. Magnetic resonance imaging: Principles and techniques: lessons for clinicians. J Clin Exp Hepatol 2015; 5(3): 246-55.
[http://dx.doi.org/10.1016/j.jceh.2015.08.001] [PMID: 26628842]

[47] Zhou Z, Lu ZR. Gadolinium-based contrast agents for magnetic resonance cancer **imaging**. Wiley Interdiscip Rev Nanomed Nanobiotechnol 2013; 5(1): 1-18.
[http://dx.doi.org/10.1002/wnan.1198] [PMID: 23047730]

[48] Estelrich J, Sánchez-Martín MJ, Busquets MA. Nanoparticles in magnetic resonance imaging: from simple to dual contrast agents. Int J Nanomedicine 2015; 10: 1727-41.
[PMID: 25834422]

[49] Suk JS, Xu Q, Kim N, Hanes J, Ensign LM. PEGylation as a strategy for improving nanoparticle-based drug and gene delivery. Adv Drug Deliv Rev 2016; 99(Pt A): 28-51.
[http://dx.doi.org/10.1016/j.addr.2015.09.012] [PMID: 26456916]

[50] Bhandari A, Bansal A, Singh A, Sinha N. Transport of liposome encapsulated drugs in voxelized

computational model of human brain tumors. IEEE Trans Nanobiosci 2017; 16(7): 634-44.
[http://dx.doi.org/10.1109/TNB.2017.2737038] [PMID: 28796620]

[51]   Pysz MA, Gambhir SS, Willmann JK. Molecular imaging: current status and emerging strategies. Clin Radiol 2010; 65(7): 500-16.
[http://dx.doi.org/10.1016/j.crad.2010.03.011] [PMID: 20541650]

[52]   Lentacker I, De Smedt SC, Sanders NN. Drug loaded microbubble design for ultrasound triggered delivery. Soft Matter 2009; 5(11): 2161-70.
[http://dx.doi.org/10.1039/b823051j]

[53]   Xing H, Hwang K, Lu Y. Recent Developments of Liposomes as Nanocarriers for Theranostic Applications. Theranostics 2016; 6(9): 1336-52.
[http://dx.doi.org/10.7150/thno.15464] [PMID: 27375783]

[54]   Zhan W. Effects of focused-ultrasound-and-microbubble-induced blood-brain barrier disruption on drug transport under liposome-mediated delivery in brain tumour: A pilot numerical simulation study. Pharmaceutics 2020; 12(1): 69.
[http://dx.doi.org/10.3390/pharmaceutics12010069] [PMID: 31952336]

[55]   Zhao G, Huang Q, Wang F, *et al.* Targeted shRNA-loaded liposome complex combined with focused ultrasound for blood brain barrier disruption and suppressing glioma growth. Cancer Lett 2018; 418: 147-58.
[http://dx.doi.org/10.1016/j.canlet.2018.01.035] [PMID: 29339208]

[56]   Aryal M, Vykhodtseva N, Zhang YZ, Park J, McDannold N. Multiple treatments with liposomal doxorubicin and ultrasound-induced disruption of blood–tumor and blood–brain barriers improve outcomes in a rat glioma model. J Control Release 2013; 169(1-2): 103-11.
[http://dx.doi.org/10.1016/j.jconrel.2013.04.007] [PMID: 23603615]

[57]   Guo Y, Wang XY, Chen YL, *et al.* A light-controllable specific drug delivery nanoplatform for targeted bimodal imaging-guided photothermal/chemo synergistic cancer therapy. Acta Biomater 2018; 80: 308-26.
[http://dx.doi.org/10.1016/j.actbio.2018.09.024] [PMID: 30240955]

[58]   Sonali , Viswanadh MK, Singh RP, *et al.* Nanotheranostics: Emerging strategies for early diagnosis and therapy of brain cancer. Nanotheranostics 2018; 2(1): 70-86.
[http://dx.doi.org/10.7150/ntno.21638] [PMID: 29291164]

[59]   Blahut J, Benda L, Kotek J, Pintacuda G, Hermann P. Paramagnetic cobalt(II) complexes with cyclam derivatives: toward 19 F MRI contrast agents. Inorg Chem 2020; 59(14): 10071-82.
[http://dx.doi.org/10.1021/acs.inorgchem.0c01216] [PMID: 32633944]

[60]   Viswanathan S, Kovacs Z, Green KN, Ratnakar SJ, Sherry AD. Alternatives to gadolinium-based metal chelates for magnetic resonance imaging. Chem Rev 2010; 110(5): 2960-3018.
[http://dx.doi.org/10.1021/cr900284a] [PMID: 20397688]

[61]   Nag OK, Naciri J, Oh E, Spillmann CM, Delehanty JB. Targeted plasma membrane delivery of a hydrophobic cargo encapsulated in a liquid crystal nanoparticle carrier. J Vis Exp 2017; 2017(120): 55181.
[http://dx.doi.org/10.3791/55181] [PMID: 28287601]

[62]   Roller BT, Munson JM, Brahma B, Santangelo PJ, Pai SB, Bellamkonda RV. Evans blue nanocarriers visually demarcate margins of invasive gliomas. Drug Deliv Transl Res 2015; 5(2): 116-24.
[http://dx.doi.org/10.1007/s13346-013-0139-x] [PMID: 25787737]

[63]   Liu X, Madhankumar AB, Miller PA, *et al.* MRI contrast agent for targeting glioma: interleukin-13 labeled liposome encapsulating gadolinium-DTPA. Neuro-oncol 2016; 18(5): 691-9.
[http://dx.doi.org/10.1093/neuonc/nov263] [PMID: 26519740]

[64]   Liu X. Ddel-13 targeted interleukin-13-liposomes-magnivest-doxorubicin for detection and treatment of glioma in early stage. Neuro-oncol 2015; 17(5): 76.

[65]   Zhang Z, Tan S, Feng SS. Vitamin E TPGS as a molecular biomaterial for drug delivery. Biomaterials 2012; 33(19): 4889-906.
[http://dx.doi.org/10.1016/j.biomaterials.2012.03.046] [PMID: 22498300]

[66]   Makino A, Kimura S. Solid tumor-targeting theranostic polymer nanoparticle in nuclear medicinal fields. ScientificWorldJournal. 2014; 2014: 424-513.

[67]   Han X, Huang J, To AKW, *et al.* CEST MRI detectable liposomal hydrogels for multiparametric monitoring in the brain at 3T. Theranostics 2020; 10(5): 2215-28.
[http://dx.doi.org/10.7150/thno.40146] [PMID: 32089739]

[68]   Saito R, Krauze MT, Bringas JR, *et al.* Gadolinium-loaded liposomes allow for real-time magnetic resonance imaging of convection-enhanced delivery in the primate brain. Exp Neurol 2005; 196(2): 381-9.
[http://dx.doi.org/10.1016/j.expneurol.2005.08.016] [PMID: 16197944]

[69]   Krauze MT, Mcknight TR, Yamashita Y, *et al.* Real-time visualization and characterization of liposomal delivery into the monkey brain by magnetic resonance imaging. Brain Res Brain Res Protoc 2005; 16(1-3): 20-6.
[http://dx.doi.org/10.1016/j.brainresprot.2005.08.003] [PMID: 16181805]

[70]   Muthu MS, Kulkarni SA, Xiong J, Feng SS. Vitamin E TPGS coated liposomes enhanced cellular uptake and cytotoxicity of docetaxel in brain cancer cells. Int J Pharm 2011; 421(2): 332-40.
[http://dx.doi.org/10.1016/j.ijpharm.2011.09.045] [PMID: 22001537]

[71]   Sonkar R, Sonali , Jha A, *et al.* Gold liposomes for brain-targeted drug delivery: Formulation and brain distribution kinetics. Mater Sci Eng C 2021; 120111652
[http://dx.doi.org/10.1016/j.msec.2020.111652] [PMID: 33545820]

[72]   Zhang LW, Wen CJ, Al-Suwayeh SA, Yen T-C, Fang J-Y. Cisplatin and quantum dots encapsulated in liposomes as multifunctional nanocarriers for theranostic use in brain and skin. J Nanopart Res 2012; 14(7): 882.
[http://dx.doi.org/10.1007/s11051-012-0882-9]

[73]   Xu L, Nirwane A, Yao Y. Basement membrane and blood–brain barrier. Stroke Vasc Neurol 2019; 4(2): 78-82.
[http://dx.doi.org/10.1136/svn-2018-000198] [PMID: 31338215]

[74]   Wang J, Wang L, Sun N, *et al.* Viscoelastic solid-repellent coatings for extreme water saving and global sanitation. Nat Sustain 2019; 2(12): 1097-105.
[http://dx.doi.org/10.1038/s41893-019-0421-0]

CHAPTER 5

Theranostics Dendrimer for Brain Tumor Diagnosis and Treatment

Aseem Setia[1], Ram Kumar Sahu[2,*], Ayodeji Folorunsho Ajayi[3] and Emmanuel Tayo Adebayo[3]

[1] *Department of Pharmacy, Shri Rawatpura Sarkar University, Raipur, Chhattisgarh - 492015, India*

[2] *Department of Pharmaceutical Sciences, Hemvati Nandan Bahuguna Garhwal University (A Central University), Chauras Campus, Tehri Garhwal-249161, Uttarakhand, India*

[3] *Reproductive Physiology and Bioinformatics Research Unit, Department of Physiology, Ladoke Akintola University of Technology, Ogbomoso, Oyo state, Nigeria*

Abstract: Brain tumors have become one of the deadliest types of cancer. Tragically, the blood-brain barrier (BBB), an astringent regulatory, well-coordinated, and effectual obstacle, prevents most substances from passing through it. As a result, breaking through this hurdle is amongst the most difficult challenges in devising effective CNS therapies. In the USA, approximately seven lakh people have a principal brain malignancy, with an ample eighty-five thousand predicted to be afflicted by 2021. Capillaries are essential for delivering oxygen and nutrients to all body tissue and vital organs. The capillaries that vascularize the CNS have a special feature known as the blood-brain barrier, which enables such vessels to firmly enforce the transfer of ions, substances, and cells in-between the blood-brain barrier. This accurate estimation of CNS homeostasis leads to proper neuronal function while also protecting neural tissue from toxic substances and microorganisms, and changes in such mechanical strength are a major aspect of the pathology and transformation of various neurological diseases. Theranostic strategies were also postulated and deemed enticing in recent times. Due to the smaller size, better topical functionalization, and capability to integrate various processing elements in one system, nanotechnology is beneficial for this system. For cancer therapy, the structure of nanotherapeutic systems focusing on diagnostic and therapeutic applications is increasing tremendously. This dual system is extremely useful for personalized medicine-based clinical applications because it seeks to analyze the position of malignancy, the biodistribution of nanosized systems, along with an advanced and efficacious therapy. Proteins, molecular markers, and genes are some of the theranostic strategies that could be used to amplify the surface of the nanotheranostics particle and make benefit of the features of the micro-environment utilising stimulus-based triggers. The current chapter focused on the theranostic approach of dendrimer for brain tumor treatment. It also enlightened about various diagnostic techniques for brain tumors with a special emphasis on nanotherapeutics.

* **Corresponding author Ram Kumar Sahu:** Department of Pharmaceutical Sciences, Hemvati Nandan Bahuguna Garhwal University (A Central University), Chauras Campus, Tehri Garhwal-249161, Uttarakhand, India E-mail: ramsahu79@gmail.com

Keywords: Blood-Brain Barrier, Brain tumor, Dendrimers, Theranostics.

INTRODUCTION

Brain diseases are the most challenging issues in healthcare because, as the global population ages, the percentage of patients with brain diseases will increase, resulting in high social repercussions due to severe morbidity and mortality [1]. Furthermore, glioma accounts for 80 percent of all melanoma and has a sudden onset and intensified belligerence [2]. Among most individuals with cerebral tumor cells, the contemporaneous treatment scheduling with radiation, surgery along with chemotherapy was found very risky, with minimum (in months) survival time [3]. Regardless of the potential bioactive agents obtained through medical updates, adequate remedies remain an unlocked therapeutic requirement because systemic administration agents are frequently ineffective due to a conventional biological obstacle: BBB (barrier between the blood and brain). A brain cancer is a malignant tissue overgrowth in the CNS region that could impede normal brain function. The cell types associated with brain tumors, as well as the tumor's location in the brain, can be identified. Gliomas are cancer cells of the brain caused by glial cells. The three subtypes of cells that produce astrocytoma, oligodendroglioma, and ependymal cells are astrocytoma, oligodendroglioma, and ependymal cells [4]. The WHO categorizes Glioma into 4 categories *i.e* grade I-IV. Grade I or II called as low grade tumours are being treated and managed by surgery and monitoring. Cancer with a greater extent of malignant glioma *viz.* III or IV grade might be harder to cure, and radiotherapy and chemotherapy are examples of alternative treatments. Targeted therapy, on the other hand, may be mandatory. Glioblastoma multi forme (GBM) is a cancerous one which is complicated to be diagnosed because of surgical resistance and invasiveness. Moreover, the poor prognosis and resistance to chemo and radiotherapy across the CNS provides limited options of therapies [5]. In US, approximately 7 lakh patients are diagnosed with primary brain tumor with an increase of around 85, 000 by the year 2021. Nearly 70% of all brain tumors are benign, with the remaining 30% being malignant. Females account for approximately 58% of all brain tumors. Males account for approximately 42% of all brain tumors [6]. The lack of particular methods for delivering therapeutic agents through the central nervous system (CNS) barriers makes the treatment of brain tumors complicated. The current practice is surgical resection, which is accompanied by multiple-therapy (chemo-radio-immuno therapy). Advantages of present therapy, on the other hand, are negligible for the patient. The term "theranostics" is a mixture of the terms identification and treatment, and it refers to techniques that have combined diagnostic along with therapeutic application (Fig. **1**). Presently interest in personalized treatment and diagnostic techniques is increasing day by day. This is a time saving approach along with the money while also limiting the negative consequences of a particular objective [7]. NPS are nanoparticles that have been used in combination with medicines and diagnostic probes, metallic nanoparticles, liposomes, polymeric combinations, dendrimers, micelles *etc*. Due to the numerous limitations of bioactive compounds, developing an optimal delivery platform for treating cancer is exceptionally hard for formulation scientists as well as clinicians in the current scenario. Furthermore, traditional chemotherapeutic agents' poor biodistribution and undesirable pharmacokinetics lead to poor treatment outcomes and serious complications affecting healthy organs. To address these constraints, efficient and useful vectors are urgently required for better targeting, efficient transit (without degradation), and optimized release of drug and at most with least toxicity [8].

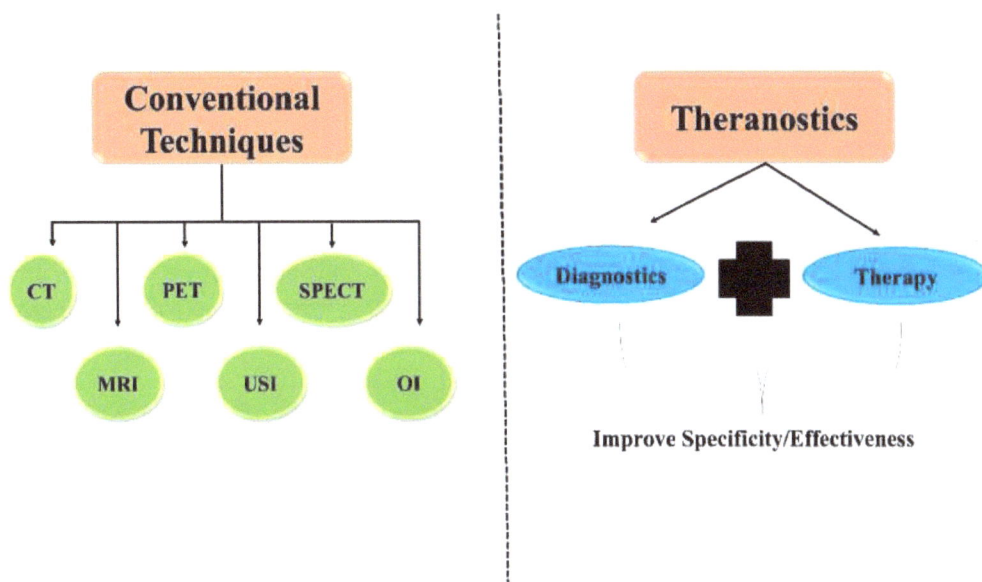

Fig. (1). Concept of conventional and theranostics technique

PHYSIOLOGY AND PHARMACOLOGY OF BLOOD-BRAIN BARRIER

BBB (Blood Brain Barrier) is an expression used to designate the special features of the CNS microvasculature. CNS consists of non-fenestrated vessels, with numerous properties that allow them to firmly enforce the drive of materials, ions, and cells between the systemic circulation and CNS [9]. Such a severely limited hurdle prompts BBB endothelial cells to closely restrict CNS homeostasis, which is required for absolute neuron functioning. Although it protects the CNS from pathogens, toxins, injuries, and diseases [10]. Various neuroactive solutes such as glutamate, epinephrine, glycine, *etc*. protect the brain. BBB, BCSFB, and the ependymal barrier separate the brain from the marginal section. The brain is a complex but well-controlled system [11]. Toxins are eliminated, allowing only essential nutrients and oxygen to flow freely. Neurotransmitters are chemical messengers that travel throughout the brain. The BBB, in specific, was intended to prevent substances from flexibly diffusing from the bloodstream to the brain parenchyma by endothelial cells (Fig. **2**). The BCSFB characterised by the choroid plexus epithelium in the ventricles curtails free passage *via* the circulatory system into CSF, whereas the ependymal, which is largely constituted of epithelial cells in the ventricles, controls diffusion from the cerebrospinal fluid into the brain [12]. As a result of the combination of these three barriers, free drug diffusion from the blood and CSF to the brain is limited, but transporters and receptors are expressed in the brain to allow preventive care and ions to enter the brain in accordance with the body's demands [13]. The BBB, which is made of endothelial cells constrained by tight junctions and creates a barrier between astrocytes, pericytes, microglia, neurons, and the extracellular matrix, is one of the most studied barriers because of its critical components and tight connections. There are other reasons why drugs are targeted at the BBB, such as the fact that it includes a large interface between the blood and the brain parenchyma (around 20 square meters) [14]. On the other hand, due to the ependymal's barrier function, there will be a continuous outflow of therapeutic substances that enter the CSF region [15]. Taut junction regulates the para-cellular transfer of soluble substances, whereas adherent junctions establish and maintain cellular processes [16]. Adjacent junctions combine to form close junctions, only cytoplasmic proteins and occluding proteins (occluding and claudin) molecules that are permeable but have a relatively small hydrodynamic diameter endothelial cells *via* the transmembrane protein intercalation [17]. More than 4 Å can transmit through the nearer aqueous pore junctions and close junction leakiness is consciously enforced, as are astrocytes, pericytes, and other cells in the area [18]. Restricting paracellular pathways prevents more than 98 percent of cancers. The cerebral cortex is penetrated by 100 percent of small and large molecular drugs. Taut junction proteins like Claudin-I, Claudin-V, and occludin downregulate sometimes. Whereas the VEGF receptor and the water channel protein aquaporin-4 were found to be up-regulated, leading to angiogenesis and increased endothelial permeability [19]. Nonetheless, the blood-brain barrier is intact in low-grade/ growing high-grade brain malignancy. Based on the preceding discussion, it is clear that an effectual technique for the future is required in brain drug delivery.

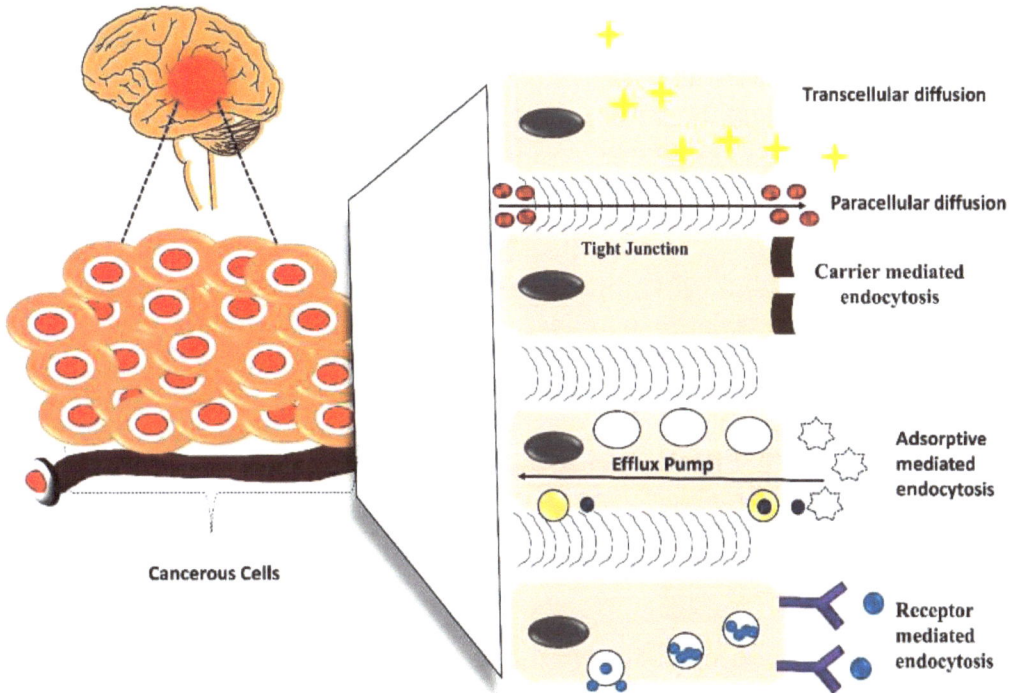

Fig. (2). Physiology & Pharmacology of BBB

Receptors of Blood-Brain Barrier

Transferrin Receptor

Transferrin receptor denoted as (TfR), has imperative responsibility in brain drug delivery. TfR has 2 (90kDa) subunits having a trans-membrane glycoprotein with (S-S) di-sulphide linkage [20]. One molecule of transferring is present in each subunit. These are abundantly found in blood-brain barrier. Through receptor-mediated transcytosis, the TfR mediates cellular uptake of iron bound to transferrin (Tf) [21]. TfR is identified in BBB endothelial cells, choroid plexus epithelial cells, and neurons. It is, conversely, found on hepatocytes, erythrocytes, intestinal cells, and monocytes. Transferrin is a vital chelator whose main purpose is serum iron transport [22]. It has special potential for reversibly binding two atoms of ferric iron (Fe^+). Following iron-binding, apotransferrin undergoes a conformational change (diferric transferrin or holotransferrin), which is important in its discriminatory detection by the transferrin receptor [23]. Clathrin-mediated endocytosis is the primary mechanism involved in transferrin-mediated iron uptake. The fate of the transferrin–transferrin receptor complex after endocytosis has been extensively studied [24]. This research has revealed two different pathways, the first entailing the complex's recycling back to the cell surface and the second contributing to its lysosomal degradation. TfRs are primarily saturable with endogenous Tf. As a result, Tf is not an excellent option for a targeting substituent to increase the brain delivery of substituted therapeutics [25]. TfR monoclonal antibodies have thus been designed to target a specific sequence within TfR's extracellular domain (ECD) while not interfering with endogenous Tf binding to TfR. Because they do not compete with circulating Tf in binding TfR, TfR monoclonal antibodies are appealing brain delivery vectors. There have been several TfR monoclonal antibodies developed with species-specific BBB permeability. Wu *et al.* (2012) investigated the effect of Tirapazamine (TPZ) in combination with cisplatin to reduce side effects and increase efficacy. For delivery systems, TPZ was covalently linked with transferrin (Tf-G-TPZ) and co-administered with cisplatin. The study' finding showed that cancer cell accretion was 2.3-fold greater than unfastened TPZ *in vivo*; there was a 53 percent tumor inhibition rate in combined effect with cisplatin, and there was limited systemic toxicity [26].

Insulin Receptor

Insulin's activities are mediated by the insulin receptor (IR), which originally belonged to the tyrosine kinase receptor family [27]. Adhesion by insulin involves sudden auto phosphorylation of the receptor, accompanied by tyrosine phosphorylation of insulin receptor substrate (IRS) proteins, which activates downstream pathways such as the PI3K and the MAPK cascades [28]. The synapse formation, neuroprotective process, and synaptic plasticity are regulated by the insulin receptor. Long-term potentiation (LTP) and depression (LTD), learning and memory, energy balance, appetite, and feeding behaviour were all found to be modulated by IR-mediated signalling [29]. Innumerable correlations have been revealed among IR-mediated signalling deficiency and neurodevelopmental disorders. The insulin receptor comprises two subunits and both are connected by a disulphide linkage. The extracellular -subunit contains a ligand-binding site [30]. The cytoplasmic portion of the transmembrane -subunit transmits tyrosine kinase activity. Pardridge and coworkers showed the data analysis procedure that generates a genetically engineered human-mouse chimeric form of the human IR monoclonal antibody (HIRMAb) through all regions of the brain of an adult anesthetized Rhesus monkey and urged its capability for drug and gene delivery across the BBB in humans *via* intravenous administration [31].

Lipoprotein Receptor

Lipidic substances are transported from the circulation to the extracellular space by means of receptors on cell surfaces, lipid carriers and transmission proteins, enzymes, and transporters on cell surfaces [32]. The transport of critical micronutrients, endogenously synthesised hormones, and lipid-modified signalling proteins and other macromolecular components across metabolically specialised tissues are considered to be its origin [33]. As a result of their ancient origin, lipoprotein receptors are among the oldest components of this complicated system. Two types of cell surface receptors are recognised by the body: those that entrap their cargo in the form of lipid-carrying lipoproteins, initiating their internalisation and inevitable delivery to the lysosomes, and those that promote lipid exchange at the plasma membrane, but do not allow the particle's protein component to be taken up by the cell. Both LDLR and LRP, a multifunctional receptor that both scavenges ligands and transmits signals, are found in the BBB (LRP1 and LRP2) [34]. BBB failure is linked with elevated LDLR expression in the hippocampus of stroke-prone spontaneously hypertensive rats. This is because LRP suppresses the inflammatory process [35]. Triacylglycerols and cholesterol (unesterified and/or esterified) have unique fates when considering lipoprotein transit and targeting *via* cell surface receptors in many instances. The brain's absorption of the nanoparticles was facilitated by LDLR-mediated endocytosis and transcytosis of ApoE or ApoB incorporated into the nanoparticles [36]. Brain, placenta, and testes have large amounts of ApoER2, whereas other LDL receptor family members are found in smaller quantities in the brain but in greater quantities elsewhere [37]. This is supported by studies that have shown the receptor is virtually likely engaged in cognitive processes involving apoE-mediated transport. It has also been shown that the 8 binding repetitions of apoER2 may be used in the brain to remove 2M/proteinase complexes from cerebrospinal fluid and neural substrate [38].

THERANOSTICS DENDRIMERS FOR BRAIN TUMOR

Brain cancer is harder to identify and recognize in its early stages. The diagnosis and detection of brain cancers are complicated because there is usually an accretion of extracellular fluid involving the tumor region [39]. Conventional prophylactic and treatment agents seemed to have impoverished biodistribution and pharmacokinetics, ensuing in cancer cell facilitation that was limited [40]. The nano theranostics strategy could be quite useful in overcoming these issues. Several appropriate nano theranostic brain cancer therapies have been identified, but more research is needed [41]. There are various strategies for the diagnosis of brain tumor (Table **1**) which include, MRI contrast agent, fluorescence imaging, CT imaging, SPECT and PET Imaging, *etc*.

MRI Contrast Agent

MRI is a popular clinical diagnostic technique. It is possible to obtain non-invasive, high resolution, three-dimensional pictures that show the condition of water molecules in three dimensions. For MRI, contrast agents that influence the relaxation time of water protons are useful [42]. Even amongst the multiple methodologies for imaging brain tumors, magnetic resonance imaging (MRI) is the most commonly traded technique for localizing the tumor site and determining tumor size [43]. This is because MRI provides delicate anatomical images and practical information with better resolution and thereby exhibits "favorable" contrast [44]. The major part of contrast agents used in the clinic today is based on Gd^{3+} ions [45]. Wiener *et al.* created the first gadolinium-infused PAMAM dendrimer for MRI imaging. MR signal intensity was enhanced by a single PAMAM dendrimer chelated with numerous Gd ions. A slowing of the molecular tumble of macromolecular Gd (III) chelates can substantially improve their relaxivity because Gd (III) chelates' relaxivity influences the water exchange rate. For MRI to be successful, contrast agents must have high relaxivity and regulated pharmacokinetics. Chelates of Gd (III) have been conjugated to the dendrimer periphery in the development of many macromolecular contrast agents. Gd (III) chelates may be conjugated to several nanoglobular (POSS core) dendrimers, including PAMAM. The pharmacokinetics and renal excretion properties of nanoglobular contrast agents play a significant role in controlling *in vivo* contrast enhancement in MRI [46]. Taratula *et al.* utilised dendrimers for cancer cell models to build synchronised systems that incorporated siRNA and MRI contrast agents (SPIO). They coupled SPIO nanoparticles with siRNA and the G5 PPI dendrimer. Once again, siRNA structures were changed using PEG-containing LHRH peptide as a targeting agent in order to add a tumor-specific targeting moiety and prevent nonspecific interactions. Hybrid nanoparticles having dendrimer/siRNA/SPIO incorporating PEG-LHRH were more effective at internalising malignant cells and suppressing targeted gene expression *in vitro*. Furthermore, the dendrimer nanodevice has the potential that will be used to co-deliver the chemotherapeutic agent, cisplatin, which exhibited enhanced *in vivo* antitumor activity [47].

Table 1. A description of theranostic dendrimers and their implementations

Types of Dendrimer	PEGylated G2.5	mPEG G 3.5 PAMAM	PAMAM	G5 PAMAM	Telodendrimer micelle	G5 PAMAM	Cationic PAMAM
Therapeutic agent	Doxorubicin	Paclitaxel	AuNPs	α-Tocopherol succinate	Paclitaxel	hNIS gene	Adenoviral NIS gene therapy
Diagnostic agent	SPIONPs	SPIONPs	AuNPs	Fluorescein isothiocyanate	^{125}I	^{123}I	^{124}I
Imaging	MRI	MRI	CT	CT	SPECT/CT	PET	PET

SPECT and PET Imaging

SPECT and PET use radioactive tracers (also known as radiopharmaceuticals) to detect, recognize, and cure a wide range of diseases and pathologies in a non-invasive manner, along with many cancer types, heart diseases, gastrointestinal, endocrine, neurological, and metabolic diseases, infection and inflammation [48]. To achieve the desired imaging and treatment protocols, the radioactive tracer agents have to be radiolabelled analogs of biomolecules that play a key role in a metabolizing or special adsorption (chemisorption) procedure, or they could be compounds with precision (*e.g.* as a ligand of a molecular receptor) to the inflamed foci, tumor, or pathogen [49]. Dendrimers' distinct properties enable the development of a wide range of PET imaging agents. It must be emphasized that to accomplish anticipated outcomes, many other important elements must be considered, such as appropriate isotopes, effective radio labelling techniques, and favorable pharmacokinetic profiles [50]. PET imaging now has access to a wide range of positron-emitting isotopes. In particular, they can be generated by medical cyclotrons or acquired from precise generators, and they are categorized into two categories based on their physical half-lives. Short-lived positron emitters with half-lives ranging from 2 to 110 minutes include ^{15}O, ^{13}N, ^{11}C, ^{18}F, and ^{68}Ga, which are suitable for measurements within an initial time frame. Long-lived positron emitters, such as ^{64}Cu, ^{76}Br, ^{89}Zr, ^{124}I, and ^{74}As, with half-lives of several hours or days, can be useful for relatively slow processes and certain effects, such as the EPR effect [51]. Nuclear medicine imaging has very high sensitivity and can be used for whole-body quantitative analysis. PET and SPECT are nuclear imaging techniques that can provide tomographic and quantitative functional information of a living subject. These imaging techniques make use of radiolabelled compounds. There are no biological counterparts to these nuclear imaging probes. PET and SPECT studies have made use of dendrimer nanodevices [52]. Grunwald *et al.* created PAMAM dendrimer-coated adenovirus vectors containing the hNIS gene (theranostic sodium iodide symporter gene). Upon intravenous injection of dendrimer-encased adenovirus vectors carrying the hNIS gene (dcAd5-CMV/NIS), hepatic allocation and liver toxicity were significantly reduced. Nevertheless, the efficacy of transduction and the accretion of dcAd5-CMV/NIS in tumor cells risen. Nonthyroidal tumors can be imaged and treated with radio-virotherapy using this delivery system. The therapeutic dose of ^{131}I induced an effective antitumor effect [53].

DENDRIMERS IN THE MANAGEMENT OF BRAIN CARCINOGENESIS

Dendrimers are globular artificial macromolecules with a repeating unit's structural system. Dendrimers have repeated dendron branches around a central core, ensuing in a proximity three-dimensional geometrical shape. The development can influence the size and molecular weight (G). The dendrimer space is accessible for drug molecule encapsulation; the peripheral functional groups are available for drug molecule modification *via* covalent bonds and complex formation [54]. Dendrimer development for various imaging platforms and drug delivery systems has received a lot of attention. Dendrimers have the size of a swarm of biological systems. Generation 5 (G5) polyamidoamine (PAMAM) dendrimers (Fig. **3**) are roughly the same size and has the shame shape as hemoglobin (5.5 nm in diameter) [55]. Tomalia *et al.* were the first to report commercially available polyamidoamine (PAMAM) dendrimers (1990) [56]. PPI and l-glutamic acid are two more dendrimers that have been studied for their possible involvement in medication delivery. Glycopeptide dendrimer vaccines have been created as preventive or therapeutic antitumor and antiviral vaccinations. POSS-core dendrimers have been employed in biological applications [57]. In comparison to traditional dendrimers, the POSS core has some structural advantages. POSS core dendrimers have a vast specific functional group content, excellently nanosized, and compact globular macromolecular architectures. Due to the extreme POSS core's eight reactive termini, they have many peripheral functional groups. The high peripheral functionality facilitates the binding of lipophilic anticancer drugs, imaging agents, and targeting agents [58]. To prepare a dendrimer, two common synthetic methods are used: divergent and convergent. Dendrimers are built from the core to the shell, generation by generation, in the divergent approach, whereas compounds are built from the periphery to the core in the convergent approach. The dendritic method could be used as a diagnostic method due to the most recent generation of nanoparticles [59]. Dendrimers are an outstanding nanocarrier for targeted drug delivery due to their monodispersibility, surface modification, and an increased number of internal pores. The main properties of dendrimer-based nanocarriers allow them to be used as drug delivery vehicles to increase anticancer drug absorption in cancer cells [60]. The EPR mechanism includes increased chemotherapeutic macromolecule permeation within the tumor cells and a reduced efflux rate from cancerous cells [61]. Dendrimers are three-dimensional structures with a heavily branched architecture, consisting of an inner initiator core, several repeated inner layers, and an external surface with multiple active sites. The amount of branching cycles conducted throughout synthesis is related to the dendrimer's size, which is assessed in generation (G). Dendrimers are monodispersed and highly capable due to their wide branching pattern. Dendrimers are created successively either with a divergent or convergent system. The former method starts with a multifunctional nucleus and is followed by repetitive monomer additions and an increase in molecular weight with an exponential rise in surface termini [62]. As a major advancement in therapy nanotechnology, dendrimeric nanocarriers were formed as a theranostic strategy as a contrast agent. Numerous dendrimers were used to transport a wide range of therapeutic drugs in order to achieve maximum therapeutic efficacy in cancer care [63]. Dendrimers can also be used in gene therapy, vaccines, antiviral therapy, and diagnostic tools.

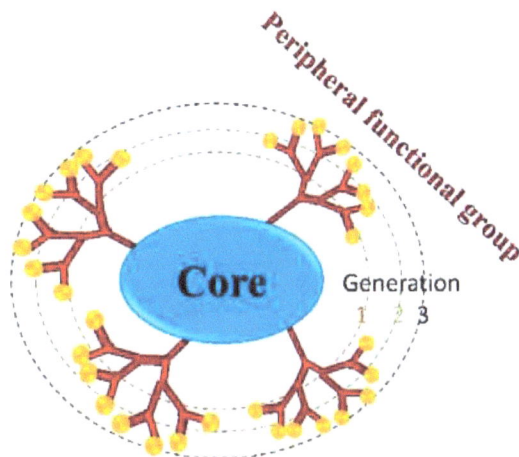

Fig. (3). Structure of Dendrimer

RECENT ADVANCEMENT IN DENDRIMER FOR BRAIN TUMOR DELIVERY

Tumor Targeting *via* PAMAM Dendrimers

Polyamidoamine dendrimers (PAMAM) are dendrimers that have a core (the earliest core was an ethylenediamine core), branches composed of amide groups arising from a branching point that develops the walls of cavities, and amine functional groups on the periphery. Consecutively, PAMAM dendrimers consist of a wide range of surface groups [64]. PAMAM dendrimers, which are one of the most extensively studied dendrimers, possess inside cavities and an ancillary molecular structure (Table **2**). They may be further modified to encompass entities for biomedical applications [65]. Bhadra *et al*. formulated 5-fluorouracil (5-FU) dendrimer and PEGylation was done *via* 4.0G PAMAM, the prepared system shows a sustained release activity for anticancer agents, causing less blood dyscrasia than non-PEGylated systems. Yuan *et al*. created a dendrimers' carrier for nucleic acid delivery and diagnosis [66]. Vincent *et al*. explored the possibility of nonviral gene transfer for treating cancer. Using antiangiogenic angiostatin (Kringle 1–3) and tissue inhibitors of metalloproteinase (TIMP) genes, Superfectants coupled to 36-mer anionic oligomers (ON36) may be utilised to inhibit cell proliferation and angiogenesis by delivering effective angiostatin and TIMP-2 genes [67].

Table 2. A list of dendrimers associated with malignant cells and BBB targeting cranial cancer therapies.

Dendrimer types	PAMAM	PAMAM	PPI	PPI	PLL
Mode of Targeting	Targeting cancerous cells	Double targeting (Blood brain barrier + tumour cell)	Targeting cancerous cells	Double targeting (Blood brain barrier + tumour cell)	-
Ligand	Cetuximab monoclonal antibody	Transferrin + Tamoxifen	Thiamine	Polysorbate 80 (P80) surfactant	T7 Peptide
Drug	Boron	Doxorubicin	Paclitaxel	Docetaxel	siRNA
Target	EGF receptors	Transferrin receptors	-	-	-

Tumor Targeting *via* Polypropyleneimine Dendrimer

Oldest used commercial dendrimers for drug delivery is the poly-propylene imine (PPI) dendrimer. The composition is based on the repetition of di-aminobutane and propylene imine unit [68]. Poly-propylene imine is also abbreviated as DAB dendrimers because diaminobutane (DAB) is an aspect of PPI. The water solubility is being provided by the amino group present at the terminal position of PPI. This enhances the water solubility of the entrapped lipophilic agent using PPI. PPI, on the other hand, has a positively charged surface that commonly disrupts the plasma membrane resulting in lysis [69]. Another issue is that PPI has a lower drug-loading capacity than PAMAM. PPI/drug complexes are less stable than PPI alone. PEGylation and acetylation of surface groups have been chosen as surface group modifications. Due to its penetration and high efficiency, the method of acetylation is preferred. Moreover, the interaction of drug molecules and the topical functional group is affected by the steric hindrance provided by the PEG chain. Kesharwani *et al.* investigated the release of various chemotherapeutic agents utilising PPI of different generations. The same group of researchers investigated the malignancy potential of 3 distinct ligand-conjugated dendrimers: dextran, galactose, and folate. In comparison to the non-targeted PPI dendrimers, receptor-conjugated PPI dendrimers not only showed superior targeted malignancy prospects but substantially lowered haemolytic toxicity. Moreover, the paclitaxel (PTX) release correlation was observed to be unrelenting when topical customized dendrimers were compared to non-targeted PPI dendrimers. The outcomes might be ascribed to the PTX being encompassed in the hydrophobic cavities of the targeted dendrimers, which behave as a sink to preserve the PTX over time. In another research, thiamine-conjugated 5.0G PPI dendrimers were found to increase PTX delivery across the BBB. According to the authors, the preferential brain uptake of PTX by the nanoconjugates might be ascribed to affiliation with thiamine transporters or enhanced passive diffusion as a result of an enhanced gradient of concentration of dendrimers at the BBB interface [70].

Tumor Targeting *via* PLL Dendrimers

Dendrimers composed of lysine residues are referred to as poly-l-lysine (PLL) dendrimers (also known as dendri-grafted poly-l-lysine or DGL) [71]. These dendrimers have higher biocompatibility, lower cytotoxicity, and easy enzymatic degradation products. Furthermore, the ability to introduce stimuli responsiveness when needed by incorporating an explicit amino acid sequence of PLL dendrimers is extremely interesting. Gene delivery has made extensive use of PLL dendrimers and their derivatives [72]. When compared to PLL dendrimers, the advanced cohort of PLL exhibits superior gene transfection, whereas conventional linear poly-lysine exhibits lesser gene transfection competence and increased cytostatic activity [73]. Recently, folate-conjugated PLL dendrimers were formulated to deliver DOX hydrochloride (anti-tumour drug). The results of the CAM assay, MTT assay, and *in vivo* evaluation all indicated that the developed systems had superior antitumor activity [74]. Another method was to deliver DOX through the lipophilic cavity of 6.0G PLL dendrimers affix with PEG-linked lipophilic Penta phenyl alanine/ Penta alanine. Tumour accumulation occurs as a result of IV administration using a nano delivery sysytem due to EPR, which eventually resulted in significant cancer proliferation suppression devoid of weight loss [75]. Al-Jamal and co-researchers designed a multifarious method containing 6.0G PLL and DOX, which improved anticancer activity in prostate 3D multicellular tumor spheroids (MTS) and solid cancers *in vivo*. These techniques overlay the way for newer antiangiogenic and/or anticancer therapeutics. PLL dendrimers, like PAMAM and PPI dendrimers, are consistently used for gene delivery. A study suggested that gene transfection efficiencies of PLL-based dendritic nanoconstructs were compared to linear and branched poly-lysine polymers. The research concluded that PLL dendrimers with 64 and 128 facade amino groups had a high propensity for gene transfection in numerous cell lines generated [76]. Ma *et al.* developed cyclodextrin derivatives containing PLL dendrons for simultaneous drug and gene delivery for tumor management. The formulated system formed colloidally stable nanocomplexes containing plasmid DNA in a watery solution and demonstrated elevated gene transfection effectiveness [77].

CONCLUSION

Traditional brain tumor treatments, including surgical intervention, radiation treatment, and immunotherapy, possess limited efficacy. Because traditional methods are ineffective, the latest methods that may be utilized as the diagnostic tool along with the anti-malignant drug delivery into tumor cells whilst also reducing allocations and toxic effects in normal cells were established. Dendrimers' precise architecture and versatile surface aid in the delivery of an increased payload of bioactive compounds, targeting ligands, and diagnostic negotiator *via* conjugation/ encapsulation for tumor diagnosis and management, as an efficient nanotechnology method, consisting of three main elements functionalization, targeting, and imaging. Theranostic nanoparticles are smart carriers capable of diagnosing, delivering, and monitoring therapeutic benefits in real time. Recognizing chemotherapeutic levels and healthy ADME profiles, along with the distribution to the targeted location accretion, by target receptor density imaging, and assessment of treatment response might aid in rational treatment and care plans. Non-invasive drug policy administration, as well as alternative therapeutic efficacy and low cytotoxicity, would all significantly contribute to nanosystems' dominance in peregrinate blood brain barrier (BBB). Furthermore, the use of esoteric apparatus for diagnosis and attempting to manipulate the CNS will keep on enhancing our knowledge in deciding in which way the human brain creates thoughts and produce actions; the massive potential of dendrimer-based nanomedicines will certainly strengthen new reliable methods of concisely delivering disparate medications to the brain.

REFERENCES

[1]   Miotto R, Wang F, Wang S, Jiang X, Dudley JT. Deep learning for healthcare: review, opportunities and challenges. Brief Bioinform 2018; 19(6): 1236-46.
[http://dx.doi.org/10.1093/bib/bbx044] [PMID: 28481991]

[2]   Jogalekar MP. Tissue engineering scaffolds and growth factors modulate cancer cell morphology and gene expression. New Mexico State University 2017.

[3]   Pitter KL. Mechanisms of glioma radiation resistance. Weill Medical College of Cornell University 2014.

[4]   Meng J, Agrahari V, Youm I. Advances in targeted drug delivery approaches for the central nervous system tumors: the inspiration of nanobiotechnology. J Neuroimmune Pharmacol 2017; 12(1): 84-98.
[http://dx.doi.org/10.1007/s11481-016-9698-1] [PMID: 27449494]

[5]   Yi S, Choi S, Shin DA, *et al.* Impact of H3. 3 K27M mutation on prognosis and survival of grade IV spinal cord glioma on the basis of new 2016 World Health Organization classification of the central nervous system. Neurosurgery 2019; 84(5): 1072-81.
[http://dx.doi.org/10.1093/neuros/nyy150] [PMID: 29718432]

[6]   Tandel GS, Tiwari A, Kakde OG. Performance optimisation of deep learning models using majority voting algorithm for brain tumour classification. Comput Biol Med 2021; 135104564
[http://dx.doi.org/10.1016/j.compbiomed.2021.104564] [PMID: 34217980]

[7]   Ogawa K. Development of Diagnostic and Therapeutic Probes with Controlled Pharmacokinetics for Use in Radiotheranostics. Chem Pharm Bull (Tokyo) 2019; 67(9): 897-903.
[http://dx.doi.org/10.1248/cpb.c19-00274] [PMID: 31474726]

[8]   Ulkoski D, Bak A, Wilson JT, Krishnamurthy VR. Recent advances in polymeric materials for the delivery of RNA therapeutics. Expert Opin Drug Deliv 2019; 16(11): 1149-67.

[http://dx.doi.org/10.1080/17425247.2019.1663822] [PMID: 31498013]

[9]   Pachter JS, de Vries HE, Fabry Z. The blood-brain barrier and its role in immune privilege in the central nervous system. J Neuropathol Exp Neurol 2003; 62(6): 593-604.
[http://dx.doi.org/10.1093/jnen/62.6.593] [PMID: 12834104]

[10]   Wekerle H, Lassmann H. The immunology of inflammatory demyelinating disease 2006.
[http://dx.doi.org/10.1016/B978-0-443-07271-0.50013-6]

[11]   Sun C, Ding Y, Zhou L, *et al.* Noninvasive nanoparticle strategies for brain tumor targeting. Nanomedicine 2017; 13(8): 2605-21.
[http://dx.doi.org/10.1016/j.nano.2017.07.009] [PMID: 28756093]

[12]   Johanson CE, Duncan JA III, Klinge PM, Brinker T, Stopa EG, Silverberg GD. Multiplicity of cerebrospinal fluid functions: New challenges in health and disease. Cerebrospinal Fluid Res 2008; 5(1): 10.
[http://dx.doi.org/10.1186/1743-8454-5-10] [PMID: 18479516]

[13]   de Boer AG, Gaillard PJ. Drug targeting to the brain. Annu Rev Pharmacol Toxicol 2007; 47(1): 323-55.
[http://dx.doi.org/10.1146/annurev.pharmtox.47.120505.105237] [PMID: 16961459]

[14]   Domínguez A, Álvarez A, Hilario E, Suarez-Merino B, Goñi-de-Cerio F. Central nervous system diseases and the role of the blood-brain barrier in their treatment. Neuroscience Discovery 2013; 1(1): 3.
[http://dx.doi.org/10.7243/2052-6946-1-3]

[15]   Erickson MA, Banks WA. Neuroimmune axes of the blood–brain barriers and blood–brain interfaces: bases for physiological regulation, disease states, and pharmacological interventions. Pharmacol Rev 2018; 70(2): 278-314.
[http://dx.doi.org/10.1124/pr.117.014647] [PMID: 29496890]

[16]   Wegener J, Seebach J. Experimental tools to monitor the dynamics of endothelial barrier function: a survey of *in vitro* approaches. Cell Tissue Res 2014; 355(3): 485-514.
[http://dx.doi.org/10.1007/s00441-014-1810-3] [PMID: 24585359]

[17]   Günzel D, Yu ASL. Claudins and the modulation of tight junction permeability. Physiol Rev 2013; 93(2): 525-69.
[http://dx.doi.org/10.1152/physrev.00019.2012] [PMID: 23589827]

[18]   Löscher W, Potschka H. Drug resistance in brain diseases and the role of drug efflux transporters. Nat Rev Neurosci 2005; 6(8): 591-602.
[http://dx.doi.org/10.1038/nrn1728] [PMID: 16025095]

[19]   Liebner S, Fischmann A, Rascher G, *et al.* Claudin-1 and claudin-5 expression and tight junction morphology are altered in blood vessels of human glioblastoma multiforme. Acta Neuropathol 2000; 100(3): 323-31.
[http://dx.doi.org/10.1007/s004010000180] [PMID: 10965803]

[20]   Widera A, Norouziyan F, Shen WC. Mechanisms of TfR-mediated transcytosis and sorting in epithelial cells and applications toward drug delivery. Adv Drug Deliv Rev 2003; 55(11): 1439-66.
[http://dx.doi.org/10.1016/j.addr.2003.07.004] [PMID: 14597140]

[21]   Zaki NM, Tirelli N. Gateways for the intracellular access of nanocarriers: a review of receptor-mediated endocytosis mechanisms and of strategies in receptor targeting. Expert Opin Drug Deliv 2010; 7(8): 895-913.
[http://dx.doi.org/10.1517/17425247.2010.501792] [PMID: 20629604]

[22]   Martinez-Finley EJ, Chakraborty S, Fretham SJB, Aschner M. Cellular transport and homeostasis of essential and nonessential metals. Metallomics 2012; 4(7): 593-605.
[http://dx.doi.org/10.1039/c2mt00185c] [PMID: 22337135]

[23]   Qian ZM, Li H, Sun H, Ho K. Targeted drug delivery *via* the transferrin receptor-mediated

endocytosis pathway. Pharmacol Rev 2002; 54(4): 561-87.
[http://dx.doi.org/10.1124/pr.54.4.561] [PMID: 12429868]

[24] Lee KW, Liu B, Ma L, *et al.* Cellular internalization of insulin-like growth factor binding protein-3: distinct endocytic pathways facilitate re-uptake and nuclear localization. J Biol Chem 2004; 279(1): 469-76.
[http://dx.doi.org/10.1074/jbc.M307316200] [PMID: 14576164]

[25] Dube BR. Formulation, Characterization and Evaluation of Nanoparticulate Therapeutic Systems for Targeting Brain Tumors (Doctoral dissertation, Maharaja Sayajirao University of Baroda (India)).

[26] Wu L, Wu J, Zhou Y, Tang X, Du Y, Hu Y. Enhanced antitumor efficacy of cisplatin by tirapazamine–transferrin conjugate. Int J Pharm 2012; 431(1-2): 190-6.
[http://dx.doi.org/10.1016/j.ijpharm.2012.04.032] [PMID: 22531857]

[27] Ganugapati J, Baldwa A, Lalani S. Molecular docking studies of banana flower flavonoids as insulin receptor tyrosine kinase activators as a cure for diabetes mellitus. Bioinformation 2012; 8(5): 216-20.
[http://dx.doi.org/10.6026/97320630008216] [PMID: 22493522]

[28] Nieto-Vazquez I, Fernández-Veledo S, Krämer DK, Vila-Bedmar R, Garcia-Guerra L, Lorenzo M. Insulin resistance associated to obesity: the link TNF-alpha. Arch Physiol Biochem 2008; 114(3): 183-94.
[http://dx.doi.org/10.1080/13813450802181047] [PMID: 18629684]

[29] Pomytkin I, Costa-Nunes JP, Kasatkin V, *et al.* Insulin receptor in the brain: Mechanisms of activation and the role in the CNS pathology and treatment. CNS Neurosci Ther 2018; 24(9): 763-74.
[http://dx.doi.org/10.1111/cns.12866] [PMID: 29691988]

[30] O'Dell SD, Day INM. Molecules in focus Insulin-like growth factor II (IGF-II). Int J Biochem Cell Biol 1998; 30(7): 767-71.
[http://dx.doi.org/10.1016/S1357-2725(98)00048-X] [PMID: 9722981]

[31] Pardridge WM. Drug transport across the blood-brain barrier. J Cereb Blood Flow Metab 2012; 32(11): 1959-72.
[http://dx.doi.org/10.1038/jcbfm.2012.126] [PMID: 22929442]

[32] Chiapparino A, Maeda K, Turei D, Saez-Rodriguez J, Gavin AC. The orchestra of lipid-transfer proteins at the crossroads between metabolism and signaling. Prog Lipid Res 2016; 61: 30-9.
[http://dx.doi.org/10.1016/j.plipres.2015.10.004] [PMID: 26658141]

[33] Lim W, Mayer B, Pawson T. Cell signaling. Taylor & Francis 2014. Jun 16.

[34] May P, Herz J, Bock HH. Molecular mechanisms of lipoprotein receptor signalling. Cell Mol Life Sci 2005; 62(19-20): 2325-38.
[http://dx.doi.org/10.1007/s00018-005-5231-z] [PMID: 16158188]

[35] Jin R, Yang G, Li G. Molecular insights and therapeutic targets for blood–brain barrier disruption in ischemic stroke: Critical role of matrix metalloproteinases and tissue-type plasminogen activator. Neurobiol Dis 2010; 38(3): 376-85.
[http://dx.doi.org/10.1016/j.nbd.2010.03.008] [PMID: 20302940]

[36] Chuang ST. Apolipoprotein E3 Mediated Targeted Brain Delivery of Reconstituted High Density Lipoprotein Bearing 3, 10, And 17 Nm Hydrophobic Core Gold Nanoparticles. Long Beach: California State University 2017.

[37] Nimpf J, Schneider WJ. From cholesterol transport to signal transduction: low density lipoprotein receptor, very low density lipoprotein receptor, and apolipoprotein E receptor-2. Biochim Biophys Acta Mol Cell Biol Lipids 2000; 1529(1-3): 287-98.
[http://dx.doi.org/10.1016/S1388-1981(00)00155-4] [PMID: 11111096]

[38] Mahley RW, Rall SC Jr. Apolipoprotein E: far more than a lipid transport protein. Annu Rev Genomics Hum Genet 2000; 1(1): 507-37.
[http://dx.doi.org/10.1146/annurev.genom.1.1.507] [PMID: 11701639]

[39]   Atlihan-Gundogdu E, Ilem-Ozdemir D, Ekinci M, *et al.* Recent developments in cancer therapy and diagnosis. J Pharm Investig 2020; 50(4): 349-61.
[http://dx.doi.org/10.1007/s40005-020-00473-0]

[40]   Aminu N, Bello I, Umar NM, Tanko N, Aminu A, Audu MM. The influence of nanoparticulate drug delivery systems in drug therapy. J Drug Deliv Sci Technol 2020; 60101961
[http://dx.doi.org/10.1016/j.jddst.2020.101961]

[41]   Kievit FM, Zhang M. Cancer nanotheranostics: improving imaging and therapy by targeted delivery across biological barriers. Adv Mater 2011; 23(36): H217-47.
[http://dx.doi.org/10.1002/adma.201102313] [PMID: 21842473]

[42]   Bull SR, Guler MO, Bras RE, Meade TJ, Stupp SI. Self-assembled peptide amphiphile nanofibers conjugated to MRI contrast agents. Nano Lett 2005; 5(1): 1-4.
[http://dx.doi.org/10.1021/nl0484898] [PMID: 15792402]

[43]   Black PM, Moriarty T, Alexander E III, *et al.* Development and implementation of intraoperative magnetic resonance imaging and its neurosurgical applications. Neurosurgery 1997; 41(4): 831-45.
[http://dx.doi.org/10.1097/00006123-199710000-00013] [PMID: 9316044]

[44]   Chen FY, Gu ZJ, Wan HP, Xu XZ, Tang Q. Manganese nanosystem for new generation of MRI contrast agent. Reviews in Nanoscience and Nanotechnology 2015; 4(2): 81-91.
[http://dx.doi.org/10.1166/rnn.2015.1066]

[45]   Morcos SK. Extracellular gadolinium contrast agents: Differences in stability. Eur J Radiol 2008; 66(2): 175-9.
[http://dx.doi.org/10.1016/j.ejrad.2008.01.025] [PMID: 18343072]

[46]   Wiener E, Brechbiel MW, Brothers H, *et al.* Dendrimer-based metal chelates: A new class of magnetic resonance imaging contrast agents. Magn Reson Med 1994; 31(1): 1-8.
[http://dx.doi.org/10.1002/mrm.1910310102] [PMID: 8121264]

[47]   Taratula O, Garbuzenko O, Savla R, Andrew Wang Y, He H, Minko T. Multifunctional nanomedicine platform for cancer specific delivery of siRNA by superparamagnetic iron oxide nanoparticles-dendrimer complexes. Curr Drug Deliv 2011; 8(1): 59-69.
[http://dx.doi.org/10.2174/156720111793663642] [PMID: 21034421]

[48]   Lu FM, Yuan Z. PET/SPECT molecular imaging in clinical neuroscience: recent advances in the investigation of CNS diseases. Quant Imaging Med Surg 2015; 5(3): 433-47.
[PMID: 26029646]

[49]   Zhu L, Ploessl K, Kung HF. PET/SPECT imaging agents for neurodegenerative diseases. Chem Soc Rev 2014; 43(19): 6683-91.
[http://dx.doi.org/10.1039/C3CS60430F] [PMID: 24676152]

[50]   Zhao L, Shi X, Zhao J. Dendrimer-based contrast agents for PET imaging. Drug Deliv 2017; 24(2): 81-93.
[http://dx.doi.org/10.1080/10717544.2017.1399299] [PMID: 29124984]

[51]   Kelloff GJ, Hoffman JM, Johnson B, *et al.* Progress and promise of FDG-PET imaging for cancer patient management and oncologic drug development. Clin Cancer Res 2005; 11(8): 2785-808.
[http://dx.doi.org/10.1158/1078-0432.CCR-04-2626] [PMID: 15837727]

[52]   Lauber DT, Fülöp A, Kovács T, Szigeti K, Máthé D, Szijártó A. State of the art *in vivo* imaging techniques for laboratory animals. Lab Anim 2017; 51(5): 465-78.
[http://dx.doi.org/10.1177/0023677217695852] [PMID: 28948893]

[53]   Grünwald GK, Vetter A, Klutz K, *et al.* Systemic image-guided liver cancer radiovirotherapy using dendrimer-coated adenovirus encoding the sodium iodide symporter as theranostic gene. J Nucl Med 2013; 54(8): 1450-7.
[http://dx.doi.org/10.2967/jnumed.112.115493] [PMID: 23843567]

[54]   Samad A, Alam M, Saxena K. Dendrimers: a class of polymers in the nanotechnology for the delivery of active pharmaceuticals. Curr Pharm Des 2009; 15(25): 2958-69.
[http://dx.doi.org/10.2174/138161209789058200] [PMID: 19754372]

[55]   Caminade AM, Turrin CO, Laurent R, Ouali A, Delavaux-Nicot B, Eds. Dendrimers: towards catalytic, material and biomedical uses. John Wiley & Sons 2011.
[http://dx.doi.org/10.1002/9781119976530]

[56]   Esfand R, Tomalia DA. Poly(amidoamine) (PAMAM) dendrimers: from biomimicry to drug delivery and biomedical applications. Drug Discov Today 2001; 6(8): 427-36.
[http://dx.doi.org/10.1016/S1359-6446(01)01757-3] [PMID: 11301287]

[57]   Huang D, Wu D. Biodegradable dendrimers for drug delivery. Mater Sci Eng C 2018; 90: 713-27.
[http://dx.doi.org/10.1016/j.msec.2018.03.002] [PMID: 29853143]

[58]   Wolinsky J, Grinstaff M. Therapeutic and diagnostic applications of dendrimers for cancer treatment. Adv Drug Deliv Rev 2008; 60(9): 1037-55.
[http://dx.doi.org/10.1016/j.addr.2008.02.012] [PMID: 18448187]

[59]   Xu Z, Kahr M, Walker KL, Wilkins CL, Moore JS. Phenylacetylene dendrimers by the divergent, convergent, and double-stage convergent methods. J Am Chem Soc 1994; 116(11): 4537-50.
[http://dx.doi.org/10.1021/ja00090a002]

[60]   Hsu HJ, Bugno J, Lee S, Hong S. Dendrimer□based nanocarriers: a versatile platform for drug delivery. Wiley Interdiscip Rev Nanomed Nanobiotechnol 2017; 9(1)e1409
[http://dx.doi.org/10.1002/wnan.1409] [PMID: 27126551]

[61]   Maeda H, Sawa T, Konno T. Mechanism of tumor-targeted delivery of macromolecular drugs, including the EPR effect in solid tumor and clinical overview of the prototype polymeric drug SMANCS. J Control Release 2001; 74(1-3): 47-61.
[http://dx.doi.org/10.1016/S0168-3659(01)00309-1] [PMID: 11489482]

[62]   Garg T, Singh O, Arora S, Murthy R. Dendrimer-a novel scaffold for drug delivery. Int J Pharm Sci Rev Res 2011; 7(2): 211-0.

[63]   Tripathy S, Das MK. Dendrimers and their applications as novel drug delivery carriers. J Appl Pharm Sci 2013; 3(09): 142-9.

[64]   Roberts JC, Bhalgat MK, Zera RT. Preliminary biological evaluation of polyamidoamine (PAMAM) StarburstTM dendrimers. J Biomed Mater Res 1996; 30(1): 53-65.
[http://dx.doi.org/10.1002/(SICI)1097-4636(199601)30:1<53::AID-JBM8>3.0.CO;2-Q]   [PMID: 8788106]

[65]   King Heiden TC, Dengler E, Kao WJ, Heideman W, Peterson RE. Developmental toxicity of low generation PAMAM dendrimers in zebrafish. Toxicol Appl Pharmacol 2007; 225(1): 70-9.
[http://dx.doi.org/10.1016/j.taap.2007.07.009] [PMID: 17764713]

[66]   Bhadra D, Bhadra S, Jain S, Jain NK. A PEGylated dendritic nanoparticulate carrier of fluorouracil. Int J Pharm 2003; 257(1-2): 111-24.
[http://dx.doi.org/10.1016/S0378-5173(03)00132-7] [PMID: 12711167]

[67]   Vincent L, Varet J, Pille JY, *et al.* Efficacy of dendrimer-mediated angiostatin and TIMP-2 gene delivery on inhibition of tumor growth and angiogenesis: *In vitro* and *in vivo* studies. Int J Cancer 2003; 105(3): 419-29.
[http://dx.doi.org/10.1002/ijc.11105] [PMID: 12704680]

[68]   Esfand R, Tomalia DA. Poly(amidoamine) (PAMAM) dendrimers: from biomimicry to drug delivery and biomedical applications. Drug Discov Today 2001; 6(8): 427-36.
[http://dx.doi.org/10.1016/S1359-6446(01)01757-3] [PMID: 11301287]

[69]   Jain V, Maingi V, Maiti PK, Bharatam PV. Molecular dynamics simulations of PPI dendrimer–drug complexes. Soft Matter 2013; 9(28): 6482-96.
[http://dx.doi.org/10.1039/c3sm50434d]

[70]   Kesharwani P, Iyer AK. Recent advances in dendrimer-based nanovectors for tumor-targeted drug and gene delivery. Drug Discov Today 2015; 20(5): 536-47.
[http://dx.doi.org/10.1016/j.drudis.2014.12.012] [PMID: 25555748]

[71]   Lúcio M, Lopes CM, Fernandes E, Gonçalves H, Oliveira ME. Organic Nanocarriers for Brain Drug Delivery 2021.
[http://dx.doi.org/10.1201/9781003119326-6]

[72]   Paleos CM, Tsiourvas D, Sideratou Z. Molecular engineering of dendritic polymers and their application as drug and gene delivery systems. Mol Pharm 2007; 4(2): 169-88.
[http://dx.doi.org/10.1021/mp060076n] [PMID: 17222053]

[73]   Chen S, Huang S, Li Y, Zhou C. Recent Advances in Epsilon-Poly-L-Lysine and L-Lysine-Based Dendrimer Synthesis, Modification, and Biomedical Applications. Front Chem 2021; 9659304
[http://dx.doi.org/10.3389/fchem.2021.659304] [PMID: 33869146]

[74]   Paleos CM, Tsiourvas D, Sideratou Z, Tziveleka LA. Drug delivery using multifunctional dendrimers and hyperbranched polymers. Expert Opin Drug Deliv 2010; 7(12): 1387-98.
[http://dx.doi.org/10.1517/17425247.2010.534981] [PMID: 21080860]

[75]   Lu J, Liong M, Li Z, Zink JI, Tamanoi F. Biocompatibility, biodistribution, and drug-delivery efficiency of mesoporous silica nanoparticles for cancer therapy in animals. Small 2010; 6(16): 1794-805.
[http://dx.doi.org/10.1002/smll.201000538] [PMID: 20623530]

[76]   Aljamal K, Ramaswamy C, Florence A. Supramolecular structures from dendrons and dendrimers. Adv Drug Deliv Rev 2005; 57(15): 2238-70.
[http://dx.doi.org/10.1016/j.addr.2005.09.015] [PMID: 16310885]

[77]   Ma H, Liu S, Luo J, *et al.* Highly efficient and thermally stable electro□optical dendrimers for photonics. Adv Funct Mater 2002; 12(9): 565-74.
[http://dx.doi.org/10.1002/1616-3028(20020916)12:9<565::AID-ADFM565>3.0.CO;2-8]

CHAPTER 6

Theranostics Nanoemulsion for Brain Tumor Diagnosis and Treatment

Deepak Prashar[1],*, **Ram Kumar Sahu[2]**, **Jiyauddin Khan[3]**, **Oluwadunsin Iyanuoluwa Adebayo[4]** and **Grace Fumilayo Adigun[4]**

[1] KC Institute of Pharmaceutical Sciences, Una-177207, H.P., India

[2] Department of Pharmaceutical Sciences, Hemvati Nandan Bahuguna Garhwal University (A Central University), Chauras Campus, Tehri Garhwal-249161, Uttarakhand, India

[3] School of Pharmacy, Management and Science University, 40100 Shah Alam, Selangor, Malaysia

[4] Reproductive Physiology and Bioinformatics Research Unit, Department of Physiology, Ladoke Akintola University of Technology, Ogbomoso, Oyo state, Nigeria

Abstract: Cancer or malignancy is the most widely occurring ailment in the recent scenario. Brain tumor is considered to be one of the most fatal among all types of tumors. The brain-related tumors are numerous and need to be treated and diagnosed in different ways. The diagnosis of brain tumor is done by various methods like MRI, CT scan and neurological testing. In the recent past, a number of nanoemulsion formulations have been formulated and developed to treat and diagnose brain cancer. The present work presents the present status of anti-cancer drugs, the parameters related to their working and the advancement in technology.

Keywords: Brain tumor, Diagnosis, Malignancy, Nanoemulsion, Treatments.

INTRODUCTION

Brain tumor is one of the critical aliments that have been associated with the medical field for the last many years. In the mid 1950-60's, this disease is considered to be the fatal disease with the least chance of survival. But with the advancement of technologies, the chances of survival and the rate of treatment have increased a lot. Still, the disease remains one of the most lethal as far as developing countries are concerned. A number of drugs are being incorporated

---

* **Corresponding author Deepak Prashar:** KC Institute of Pharmaceutical Sciences, Una-177207, H.P., India; E-mail:prashardeepak99@yahoo.in

into the treatment of brain tumors (Table **1**) approved drugs (by the National Cancer Institute) and their combinations are highlighted.

Table 1. FDA Approved Drugs for Cancer Treatment [1]

S. No.	Drug Name	Brand Name	FDA Approval Status	Therapeutic Uses
1.	Everolimus	Afinitor Afinitor Disperz Zortress	Yes	• Breast carcinoma • Pancreatic Carcinoma • Gastrointestinal cancer • Pulmonary cancer • Renal cell carcinoma Astrocytoma
2.	Bevacizumab	Avastin Mvasi Zirabev	Yes	• Cervical cancer • Colorectal cancer • Glioblastoma (a type of brain cancer) • Hepatocellular carcinoma (a type of liver cancer) • Nonsquamous non small cell pulmonary carcinoma • Ovarian carcinoma • Oviduct carcinoma • Peritoneal carcinoma (primary) •Kidney cancer
3.	Carmustine	BiCNU	Yes	• Brain tumor • Hodgkin lymphoma • Non Hodgkin lymphoma • Multiple myeloma
4.	Carmustine	Gliadel Wafer	Yes	• Glioblastoma multiforme •Malignantglioma
5.	Naxitamab-gqgk	Danyelza	Yes	• Neuroblastoma
6.	Lomustine	Gleostine	Yes	• Brain tumors • Hodgkin lymphoma
7.	Temozolomide	Temodar	Yes	• Anaplastic astrocytoma • Glioblastoma multiforme (GBM)
8.	PCV combination	P = Procarbazine Hydrochloride C = Lomustine (CCNU) V = Vincristine sulphate	Yes	• Brain tumors

Nanoemulsions are drug carriers which are colloidal particles system of sub micron size. They are been widely employed in the delivery of drugs for the treatment of ailments. The size range in which they are available is from 10-1000nm. Structure wise, these are the solid spherical particles with negative charge supported by amorphous and lipophilic surfaces. Nanoemulsions are the mini-emulsions that are basically the oil/water or water /oil dispersion. They are stabilized by an interfacial film of surfactant molecules having a droplet size range 20- 600nm. This small size of nanoemulsion provides it the transparent nature. Practically, three types of the nanoemulsion can be formulated (Fig. **1**).

1. o/w nanoemulsion (dispersed phase oil and continuous phase water/aqueous)

   a. Oil in water nano-emulsion (Neutral)
   b. Oil in water nano-emulsion (Cationic)
   c. Oil in water nano-emulsion (Anionic)

2. w/o nanoemulsion (dispersed phase is water and continuous phase is oil)

3. Bi-continuous Nanoemulsion

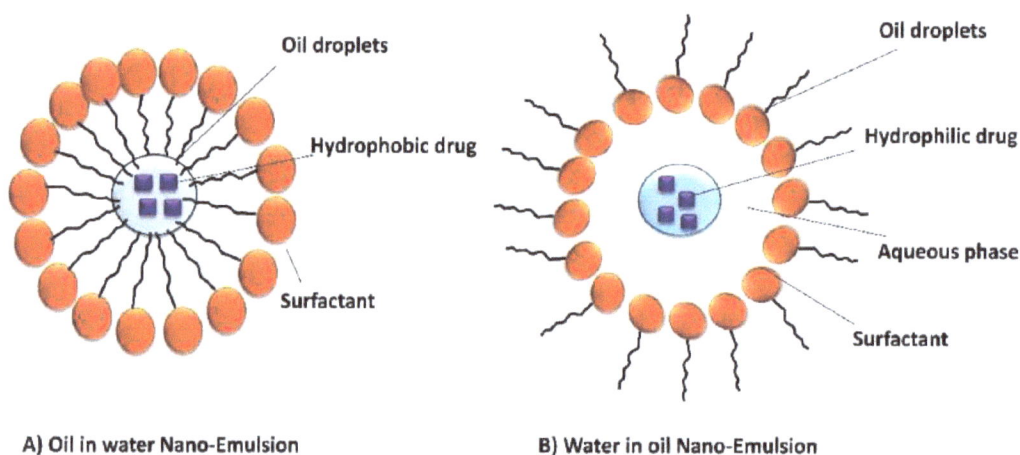

A) Oil in water Nano-Emulsion   B) Water in oil Nano-Emulsion

Fig. (1). (A) Oil In Water Nano-Emulsion (B) Water In Oil Nano-Emulsion

BASICS OF NANOEMULSION

Nanoemulsion is being utilized in numerous fields as the drug delivery carrier. The fields in which nanoemulsion is required include parenteral delivery, oral delivery, ocular delivery, transdermal delivery, and topical delivery of the drugs. Moreover, these nanoemulsions have also shown their applicability in biotechnology and targeted drug delivery. The merits of the nanoemulsion are quite large in number too. In site-specific drug delivery, a large quantity of hydrophobic drugs can be dissolved, protecting the drug from degradation with longer stability, serving as a good substitute for liposomes to enhance bioavailability. They also have the ability to make multiple formulations having a taste masking effect and small size with a better rate of absorption. For these formulations, there are many options available for the nanoemulsion creation. These methods of preparation of nanoemulsion include ultrasonication, microfludization, high pressure homogenization (High energies approaches), phase inversion temperature, membrane emulsification, spontaneous emulsification, and emulsion inversion point (low energy approaches). Furthermore, the nanoemulsions can be characterized by different methods. This characterization of the product helps in deciding the quality and stability of the final material (Table **2**). Apart from these parameters, there are some other methods available for the determination of stability of the nanoemulsions [2 - 8].

Table 2. Parameters for the determination of nanoemulsion stability

S. No.	Method of Characterization	Detail
1.	Droplet size	It can be carried out using electron microscopy or light scattering technique.
2.	Surface Charge	It is done by determining zeta potential (around 30mV for stable formulation). The Zetasizer Nano Z is the equipment used for this purpose.
3.	Viscosity	For this purpose, Brookfold viscometer is used. Most of the times with an increase in water content and the viscosity of the emulsion decreases.
4.	Electrical conductivity measurement	It is done using a conductivity meter. The triplet studies of the sample are carried out to obtain the best possible results.
5.	Refractive index	Refractrometer is used in this case at 25±0.5 °C.
6.	Percentage Transmittance studies	The transmittance studies are carried out using a spectrophotometer. If the percentage transmittance is high and close to 100%, it indicates the transparent nanoemulsion.
7.	pH	Using the pH meter, the value of pH can be precisely determined and can be further adjusted if required.
8.	TEM (Transmission electron microscopy)	Through this method, the morphology and structure of the nanoemulsions can be determined.
9.	Drug content	By using the reverse phase HPLC method (C18 column), the drug content can be determined in nanoemulsions formulations.
10.	Thremodynamic stability studies	In this case, the nanoemulsions are exposed to different stress conditions. a) Heat cooling cycle: In this, the formulations are alternatively subjected to 6 cycles of 4°C and then to 45°C to observe stability. b) Centrifugation: In this, the formulations are centrifuged at 3500 rpm and if no phase separation occurs, then further stress is applied. c) Freeze thaw cycle: Here the formulations after centrifugation are alternatively subjected to a cyclic exposure of 21°C and 25°C (above) for least 3 months to observe any undue changes.

(Table 2) cont.....

S. No.	Method of Characterization	Detail
11.	Accelerated stability studies	The accelerated stability studies for the formulation were also carried out at 30, 40, 50, and 60 °C at ambient humidity conditions.
12.	*In vitro* skin permeation studies	Keshary Chien diffusion cell is used for the study of *in vitro* skin permeation study. The process is being carried out using abdominal skin of male rats weighing 250±10 gm. The process is carried out using re-circulating water bath and 12 diffusion cells.

Nanoemulsion formulations can be made using active pharmaceutical ingredients, additives and emulsifiers. All these raw materials are required for the formulation of a stable emulsion. The use of a proper quantity of materials will allow better and stable nanoemulsions with enhanced bioavailability. The materials being used for the formulation of nanoemulsions are as follows:

1. Oils: Peanuts oil, Castor oil, Corn oil, Primrose oil, Coconut oil, Linseed oil and mineral oil *etc*.

2. Emulsifiers: Phosphlipids, Natural Lecithin, Castor Oil Derivatives, Polysorbates, Sterylamine.

3. Excipients: Ethanol, Propylene Glycol, Glucose, Sucrose, Fructose, Maltose *etc*.

4. Surfactants: PEG 300, Caprylic glyceride, Polysorbate 20and 80, Polyoxy 60, sorbitan monooleate.

5. Co surfactants: PEG 300, PEG 400, Propylene glycol, poloxamer, Glycerine, Ethanol.

6. Antioxidants: α- Tocopherol, Ascorbic acid

7. pH adjuster: Sodium Hydroxide, Hydrogen chloride

8. Tonicity modifier: Xylitol, sorbitol, glycerol

9. Presevative: Benzalkonium Chloride (0.01%w/v), Parabens (Methyl and Propyl)

In the past and in the present, numerous advances are observed in the administration of drugs in nanoemulsions. Drugs of various categories are administered with the help of nanoemulsions. Various carriers and also almost all methods are used for the formulation of these drugs (Table **3**). Improving bioavailability is one of the main criteria for formulation with nanoemulsions.

Brain Tumor Nanoemulsion

Among the CNS disorders, brain tumor is the most difficult to treat [1]. According to the report of World Health Organization, almost 2, 38,000 diagnoses of brain and CNS are carried out for the detection of tumor. Out of this large number, gliomas (tumor of glial cells) constitute about 80% of brain tumors. This is the malignant type of tumors [2]. Brain tumor can be of different types with diverse characteristics (Table **4**). According to the WHO updates in 2016 [3], brain related tumors can be classified as follows:

Table 3. Advancement in drug delivery based on nanoemulsions scenario [9 - 15]

S. No.	Active Pharmaceutical Ingredient	Method of Preparation	Surfactant/Emulsifier Used	Detailed Application
1.	Prednicarbat	High-pressure Homogenisation	Phytosphingosine	Atopic Dermatitis
2.	Resperidone	Brain targeting (nasal route)	PEG 400	Antipsychotic
3.	Celecoxib	Spontaneous emulsification	Diethyl glycol	Arthritis and osteoarthritis.
4.	Praziquantel	Spontaneous emulsification	Poloxamer	Increase Schistosomicidal effect.
5.	Benzathine	Spontaneous emulsification	Penicillin G Poloxamer	Formulation to encapsulate more soluble drugs.
6.	Ampicillin	Solid dispersion	PEG 400	Protein drug delivery inside oil phase.
7.	Polyanionic	High power homogenisation	Poloxamer 188	Cancer treatment
8.	Primaquine	High power homogenisation	Poloxamer 188	Latent stages of malaria.
9.	Ramipril	Spontaneous emulsification	Caprylo caproyl macrogol-8- glyceride	Liquid formulation for children and old patients.
10.	Acelofenac	Spontaneous emulsification	PEG 400	Improved Transdermal delivery
11.	Ramipril	Spontaneous emulsification	Cabitol	Enhanced bioavailability.
12.	Citronella oil	High power homogenisation	Glycerol	Mosquito repellant
13.	Celecoxib	Low power homogenisation	Propylene mono caprylic ester	Evaluation of stability

(Table 3) cont.....

S. No.	Active Pharmaceutical Ingredient	Method of Preparation	Surfactant/Emulsifier Used	Detailed Application
14.	Saquinavir	----------	PUFA	Enhanced bioavailability and brain disposition.
15.	Domperidone	Pseudoternary phase diagrams	Polysorbate 20	Enhanced percutaneous absorption.
16.	Lipidic	Intravenous injection	• G1 into the mammary tissue • .G2 into the peritumoral • G3 into the tumoral tissue	Decreases toxicity without decreasing the anticancer action.
17.	Phytosphingosine	Homogenisation And Emulsification	---------------	Dermal application of ceramide.
18.	Antisense oligonucleotides	Inhibits HUVEC proliferation *in vitro*	VEGFR-2 (17 MER)	Triglycerides cationic nanoemulsion was non-toxic on HUVEC and retinal cells
19.	Positively charged (o/w) nanoemulsion	High pressure Homogenisation	Carbopol 940	Increased skin elasticity and hydration.
20.	Progestrone	Homogenisation	Sucrose ester	Increased skin permeation.
21.	β -carotene	High pressure Homogenisation	Tween 20	Produces stable o/w nanoemulsions of β - carotene
22.	β -carotene	High-energy emulsification-evaporation technique	Tween 20	Influences the stability of nanoemulsions
23.	Caffeine	Oil phase titration	Tween 80	Transdermal delivery of anticancer drugs.
24.	Besifloxacin	Pseudo ternary phase diagrams	Cremophor® RH 40	Better alternate for marketed suspension for eye infection.
25.	Osthole (OST)	pseudoternary phase diagram method	polyethylene glycol and polyoxyethylene 35	Improves bioavailability in treatment of Alzheimer's disease
26.	Ciprofloxacin	hot homogenization and ultrasonication	Tween 80	Improves the effect of drug in treatment of Bacterial keratitis
27.	Sesame oil	ultrasonic emulsification	Tween 20	Enhanced physical stability

Advancements in Nanoemulsions For Tumor Diagnosis and Treatment

Theranostics has the opportunity to modernize the methods of diagnosis, treatment and prognosis of malignant diseases. Modern approaches to drug delivery could be used to develop the same for early detection of malignancies. The previous research and reviews suggest that the drugs encapsulated in nanoemulsions are formulated for this purpose of detection and treatment.

Table 4. Detail specifications of tumors and its treatment

S. NO.	Tumor	Characteristics	Symptoms	Possible Recommended treatment
1.	Acoustic Neuroma	It grows around the 8th cranial nerve along with some signs in other nerves too.	Hearing loss, Vertigo, Dizziness, Tinnitus, Numbness of face, Body imbalance with loss of co-ordination	Radio surgery
2.	Chordoma	Affected areas are the sacrum, the base of the skull, and lower tip of the spine. It arises from the cells left over from early fetus development. It can lead to hydrocephalus and also invade bones and soft tissues of the brain.	Double vision and headache Headaches	Surgery and radiotherapy are the common forms of treatment. If the tumour is localised to the spine, surgery is performed
3.	CNS Lymphoma	Usually occurs in patients with weak immunity and affects the whole central nervous system. Most common in men and women in the 60-80 age group, with men more commonly affected than women. Accounts for 2% of all brain tumors.	Partial paralysis of one side of body, headache, visual disturbances, speech distortion and epilepsy	Radiation therapy, chemotherapy and steroids are the most common form of treatment.
4.	Craniopharyngioma	It commonly occurs in the parasellar region, at the base of the brain and near optic nerve. It arises from cells of early fetal development and is associated with a cyst. Occurs in all sexes in the peak at the age of 50-60 years.	Delayed child development, headache, weight gain, visual disturbances.	Surgery is the most common treatment. Radiation therapy may be used.

(Table 4) cont.....

S. NO.	Tumor	Characteristics	Symptoms	Possible Recommended treatment
5.	Brain Stem Glioma	Located in the base of the brain ranging from high to low grade. Predominantly seen in the children between 3-10 years of age, but may also occur in adults too.	Speech disturbances, difficulty in swallowing, numbness of limbs double vision, headaches and facial weakness.	Radiation therapy is the only option to delay its occurrence. Surgery cannot be carried in this case.
6.	Ependymoma	It is located in the specified area of the brain (centre of the brain), extends to the spinal cord, and can grow both slowly and rapidly. It can cause blockage of the ventricles, resulting in hydrocephalus. The age group affected is 40-50 years old, with the first signs appearing after the age of 35. Common in all age groups with a frequency of 2%.	Visual disturbances, neck pain and stiffness, fatigue, body co-ordination, weakness, nausea, vomiting and severe headache.	If spread to the spinal cord, the diagnosis is made and then surgery followed by radiation therapy is performed.
7.	Mixed Glioma	Most aggressive tumor comprises 2 or more types of gliomacells. Occurs at the age of 20-50 years and accounts for about 1% of total cases.	Vision defects, nausea, seizures and behaviour disturbances.	Treatment based nature of tumor.
8.	Optic Nerve Glioma	Occurs in the nerve pathway of the eye and brain predominantly in infants, but can occur in adults too.	Time-related loss of vision, headache, double vision.	Surgery, chemotherapy and radiation therapy in young patients.
9.	Subependymoma	Slow growing tumor in the 4th lateral ventricle affecting males more than females	Headache, nausea, loss of balance.	Surgery and radiotherapy.
10.	Medullo-blastoma	The location is near the brain stem or cerebellum which can later spread to the spinal cord through CSF. It is also called PNET (primitive neuro ectodermal tumor). Hydrocephalus can also occur with the obstruction of 4th ventricle predominates in children below 10 years of age	Double vision, lethargy, headache, morning sickness, lack of co-ordination, and behavioral changes. Pressure behind the eye is predominant symptoms.	Standard treatment is surgery and other options are chemotherapy and radiation therapy (brain and spine).

(Table 4) cont.....

S. NO.	Tumor	Characteristics	Symptoms	Possible Recommended treatment
11.	Meningioma	It occurs on continues exposure to radiation especially X-rays. Common in the age group of 40- 50 years. It is twice as likely to occur in women as in men, with an incidence of about 35%. It can also enter the female body during pregnancy.	Vision defects, nausea, seizures and behaviour disturbances.	The cancer is detected by an MRI scan and treatment includes surgery and chemotherapy. The probability of recurrence is quite high even after decades of treatment
12.	Metastatic Brain Tumors	Common in later stages of life affecting some visceral organs like breast, lungs, kidney, colon skin. Localised in the cerebrum in most cases and in a few cases in the cerebellum	Epilepsy, non co-ordination, headache, behavioral changes	Radiosurgery and surgery are the standard treatment options, followed by WBRT (whole brain radiation therapy). Chemotherapy is preferred for metastatic tumors in certain areas of the brain
13.	Oligodendroglioma	They target the frontal or temporal lobes of the brain and occur mainly in children and between the ages of 20-40 years. Occurs more often in males than females and accounts for about 2% of total cases. 1p or 19q chromosome loss is the main cause	Seizures, paralysis and body weakness	Treatment depends on the extent of oligodendroglioma, but radiotherapy is the standard treatment option. MRI is performed as a diagnostic technique. Gene profiling is also used to accurately identify the tumor.
14.	Pituitary Tumors	Located near the pituitary gland above the nose and ranges from low to high grade. Occurs at age 50+ with excessive hormone release. It accounts for about 15% of all cases of brain tumors	Glactorrhea, vision loss, amenorrhea, histurism, headache, importence, abnormal digits, behavior changes and weight gain	Transphenoidal surgery for large tumor, and for standard treatment drugs are preferred with hormonal maintenance
15.	Primitive Neuroectodermal (PNET)	Arises from underdeveloped brain cells in the form of cysts and calcifications that spreadto all parts of the brain	Morning headache, nausea, vomiting, epilepsy, weakness, fatigue, weight loss, bipolar nature	Surgery followed by radiotherapy and chemotherapy
16.	Schwannoma	Occurs on the 8th cranial nerve and arises from protective sheath around he end of the nerve	Body imbalance, tinnitus, and one ear hearing loss	Surgery and radiotherapy but the chances of reoccurrence are there.

Qu et al., 2021 formulated the disulfiram nanoemulsion (nose to brain) as *in situ* gel. The gel was being formulated for the treatment of glioblastoma. The results suggested that the DSF-INEG/Cu has the ability to inhibit tumour growth by effectively inhibiting the proliferation of C6 and U87 cells [16].

Desai and Thakker 2019 designed the lipid based nanoemulsion of Darunavir to enhance its bioavailability and overcome the side effects associated with drug administration in the brain. The formulation was prepared using Tween 80, Lecithin and soya bean oil. The enhancement in bioavailability was observed along with the fewer dose-related side effects. Moreover, better organ distribution was observed with the formulation too [17].

Savale 2017 formulated and evaluated the nanoemulsion of Quercetin (QUR) for treatment of brain tumor by the intranasal route. The problem of low blood-brain barrier (BBB) permeability associated with quercetin was effectively overcome by this method. The developed nanoemulsion loaded with QUR proves to be a capable solvent in terms of CNS release [18].

Li et al., 2014 developed a nano-theranostic multifunctional polymer system to deliver doxorubicin along with a brain imaging agent. The formulation was intended for metastatic brain tumor, which is difficult to identify due to its aggressiveness and location. Instead, such nanoformulation approaches can be used for it. The starch grafted with poly(methacrylic acid) polysorbate 80 was used for the formulation. This formulation was found to be effective in inhibiting brain metastasis, which is confirmed by the *in vivo* imaging method [19]

Shinde et al., 2011, presented a systematic review on the role of microemulsions and nanoemulsions in targeting drug delivery to the brain. The role of multifunctional excipients and potential routes of drug delivery in brain cancer have been discussed and evaluated [20].

Desai et al., 2008 conducted a study to improve drug combinations in brain tumors. Paclitaxel and Ceramide were administered together in the form of a nanoemulsion. The combination of these two drugs proved to be therapeutically beneficial in human gliobastoma. Single drug therapy was not suitable in this case and the problem is overtaken by combination therapy [21].

Benefits and Limitations of Nanotechnology in Cancer Treatment

Nanotechnologies have effectively improved the safety criteria of nanocarriers for cancer therapy, such as drug delivery. The permeability retention effect for suitable chemotherapeutic passive targeting can be easily achieved by the nano size. Similarly controlled delivery can be achieved through the uptake of specific cell types and active targeting through receptors [22]. Apart from this, the nanotechnology also provides increased stability of the drug, controlled release, and better water solubility, which are the main problems in drug delivery in the brain [23]. Nanoemulsion also provides increased encapsulation capacity, better bioavailability and potentially improved physiochemical stability [24 - 27]. Some studies also show that nanoemulsion can be effectively used for the delivery of photosensitive drugs [28]. Similarly, nebulizer lipid-based nanoemulsion can also be formulated for the treatment of lung cancer with resistance to water and enzyme degradation [29].

Literature indicates that a number of formulations have been developed to provide reduced toxicity and safer drug delivery. However, the main problem with nanoemulsions is that very few formulations are currently approved by the Food and Drug Administration (FDA). This has limited their commercial use [30]. The conditions required for such formulations are high temperature and pressure which might not be suitable for thermolabile drugs and excipients. Similarly, the formulation and development of multifunctional nanoemulsion also pose the problem of large-scale manufacturing and altering the production variables. Moreover, pharmacokinetic parameters also need to be evaluated each time along with the *in vivo* metabolic parameters which is a very difficult criteria. The low clinical relevance of nanoemulsion for cancer therapy is the major limitation for its effective and widespread commercial use [31].

FUTURE PERSPECTIVE

Nanoemulsions are capable of encapsulating lipophilic and lipophobic drug components and can therefore be used for a variety of nanoformulations [30]. The main challenge in the future development of nanoemulsions is to modify them each time to improve their efficacy. In addition, the mechanism must also be modified to provide an advantage over the other commercial formulations. As part of the continuous improvement process, ingredient compatibilities must also be explored to develop a better formulation. Drug stability, drug targeting approach and mechanism of action improvement need to be improved and are the most important study point for future drug development. In addition to production, the PK /PD modeling system also needs to be optimized for better results. Similarly, research is needed to identify the different delivery routes for nanoemulsion-based anticancer drugs. The use of nanoemulsions as imaging agents is emerging as they allow real-time monitoring of the tumor with minimal destruction and invasion. For better and safer cancer drug delivery, all aspects of nanoemulsion need to be further developed.

CONCLUSION

This chapter addresses the status of anticancer drugs and the current status of the FDA. Ongoing work in the field of nanotechnology suggests that nanoemulsion may be a fruitful option for the treatment of brain tumors. The drugs, which pose a number of complications in the treatment of brain diseases, can be administered or co-administered to patients in the form of nanoemulsion. Similarly, the dyes contained in the nanoemulsions can also be used to diagnose diseases of the brain, especially cancer. The future prospects of nanoformulation are quite promising as far as the diagnosis and treatment of brain tumors are concerned.

ACKNOWLEDGEMENTS

The authors wish to thank the other supporting members of the group for their help throughout the course of this work. Further we wish to thank the technical team to help us in all prospects. Special thanks to (Prof) Dr B.S Kaith, National Institute of Technology, Jalandhar, Punjab for guiding in transforming the thoughts into a meaningful work.

REFERENCES

[1]   Available from: https://www.cancer.gov/about-cancer/treatment/drugs/brain

[2]   Sukanya G, Mantry S, Anjum S. Review on nanoemulsions. International Journal of Innovative Pharmaceutical Sciences and Research 2013; 1(2): 192-205.

[3]   Reddy CS, Kumar MP. Current review on nanoemulsion. J Glob Trends Pharm Sci 2017; 8: 3634-43.

[4]   Bhatt P, Madhav S. A detailed review on nanoemulsion drug delivery system. Int J Pharm Sci Res 2011; 2: 2482-9.

[5]   Sangwan Y, Hooda T, Kumar H. Nanoemulsions: A Pharmaceutical Review. Int J Pharm Pharm Res 2014; 5: 1031-8.

[6]   Mangale MR, Pathak SS, Mene HR, More BA. Nanoemulsion: as pharmaceutical overview. Int J Pharm Sci Rev Res 2015; 33: 244-52.

[7]   Singh KK, Vingkar SK. Formulation, antimalarial activity and biodistribution of oral lipid nanoemulsion of primaquine. Int J Pharm 2008; 347(1-2): 136-43.
        [http://dx.doi.org/10.1016/j.ijpharm.2007.06.035] [PMID: 17709216]

[8]   Akhter S, Jain G, Ahmad F, *et al.* Investigation of Nanoemulsion System for Transdermal Delivery of Domperidone: *Ex vivo* and *in vivo* Studies. Curr Nanosci 2008; 4(4): 381-90.
        [http://dx.doi.org/10.2174/157341308786306071]

[9]   Kassaee SN, Mahboobian MM. Besifloxacin-loaded ocular nanoemulsions: design, formulation and efficacy evaluation. Drug Deliv Transl Res 2021.
        [http://dx.doi.org/10.1007/s13346-021-00902-z] [PMID: 33575973]

[10]   Song Y, Wang X, Wang X, *et al.* Osthole-Loaded Nanoemulsion Enhances Brain Target in the Treatment of Alzheimer's Disease *via* Intranasal Administration. Oxid Med Cell Longev 2021; 2021: 1-16.
        [http://dx.doi.org/10.1155/2021/8844455] [PMID: 33564364]

[11]   Youssef AAA, Cai C, Dudhipala N, Majumdar S. Design of Topical Ocular Ciprofloxacin Nanoemulsion for the Management of Bacterial Keratitis. Pharmaceuticals (Basel) 2021; 14(3): 210.

[http://dx.doi.org/10.3390/ph14030210] [PMID: 33802394]

[12]   Available from: https://iopscience.iop.org/article/10.1088/1757-899X/1114/1/012085/pdf

[13]   Béduneau A, Saulnier P, Benoit JP. Active targeting of brain tumors using nanocarriers. Biomaterials 2007; 28(33): 4947-67.
[http://dx.doi.org/10.1016/j.biomaterials.2007.06.011] [PMID: 17716726]

[14]   Burgo LSD, Hernandez RM, Orive G, Pedraz JL. Nanotherapeutic approaches for brain cancer management Nanomedicine: Nanotechnology. Biol Med (Aligarh) 2014; 10(5): e905-19.

[15]   Available from: https://braintumor.org/brain-tumor-information/understanding-brain-tumors/t-mor-types/

[16]   Qu Y, Li A, Ma L, *et al.* Nose-to-brain delivery of disulfiram nanoemulsion in situ gel formulation for glioblastoma targeting therapy. Int J Pharm 2021; 597120250
[http://dx.doi.org/10.1016/j.ijpharm.2021.120250] [PMID: 33486040]

[17]   Desai J, Thakkar H. Enhanced oral bioavailability and brain uptake of Darunavir using lipid nanoemulsion formulation. Colloids Surf B Biointerfaces 2019; 175: 143-9.
[http://dx.doi.org/10.1016/j.colsurfb.2018.11.057] [PMID: 30529999]

[18]   Savale SK. Formulation and Evaluation of Quercetin Nanoemulsions for Treatment of Brain Tumor *via* Intranasal pathway. Asian Journal of Biomaterial Research 2017; 3(6): 28-32.

[19]   Li J, Cai P, Shalviri A, *et al.* A multifunctional polymeric nanotheranostic system delivers doxorubicin and imaging agents across the blood-brain barrier targeting brain metastases of breast cancer. ACS Nano 2014; 8(10): 9925-40.
[http://dx.doi.org/10.1021/nn501069c] [PMID: 25307677]

[20]   Shinde L, Jindal RB, Devarajan AV. Padma. Microemulsions and Nanoemulsions for Targeted Drug Delivery to the Brain. Curr Nanosci 2011; 7(1): 119-33.
[http://dx.doi.org/10.2174/157341311794480282]

[21]   Desai A, Vyas T, Amiji M. Cytotoxicity and apoptosis enhancement in brain tumor cells upon coadministration of paclitaxel and ceramide in nanoemulsion formulations. J Pharm Sci 2008; 97(7): 2745-56.
[http://dx.doi.org/10.1002/jps.21182] [PMID: 17854074]

[22]   Senapati S, Mahanta AK, Kumar S, Maiti P. Controlled drug delivery vehicles for cancer treatment and their performance. Signal Transduct Target Ther 2018; 3(1): 7.
[http://dx.doi.org/10.1038/s41392-017-0004-3] [PMID: 29560283]

[23]   Ngandeu Neubi GM, Opoku-Damoah Y, Gu X, *et al.* Bio-inspired drug delivery systems: an emerging platform for targeted cancer therapy. Biomater Sci 2018; 6(5): 958-73.
[http://dx.doi.org/10.1039/C8BM00175H] [PMID: 29564432]

[24]   Mahato R. Nanoemulsion as Targeted Drug Delivery System for Cancer Therapeutics. J Pharm Sci Pharmacol 2017; 3(2): 83-97.
[http://dx.doi.org/10.1166/jpsp.2017.1082]

[25]   Chrastina A, Baron VT, Abedinpour P, Rondeau G, Welsh J, Borgström P. Plumbagin-Loaded Nanoemulsion Drug Delivery Formulation and Evaluation of Antiproliferative Effect on Prostate Cancer Cells. BioMed Res Int 2018; 2018: 1-7.
[http://dx.doi.org/10.1155/2018/9035452] [PMID: 30534567]

[26]   Deli G, Hatziantoniou S, Nikas Y, Demetzos C. Solid lipid nanoparticles and nanoemulsions containing ceramides: Preparation and physicochemical characterization. J Liposome Res 2009; 19(3): 180-8.
[http://dx.doi.org/10.1080/08982100802702046] [PMID: 19552579]

[27]   Periasamy VS, Athinarayanan J, Alshatwi AA. Anticancer activity of an ultrasonic nanoemulsion formulation of Nigella sativa L. essential oil on human breast cancer cells. Ultrason Sonochem 2016;

31: 449-55.
[http://dx.doi.org/10.1016/j.ultsonch.2016.01.035] [PMID: 26964971]

[28]   Clares B, Calpena AC, Parra A, *et al.* Nanoemulsions (NEs), liposomes (LPs) and solid lipid nanoparticles (SLNs) for retinyl palmitate: Effect on skin permeation. Int J Pharm 2014; 473(1-2): 591-8.
[http://dx.doi.org/10.1016/j.ijpharm.2014.08.001] [PMID: 25102113]

[29]   Asmawi AA, Salim N, Ngan CL, *et al.* Excipient selection and aerodynamic characterization of nebulized lipid-based nanoemulsion loaded with docetaxel for lung cancer treatment. Drug Deliv Transl Res 2019; 9(2): 543-54.
[http://dx.doi.org/10.1007/s13346-018-0526-4] [PMID: 29691812]

[30]   McClements DJ. Nanoemulsions versus microemulsions: terminology, differences, and similarities. Soft Matter 2012; 8(6): 1719-29.
[http://dx.doi.org/10.1039/C2SM06903B]

[31]   Wilhelm S, Tavares AJ, Dai Q, *et al.* Analysis of nanoparticle delivery to tumours. Nat Rev Mater 2016; 1(5): 16014.
[http://dx.doi.org/10.1038/natrevmats.2016.14]

CHAPTER 7

Theranostics Micelles for Brain Tumor Diagnosis and Treatment

Nidhal Khazaal Maraie[1,*], Zainab H. Mahdi[2] and Zahraa Amer Al-Juboori[3]

[1] *Department of Pharmaceutics, College of Pharmacy, Al-Farahidi University, Baghdad, Iraq*

[2] *Department of Pharmaceutics, College of Pharmacy, Applied Science Private University, Amman, Jordan*

[3] *Department of Pharmaceutics, College of Pharmacy, Mustansiriyah University, Baghdad, Iraq*

Abstract: Brain cancer is considered one of the most vicious and devastating tumors owing to its poor prognosis and high mortality rate. Common strategies for treatment include surgery, radiation, and chemotherapy. Unfortunately, these are limited due to their invasive nature and the inherent difficulties of brain surgery, given there is a high possibility of tumor relapse. Further, radiation and chemotherapy have a non-selective harmful effect on normal tissues, accompanied by limited drug delivery due to the presence of various barriers, including the blood-brain barrier. For this reason, the theranostic approach was developed by incorporating one or more therapeutic and diagnostic agents in a single nanocarrier moiety which could be modulated at its surface with certain proteins, legend, surface markers, or a stimuli-responsive agent that is capable of selectively targeting the tumor site after passing through the blood-brain barrier. This new field will permit the early and precise detection of cancer tissue, facilitate the process of drug delivery and assist in monitoring treatment outcomes. Micelles are considered one of the most commonly used nanocarriers due to their high stability and loading capacity, along with efficient release controlling properties. This chapter will present brief information about brain anatomy and cancer, and will discuss the main strategies implemented in the diagnosis and treatment of brain cancers. Furthermore, it will introduce the theranostic micelle approach by highlighting micelles types and preparation techniques, as well as explain the different barriers and approaches to targeting.

Keywords: Active targeting, Blood-brain barrier, Blood-brain tumor barrier, Brain cancer, Brain tumor stem cells, Chemotherapy, Computed tomography, Focused ultrasound, Gene therapy, Magnetic resonance imaging, Optical imaging, Paracellular, Passive targeting, Photodynamic therapy, Photothermal therapy, Polymeric micelles, Stimuli-responsive targeting, Theranostic, Transcellular, Tumor microenvironment.

---

* **Corresponding author Nidhal Khazaal Maraie:** Department of Pharmaceutics, College of Pharmacy, Al-Farahidi University, Baghdad, Iraq, E-mails: dr_nidhal_khazaal@yahoo.com, , drnidhalkhazaal@uoalfarahidi.edu.iq.

INTRODUCTION

The brain is a unique organ isolated in a chamber distant from other organs, yet it controls every other organ in the human body. However, like any other organ, it is susceptible to different diseases. Brain tumors are considered the most vicious and dreadful type of tumor, ranging from benign to malignant, often ending up being metastatic [1]. Central nervous system tumors account for 2-5% of all tumors, as brain involvement is 80% while 20% for the spinal cord. The majority of brain tumors are primary, although 20-40% can develop metastasis. These tumors cause 2% of deaths from the total percentage of deaths resulting from all cancers, and they account for 20% of all cancers in children [2].

Brain tumors include gliomas, meningiomas, and pituitary tumors. The most common brain tumors are malignant gliomas, which are divided into oligodendrogliomas, astrocytomas, ependymomas, and oligoastrocytomas. The benign form of this tumor is characterized by slow growth, and it can be removed easily by surgery with or without the aid of radiotherapy [3]. However, the malignant form is characterized by rapid growth and lower survival rate, while medulloblastoma and ependymoblastoma are considered lethal forms of this tumor [4].

According to the World Health Organization, a grade from I-IV is given to brain tumors based on the severity of cancer according to their various catastrophic outcomes. Grades I and II are designated to tumors with a good prognosis, while by contrast, the higher grades III and IV are designated to malignant tumors with severe complications [5].

Based on population studies, primary CNS tumors affect more than 60,000 people per year in the USA; one-third of these cases are estimated to develop into a malignant type [6]. The mortality rate of brain tumors is estimated at 3 per 100,000 worldwide. 11 new cases are diagnosed on daily basis in the UK, while only two are expected to survive. The global prevalence of brain tumors among males and females is 3.6 and 2.5 per 100,000, respectively, and this rate has been increasing over the years [7]. Despite the low incidence of primary brain tumors compared with other types, this type gives rise to an inconsistent level of morbidity and mortality. In addition, it interferes with the patient's ability to move and speak, which requires more attention and clinical interventions [8].

The rate of prevalence of brain tumors in developing countries is ambiguous due to a lack of advanced diagnosis techniques. Such undiagnosed cases are associated with a lower level of reporting in these countries [9].

The risk factors associated with the development of brain tumors are not fully clear, however, according to different researchers, the sum of all the possible factors associated with primary tumors are listed in Table **1**, and by contrast, glial and meningeal neoplasms definitely arose due to ionizing radiation [10]. Generally, the most agreed-upon risk factors that are associated with brain tumors are genetic causes; several genetic syndromes have been reported to correlate with primary brain tumor development. Moreover, viral infection is a potential risk factor, although the correlation is unclear. However, several viral families have been reported to be associated with brain cancer development, such as polyomaviruses and herpesviruses [11].

Table 1. Risk factors associated with brain tumors [11]

Potential Risk Factors
Radiation: Ionizing
Head trauma
Allergies
Diet and vitamins N-nitroso compounds Fat intake Aspartame ingestion Tobacco Alcohol
Chemicals Hair dyes and sprays Traffic-related air pollution
Infection Simian Virus 40 Human Cytomegalovirus Polyomaviruses (e.g. JC and BK) Toxoplasma infection Varicella-zoster – protective role
Genetics Neurofibromatosis type 1 Neurofibromatosis type 2
Occupational Exposure Electrical workers and electromagnetic fields Agriculture workers are exposed to pesticides, herbicides, and fungicides Other industries (vinyl chloride, petrochemical, and rubber industries

TREATMENT PROTOCOLS IN BRAIN CANCERS

Due to the anatomical and physiological nature of the brain, brain cancers differ from other types of cancer affecting the rest of the body. This is because distinguishing between malignant and benign tumors is difficult, and the treatment of brain cancer is challenging as the anticancer agent should dodge several obstacles to reach the tumor, such as the blood-brain barrier, and the cerebrospinal fluid barrier [12]. It has been found that only 5% of drugs can penetrate these barriers owing to their physicochemical properties as well as molecular characteristics [13].

The blood-brain barrier is surrounding the capillary lumen and is anatomically composed of astrocytes, endothelial cells, and pericytes. The endothelial cells have a tight sealed connection or junction between them which hinders the penetration of vast molecules to the brain, such as proteins, peptides, antibodies, and oligonucleotides. Furthermore, the endothelial cells are composed of efflux transport pathways (e.g. p- glycoprotein) that remove the undesired material and bring them back into circulation [14].

Therefore, it is necessary to choose an anticancer agent that is capable of penetration to reach the tumor. The level of penetration can be modified *via* the employment of different technologies, such as nanotechnology or the modification of the drug's electrical nature or solubility, given a more water-soluble drug tends to penetrate these barriers by passive diffusion, while amphiphilic lipidic molecules penetrate with the aid of carrier-mediated transport [15]. However, the complex mechanism of receptor-mediated transcytosis and non-specific absorptive-mediated transcytosis was responsible for the transportation of larger molecules. On the other hand, it has been found that penetration can be enhanced *via* temporary disruption of the barrier. The employment of polymers was quite beneficial, as polymer-based systems are a potential option to deliver drugs while targeting brain cancer [16].

The current strategies to treat brain cancer involve surgery, radiation, and chemotherapy. Unfortunately, these therapeutic strategies even when combined are not successful due to the high relapsing rate of glioblastoma, reoccurring within a year, while the reccurrence rate of astrocytoma is three years [17].

Surgery

The eradication of tumors has been accomplished by surgery, *via* biopsy and resection, which can both be conducted to effectively eliminate brain tumors. Despite it being an invasive procedure, it was reported that the surgical removal of tumors prolongs life up to 6 months [18].

The success of this method of treatment requires well-defined tumor edges, which are less likely to be found if its extension occurs in normal brain tissues. However, partial removal can be considered useful as it reduces brain pressure and improves body function. Surgery can be used to place shunts in the brain that reduce brain pressure by draining the excess fluids, while biopsy aids in providing complete information regarding the tumor, paving the way for the proper selection of therapeutic strategies [19].

Chemotherapy

Different agents have been developed to treat brain tumors or are otherwise still under development, such as carmustine, lomustine, and nimustine are alkylating agents that produce their cytotoxic effect by methylation of DNA at the O6 position of quinine. They are used to treat malignant astrocytomas [20]. Side effects associated with the use of these agents include myelosuppression, nephrotoxicity, and GIT disturbances. Temozolomide 1, the latest alkylating agent approved by the FDA, is capable of penetrating the blood-brain barrier and is also capable of a high absolute bioavailability post oral administration, with a short half-life (1.8 h). Therefore, it needs to be administered in very systemic doses to compensate for the clearance [21]. For the treatment of glioblastoma, a dose of 75 mg/m2 per day is given as a single dose used during radiation therapy followed by a 5-day regimen over the following months.

Other anticancer agents that are being used to treat brain cancer include paclitaxel, anthracyclines, etoposide, topotecan, irinotecan, and methotrexate. Unfortunately, they cannot penetrate through the blood-brain barrier, which imposes the use of systemically higher doses to achieve the proper brain tumor concentration or modification of molecules *via* nanoparticle conjugates [22].

Gene Therapy

This approach of treatment utilizes genetic elements to treat or prevent disease conditions, where either a whole gene or regulatory factors can be delivered to the targeted cell *via* a mechanical procedure or a delivery vehicle to correct the preexisting defect, hence providing a higher level of therapeutic efficacy with local administration. Gene therapy can be associated indirectly with the treatment of brain cancer *via* the genetic modification of viruses that can target glioma and kill cancer cells without affecting normal cells [23].

Both viral and nonviral vectors are utilized to deliver the genetic material to the desired target site. The viral vector (adenoviral vector), adenovirus, is a double-stranded DNA virus with no envelope that shows various advantages such as high possibilities for genetic modifications, and low biosafety concerns, as its genomic material is episomal, which hinders insertional mutations. The virus has a marvelous safety profile when delivered to the tissues especially the brain, the vector enters the cell *via* two ways: by attachment of its domain and adenovirus receptor, and by endocytosis as well [24].

Non-viral vectors (non-polymeric delivery system): the liposomes and nanoparticles are famous delivery vehicles in the formulation field, due to many advantages such as their micro size, lipophilic nature, and ability to mimic the cellular membrane. The pegylated formula of liposome has extra advantages as it can conjugate with monoclonal antibodies, showing higher efficiency in targeting the glioma cells in cancer and an efficient delivery of genomic material to the brain [25].

However, several challenges for gene therapy may arise in the treatment of brain cancer. These are represented by the heterogeneity of different brain tumors like glioblastoma, which produces various genetic alterations in receptor expression for the used vectors, which in turn hinders the binding and infectivity to tumor cells [26]. Regarding the dependence on the chemical and physical properties of the materials to be injected [27], the activation of antibodies is responsible for the scavenging of those vectors [28], in addition to the resistance developed by targeted tumor cells due to different genetic alterations to increase the survival of these cells [29].

Photodynamic Therapy (PDT)

PDT involves the photo-activation of selective tumor-binding photosensitizer molecules that are activated upon exposure to photoirradiation by energy transfer. This results in oxygen excitation to either singlet state where energy is converted into heat/light that can diffuse for a short distance, therefore, minimizing the risk of normal tissue damage, or triplet state, where energy generates oxygen free radicals which bind to macromolecules such as proteins, fatty acids, and cholesterol [30]. This binding causes damage to the cellular membrane and cellular component, particularly in mitochondria, resulting in cellular death *via* the activation of apoptosis or necrotic pathways [31].

Singlet oxygen was reported to exist for about 0.04 µs - 4 µs while being capable of traveling for a distance estimated at 0.02 µm- 1 µm making this procedure of treatment the safest method to treat brain cancer. Effective PDT depends on the type of photosensitizer being used that will determine the extent of cellular damage and the oxygenation level within tumor cells to produce the required free radicals [32].

The light source is adjusted so that the wavelength, known as the photodynamic dose, is adjusted according to the absorption spectrum of the photosensitizer. This is generally between 400 and 900 nm, however, the longer wavelength is preferred as it is capable of penetrating the tissue deeply with high energetic photons which activate the photosensitizer. For better results, light activation is applied in a pulsed fashion (rather than continuous) to allow for tumor reoxygenation, thus resulting in higher levels of free radicals [33].

Different photosensitizers have been employed in the treatment of brain cancer. They can be systemically nontoxic while accumulating in high concentration in the target tissue. Moreover, they can be easily activated by a specific wavelength with minimum side effects on the adjacent tissues. Generally, they are classified into three-generations: first, second and third. The first generation involves naturally occurring porphyrins such as hematoporphyrin, which have strong absorption restricted to about 400 nm with limited excitation with a longer wavelength. The second-generation (such as chlorins and 5 – aminolevulinic acid) is developed to overcome the limitations of the previous generation of sensitizers; they are activated with a higher wavelength (>600 nm) and generate singlet oxygen [34]. Chlorins (talaporfin sodium and temoporfin) are used to treat dermatological diseases. However, temoporfin is considered the most potent photosensitizer with good toleration. Finally, third generation photosensitizers are highly selective towards cancer cells by prodrug means, or *via* conjugation with nanoparticles and antibodies. Eventually, the off-target effect will be reduced and the overall therapeutic effect is enhanced. However, no third-generation photosensitizer has been approved for human use as of yet [35].

Side effects vary according to the photosensitizer and the method of administration, however, generally a common side effect is retinal and cutaneous photosensitivity, the duration of this effect varies depending on the type of photosensitizer (e.g. in the case of temoporfin up to 6 weeks). Therefore the patient should be advised to avoid exposure to sunlight, and stiff neck, fever, and headache are side effects too that are yet less reported [36].

The goal of radiotherapy is to remove tumor mass in the non-operable region of the brain. Normal cells are capable of bearing 60 grays (Gy) doses of antitumor radiation, which is lower than the threshold required to kill tumor cells. For example, glioblastoma requires 180-200 centigray (cGy) for five consecutive days per week for at least six weeks [37]. Occasionally, hyper fractionated radiation is used to minimize brain damage induced by high doses of radiation. The high dose (about 6000 cGy) is fractionated into smaller doses and delivered over smaller areas. The side effect of radiation therapy includes brain swelling [38]. A new technique named stereotactic radiosurgery is used nowadays for the treatment of brain cancer, where radiation is delivered to the tumor with a diameter of less than 3 cm with the aid of computer imaging. Therefore, lesser harmful effects on normal brain tissues will be achieved [39].

Photothermal Therapy (PTT)

PTT is a noninvasive procedure used to treat brain cancer *via* the employment of topical or interstitial (optic fiber) external near-infrared laser (NIR) that irradiates the tissue. This radiation is accumulated within a photo-absorbing agent (PTA) (e.g. cyanine derivatives) which in turn converts the radiation into heat, releasing it within the tumor. For NIR irradiation to reach PTA, irradiation must cross multilayers starting from the scalp and skull through healthy tissues reaching the tumor tissue. Therefore, the power density should be calculated to be within the safety margins (maximum permissible exposure: 1.0 W/cm2 and 0.33 W/cm2 for 1,064 and 808 nm lasers, respectively) [40].

The NIR wavelength is approximately 650-900 nm and can penetrate through soft tissues. This strategy is promising for brain cancer, since as a method of nonmechanical management, it is quite advantageous in terms of avoidance of drug resistance and side effects on healthy tissues. However, such therapy should be monitored *via* imaging techniques to monitor the increase in temperature within the brain [41].

Nanotechnology has been employed to deliver the PTA solely to the tumor *via* conjugation with nanoparticles (NP), which allows the PTA to cross the blood-brain barriers post-systemic administration. Thus, conjugation avoids the excessive heating of normal tissues. The tumors are associated with angiogenesis (generation of vascular supply to the tumor), which provides the tumor with the required nutrients. Moreover, those vessels have large intercellular gaps that allow the passage of macromolecules. The nanoparticles can penetrate through these gaps and retain there rather than normal tissues. This accumulation inside the tumor requires the protection of these particles from ingestion by macrophages, hence coating the surfaces of these particles with polyethylene glycol would overcome this problem [42].

DIAGNOSTIC TECHNIQUES FOR BRAIN CANCERS

The motor drive for brain tumor diagnosis involves symptoms such as headache, nausea, seizures, changes in personality, loss of libido, dementia, and focal neurological impairment. An extra set of tests can be performed to exclude or confirm cancer such as magnetic resonance imaging (MRI) and computed tomography (CT), which are considered the most preferable tools to detect the brain tumors and their grade to establish the proper treatment and assess the prognosis of the treatment. The WHO introduced a histological classification of tumors based on the cell type. The grade of a tumor is based on the level of necrosis, endothelial cell proliferation, and mitotic activity. Furthermore, molecular markers have been used to identify cancer including 1p/19q codeletion O6-methylguanine, methyltransferase promoter methylation, and isocitrate dehydrogenase-1 mutations, yet these markers are identified as an invasive tool that requires a biopsy from the tumor tissue to be detected [43].

Single-Photon Emission Computed Tomography (SPECT)

SPECT is a nuclear medicine tomographic imaging technique employing gamma rays with a net result of three-dimensional information. It is characterized by rather poor spatial resolution, yet is more sensitive and has a low cost. During SPECT imaging, four nuclides are utilized: thallium 201, technetium 99, iodine 123, and indium 111. The SPECT tracers are either radionuclides or a metabolism substrate labeled with radionuclides. Those tracers diagnose grade gliomas and are used to monitor the patient during treatment to assess the prognosis. Nowadays, SPECT tracers are chelated with radionuclides, which limits their use to identify certain tumors [44].

Magnetic Resonance Imaging (MRI)

MRI was introduced in the 1970s, and is nowadays considered an essential tool in clinical research settings. It is based on basic nuclear magnetic resonance NMR. This technique is suitable for the examination of soft tissues and can be used to detect brain injuries and tumors.

The signaling in this tool relies on the exten,t of contrast gained from the examined sample including spin-lattice/longitudinal relaxation time (T1), transverse relaxation time (T2), and spin density (r). Those factors are variable according to the tissue type, therefore, the final image would have different contrasts (bright/ dark) representing the different tissues. However, to highlight the tumor distinctively, a contrast agent is often injected, such as gadolinium chelates and iron particles. This contrast agent aids in altering the T1 and/ or T2 of the protons in the vicinity of the agent, which in turn generates a suitable contrast to facilitate diagnosis [45].

Optical Imaging

Tumors are associated with alteration in physiological processes within the cancer cells, leading to the production of a large number of molecules. These molecules and pathways are being tracked *via* optical imaging, which is a sensitive and non-invasive technique that represents molecular imaging being used in clinical settings. This method involves bioluminescence and fluorescence. When the latter requires a probe, the body tissues have a minor autofluorescence, therefore, the optical imaging results in an elevated signal-to-noise ratio, thus picomolar or femtomolar concentrations for optical reports or contrast, molecules modified with a fluorescent group such as green fluorescent protein, are required. These agents can be absorbed by the blood cell, thus reducing tissue penetration and leading to a decline in the optical signals by 10 folds per cm of tissue. Tissue differential absorption of light produces images that are weighted toward optical reporter and probes. These are placed on the surface of the subject, which is considered a limitation of this technique that is overcome by 3D imaging and analysis procedures e.g fluorescence molecular tomography (FMT). This technique aims at rather relative than absolute quantification of imaging signals. Moreover, it is quite important in molecular imagining for research purposes [46].

Dyes

Organic near-infrared fluorescent dyes have gained significant attention as a tool for imaging, as they have an improved photophysical property. Moreover, their abundance is suitable for large scale synthesis, and due to their binding capacity with a variety of molecules such as amino acids, nucleotides, DNA primers, and dsDNA, which in turn had been applied in molecular imaging. These dyes are considered a promising approach for cancer detection due to their ability to bind to cancer tissues *via* covenant and noncovalent bonds. Nonetheless, some of these dyes tend to accumulate within tumor cells without the aid of a tumor-targeting ligand. These dyes are conjugated with special ligands (e.g. Cy5.5 with RGD which is used in glioma imaging), after which the complex will lead to an elevated cell-associated fluorescence on tumor cells, which expresses integrin and endothelial cells. This conjugate is uptaken by the tumor within 2 hours and eliminated slowly. The conjugate can be encapsulated to modify the uptake and targeting, thus resulting in better imaging for gliomas and theragnosis, especially if the drug was loaded with dyes [47].

THERANOSTIC MICELLES: A PROMISING TOOL FOR DIAGNOSIS AND MANAGEMENT OF BRAIN TUMORS

The term theranostic is derived from two terms: therapeutics and diagnostics, therefore the term refers to a strategy that involves simultaneously conducting both diagnosis and treatment. Consequently, a theranostic method is a time and cost saver, and it has gained increasing attention from researchers due to its better outcomes. This technique is facilitated by nanoplatforms, which are a complex drug delivery system composed of nanoparticles, drugs, and imaging probes. A nanoplatform (NPS) consists of a variety of techniques such as polymer micelles, liposomes, metal nanoparticles, and polymer-drug conjugates. Overall, it manifests many advantages including increasing drug solubility, improving drug pharmacokinetics and pharmacodynamics, delivering the proper dose of cytotoxic agents to the target tissues with minimal side effects and accumulation in the tumor through enhanced permeability and retention effect (EPR). It also offers drug release control through environmentally responsive detectors such as pH, light, ultrasound, temperature, or enzymatic activation.

The EPR has demonstrated various effects among patients, tumor types, tumors of the same origin, and metastases of the same patients, which resulted in different responses during the treatment of gliomas and other brain tumors, largely due to the limitation of transportation through the blood-brain barrier causing an accumulation of the product in other systems across the body, such as lymph nodes [48].

Micelles Composition

Micelles are a colloidally assembled preparation dispersed into a given system. They vary in terms of size (usually ranging from 5 – 100 nm), and composition (as they can be prepared from fatty acid, salts of fatty acid, and phospholipids). They are defined as aggregates of surfactants that aggregate in response to the surrounding environment (e.g. polar, non-polar). The surfactant structure is divided into head and tail, where the tail is a metaphor for the -nonpolar hydrocarbon chain, while the head is the polar side of the structure, so that in a polar media, the tails are arranged to the center forming a spherical shaped structure. Whenever the concentration of a micellar component in the media is reduced, these components occur as monomers, however, by increasing the concentration, aggregation will take place. The required concentration for aggregation is called critical micelle concentration (CMC) and the aggregation is governed by Vader Waals forces at the tail, while hydrogen bonding crosslinks the outer shell with the surrounding polar media. While being dispersed into the water, the head polar structure shows an interaction with the surrounding water leading to perforating the micelle, which can be employed as a drug delivery system as it increases the solubility of the drug thus reducing dose and toxicity, along with the elongation of the half-life of the drug due to increased volume of distribution with a potential targeting capability [49].

Micelles can be considered a trojan that protects the drug from ingestion by macrophages and degradation. The micelle generally resembles a spherical shape and can be assembled into different shapes, such as rods, lamellae, or vesicles. These different morphologies depend on solvents, length of chain, as well as the temperature, and the shape, which are confirmed by nuclear magnetic resonance, x-ray diffraction, electron spin resonance, and many others. Micelles are more recently modified using different polymers, which results in enhancing their biological properties. Polyethylene glycol is one of these polymers; it is a hydrophilic biocompatible anon toxic polymer used to stabilize the steric structure of the micelle. Meanwhile, polyesters and polyaminoacids are polymers that enhance the hydrophobic core structure [50].

Classification of Micelles

Charged polymers have been investigated to produce micelles as they are capable of binding to biological molecules such as lipids and proteins. These electrostatic charges will result in an assembly characterized by the degree of hydrophobicity of the used polymers. So for an amphiphilic polymer, the resultant formation is nanomicelles (NdialysisM) consisting of the hydrophilic shell while the core is hydrophobic. The nanomicelles are quite advantageous as their composition allows for the encapsulation of lipid-soluble drugs, thus carrying the drug through circulation to the targeted tissue. This is associated with the prolongation of the drug's half-life [51].

The initial types of these micelles were formed by the conjugation of PEG and diacyl- lipids which are a long chain of a fatty group providing extremely hydrophobic blocks, and later, oleic acid. This is a monounsaturated fatty acid that is conjugated *via* amid linkage to chitosan, which has no amphiphilic properties, resulting in the impairment of micelle formation in aqueous media. Yet, when chitosan chains bind to oleic acid, the water solubilization enhances due to the amide bond, and the polymer will assemble into a nano self-aggregating micelle while in water, these micelles are used to treat cancer after being coated with folic acid and albumin [52].

Preparation Methods

The micelles are loaded with a drug by chemical means *via* chemical conjugation or by physical means *via* entrapment of the drug. The most well-known methods of drug incorporation inside the micelles are myriad, however they can be summarized as follows: emulsion techniques (oil in water, water in oil in water), dialysis, co-solvation, and lyophilization and the direct dissolution method. The emulsion techniques are used for hydrophobic drugs that exhibit very low water solubility [53].

The dialysis method involves dissolving both the drug and the amphiphilic polymer in a water-miscible organic solvent (e.g. dimethylformamide). The mixture is subjected to dialysis *via* the employment of a dialysis bag against water, and the water then washes out the solvent gradually. Thus, the amphiphilic polymer will aggregate around drug molecules due to drops in organic solvent concentration forming a larger micelle than the dialysis membrane pores, while the unloaded drug will be removed during the dialysis [54].

Solvent evaporation involves the employment of a water-miscible organic solvent to dissolve the drug and block the polymer. The mixture is set to evaporate the solvent resulting in a thin film on the wall of the container, which in turn is subjected to reconstitution with water, hence the production of micelles [55].

The direct dissolution method involves dissolving both the amphiphilic polymer and the drug in an aqueous solvent. This method is associated with low drug loading inside the micelles, however, the loading increases when the solution is heated or stirred [56].

The pharmaceutical preparation of polymeric micelles depends on the stability of micelles in the final formulation under given thermodynamic and kinetic conditions, which ensure not only the stability in the dosage form but also avoid the release of the drug in tissues other than the targeted tissue [57].

BARRIERS OF MICELLAR DRUG DELIVERY IN BRAIN TUMORS: OBSTACLES AND SOLUTIONS

To achieve a successful theranostic micellar delivery in brain tumors, it is important to guarantee the localization of the nanocarrier system at the site of action. For this reason, it is important to identify the main barriers to micellar drug delivery in brain tumors and determine how to overcome them. These are represented by the blood-brain barrier (BBB), blood-brain tumor barrier (BBTB), tumor heterogeneous microenvironment, and therapeutic resistance owing to glioma stem cells [58, 59].

Blood-Brain Barrier (BBB)

The BBB is a highly specialized system of brain capillary endothelial cells (BCECs) and surrounding structures that deliver essential nutrients to the brain and prevent the passage of harmful toxins from the blood. This results in a significant challenge for drug delivery in the case of a brain tumor [60]. The BBB was first identified in 1885 by Ehrlich after observing the staining effect of intravenous dyes on most organs except the brain [61]. However, the actual structure of the BBB was identified in 1937 after the invention of the scanning electron microscope [62]. Generally, it consists of four essential cellular structures (i) Astrocytic perivascular endfeet, (ii) Microglial cells (iii) Pericytes, and (iv) The brain capillary endothelial cells (BCECs), as illustrated in Fig. (**1**).

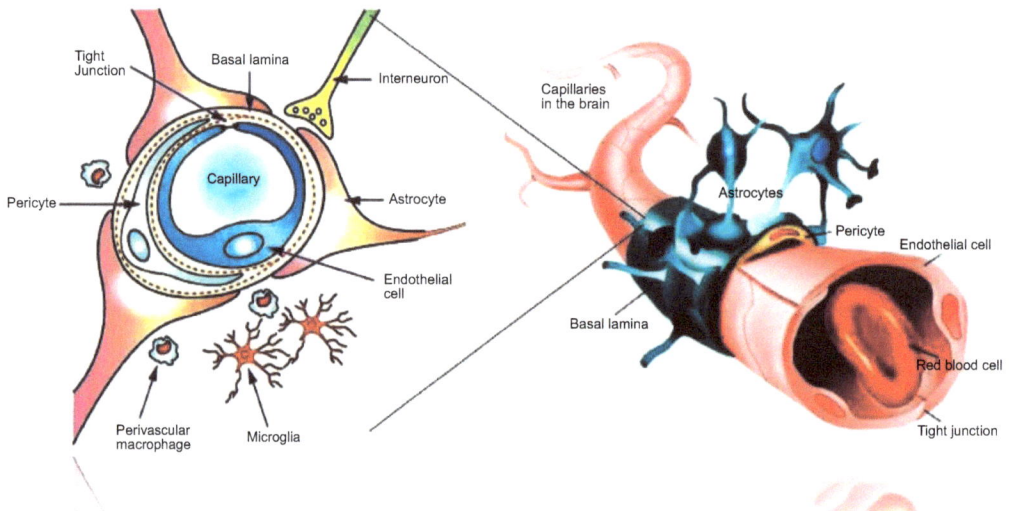

Fig. (1). The basic structure of the blood-brain barrier (BBB)

The astrocytic endfeet are the last part of the astrocytes that are closely connected to the endothelial cells, which cover about 99% of the capillaries and are essential in the formation and maintenance of BBB integrity [63, 64]. Microglia are localized immune cells in the brain that in combination with macrophages are the first defense line in the central nervous system (CNS) against blood-born foreign bodies and are also responsible for vascular growth regulation [65, 66]. Furthermore, pericytes are multi-functional cells responsible for vascular function and BBB permeability [67, 68]. These structures collectively surround the BCECs through the basal lamina to form the impermeable BBB [69]. The BCECs consist of monolayer non-fenestrated blood vessel endothelial cells that are closely attached *via* tight junctions (TJs) [70]. The lipidic nature of the endothelial cells permits the transcellular diffusion of only a few small lipophilic molecules (less than 400 Da), which form less than 8 hydrogen bonds [71, 72]. Moreover, the presence of tight junctions (TJs) in the BCECs greatly restricts the paracellular diffusion to small hydrophilic molecules [73]. Occludins, claudins, tricellulins, and junctional adhesion molecules are the main TJs proteins [67].

In addition to the previously mentioned physical barriers in BBB, there are also physiological barriers, including metabolic or enzymatic barriers [74]. Metabolic barriers in CNS are represented by the efflux transporters expressed in the endothelial cells that bind to many drugs and hamper their accumulation in the brain. These efflux transporters include various multidrug resistance families which usually belong to the class of ATP-binding cassette (ABC) transporters, in which P glycoprotein (P-gp) multidrug resistance receptors (MDR1, ABCB1) are the most abundant types [75 - 77]. Unfortunately, the expression of these ABC transporters is usually increased in brain cancer and after radiotherapy or chemotherapy, it further complicates the process of drug delivery in the case of a brain tumor [78, 79].

Consequently, the BBB provides a physical and biochemical barrier for the passage of more than 98% of small molecules and 100% of large ones. However, in addition to the paracellular and transcellular lipophilic pathways, other transport pathways are available through the BBB including carrier-mediated transcytosis (CMT), receptor-mediated transcytosis (RMT), adsorptive-mediated transcytosis (AMT), and cell-mediated transport in addition to BBB disruption enhanced transport, which has recently been investigated and employed for targeting brain cancers *via* the "Trojan horse" strategy [59, 80] as shown in Fig. (2).

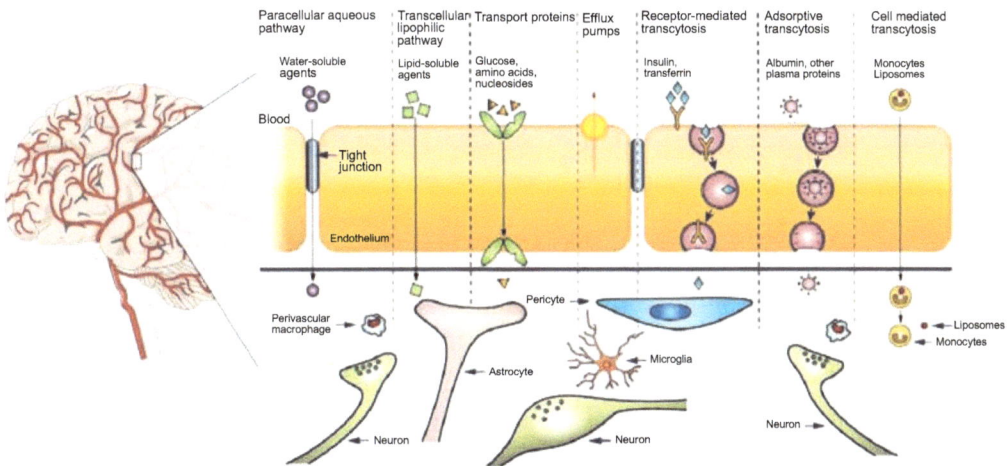

Fig. (2). Main transport pathways *via* blood-brain barrier (BBB)

Carrier-Mediated Transcytosis (CMT)

This transport system is responsible for the passive delivery of small essential nutrients and endogenous substrates to the brain, such as glucose, amino acids, hormones, monocarboxylic acids, and bile salts. It is stereo-specific, so it is suitable only for a limited number of drugs with structural similarity to the endogenous substrates [71, 81]. Different nutrient transport systems are illustrated in Table **2**. However, the glucose transporter (GLUT1) is the most abundant one and is highly expressed in capillary endothelial cells compared to other transport systems [82].

Table 2. Different transporters in brain capillary endothelial cells (BCECs)

Transport system	Ligand type	Reference
Glucose transporters(GLUT)	Glucose; Mannose	[83 - 86]
Choline transporter (ChT)	Choline; Thiamine	[87, 88]
Cationic amino acids transporter (CAATs)	Arginine; Lysine	[89]
Anionic amino acids transporters (AAATs)	L-glutamate; L-aspartate	[90, 91]
ﻟﻚeta amino acid transporter)ﻟﻚAATs)	Beta)ﻟﻚ)-alanine	[90]
Nucleoside transporters (NTs)	Nucleoside transporters (ENT1, ENT2, ENT3, and ENT4); Concentration nucleoside transporters (CNT2)	[92]
Fatty acid transporters (FAT)	Fatty acids	[93, 94]
Monocarboxylate transporter (MCT)	Lactate; Short-chain fatty acids; Biotin; Salicylic acid; Valproic acid; Phenylbutyrate; 3,5,3'-triiodo-L-thyronine	[95]

Receptor-Mediated Transcytosis (RMT)

The RMT is responsible for transferring large molecules across BBB and is considered one of the most optimum strategies for drug delivery in brain cancer because of its higher selectivity, affinity, and specificity [96, 97]. During this process, the macromolecule or ligand-carrying nanoparticles bind to a specific receptor in the BCECs to be transferred inside a vesicle to the basolateral membrane to reach the brain [98]. Different receptors are commonly expressed in the endothelial cells including the low-density lipoprotein receptor (LDLR), the transferrin receptor (TfR), the lactoferrin (Lf) receptor, the insulin receptor (IR), and the nicotinic acetylcholine receptors (nAChRs) [99, 100], as illustrated in Table **3**. However, the main limitation of this system is represented by the competitive effect of the endogenous molecules, which might reduce the binding efficiency of the exogenous ligand [101]. The transferrin receptor (TfR1) which is responsible for iron transportation in the CNS, is considered one of the most promising methods for brain delivery due to its overexpression in BBB and different types of brain tumors [102, 103]. Furthermore, a monoclonal antibody technology was extensively studied and adapted to avoid the saturation of the TfR1 with the endogenous transferrin (Tf) by delivering the monoclonal antibodies (OX26 or RI7217) against the endogenous Tf [104, 105].

Table 3. Various receptors in brain endothelial cells

Receptor type	Ligands	References
Transferrin receptor (TfR1)	Ferritin nanocage	[106, 107]
Low-density lipoprotein receptor (LDLR), LDLR-related protein 1 (LRP1), and LRP2)	Angiopep-2(ANG), apolipoprotein B or E (ApoB or ApoE),	[108 - 110]
Lactoferrin (Lf)	lactoferrin	[111]
Nicotinic acetylcholine receptors (nAChRs)	rabies virus glycoprotein-RVG29	[112, 113]
Insulin receptor (IR)	Insulin	[114, 115]

Adsorptive-Mediated Transcytosis (AMT)

AMT is a non-specific method with lower binding affinity and greater capacity compared to RMT [116]; it is used for the transportation of large molecules like albumin and plasma protein *via* BBB through the electrostatic interaction between the negatively charged endothelial membrane and the positively charged macromolecule [117]. Different cationic proteins or cell-penetrating peptides (CPP) can be used to transport different types of proteins by AMT [117, 118]. However, it must be kept in mind that this electrostatic interaction of these cationic macromolecules with BCECs is not always consistent due to their higher tendency for the adsorption of serum proteins or other circulating biomolecules, which alter the surface structure and form a protein corona, which in turn might alter the pharmacokinetic properties of the macromolecule [119, 120], an effect which can be reduced by coating with PEG or poly(lactic acid) (PLA) due to the reduction of non-specific protein absorption [121].

The most common example of cationic proteins is the cationic bovine serum albumin (CBSA), which is obtained from the reaction of the carboxylic group with a cationic amine reagent [117]. This CBSA could then be conjugated with different nanoparticles to enhance brain drug delivery *via* AMT [122, 123]. Meanwhile a cell-penetrating peptide (CPP) is a non-immunogenic cationic or amphipathic peptide with different sequences and sizes and a high capability for physical or covalent binding with other molecules to deliver them *via* the lipophilic brain barrier [124]. One of the early-discovered CPPs is a trans-activator of transcription (TAT) with an amino acid sequence (YGRKKRRQRRR), which was derived from the human immunodeficiency virus-1 (HIV-1) and is susceptible to conjugation with different cargoes to enhance their brain penetration [125, 126]. Some other examples of CPP, along with their amino acid sequence, are listed below in Table **4**. Nevertheless, it is worth noting that an efficient cell-penetrating property does not ensure a good influx to the brain because of the presence of the P-glycoprotein (P-gp) efflux pumps. For this reason, it is important to carefully select the CPP targeted nanosystem for successful drug delivery in a brain tumor [80]. Different approaches are adapted to enhance the brain penetration ability of CPP, such as the use of activable cell-penetrating peptides (ACPPs) that are activated under certain triggers at the site of action, such as UV light, pH, or enzymatic activity [127 - 129]. Another approach is the conjugation of CPP with a tumor-targeting peptide (TTP) that specifically interacts with special receptors overexpressed on the tumor cells [130, 131].

Table 4. Examples of cell-penetrating peptides (CPP) along with their amino acid sequence

CPP	Sequence	Reference
Trans-activator of transcription (TAT)	AYGRKKRRQRRR	[126, 132]
Low molecular weight protamine (LMWP)	CVSRRRRRRGGRRRR	[133]
Vascular endothelial-cadherin protein (pVEC)	LLIILRRRIRKQAHAHSK	[131, 134]
Penetratin	CKRRMKWKK	[135, 136]
Transportan 10 (TP10)	AGYLLGKINLKAL AALAKKIL	[137]
SynB1 SynB3	RGGRLSYSRRRFSTS TGR RRLSYSRRRF	[138] [139]

Cell-Mediated Transport

Despite promising studies on CMT, RMT, and AMT, they have certain constraints characterized by the non-selective nature of the transporters or carriers to the brain, in addition to the possible instability or immunogenicity of the peptides or antibodies [80]. Hence, cell-mediated transport can be implemented using mesenchymal stem cells (MSCs) [140, 141], neural stem cells (NSCs) [142, 143], macrophages [144, 145], exosomes [146, 147], red blood cells (RBCs) [148], and neutrophils [149]. In this approach, different nanoparticles carrying therapeutic and diagnostic agents could be conjugated or internalized by certain techniques to enhance their brain-crossing capabilities [150].

BBB Disruption- Enhanced Transport

Besides the previously mentioned approach, the delivery of the theranostic moieties can be enhanced by increasing the permeability of the BCECs due to BBB disruption. This can be accomplished by using chemical, biological or physical stimuli [151]. Chemical stimuli, such as the hyperosmotic solution of mannitol, or arabinose, which could be infused in the cerebral artery followed by intra-arterial drug delivery, can cause a reversible, dose-dependent shrinkage in the endothelial cells resulting in the transient opening of the BBB [152]. Other examples include cyclodextrins, oleic acid, lysophosphatidic acid, sodium dodecyl sulphate [151], and autocatalytic agents, which can all be used for a brain tumor [153]. Furthermore, biological agents that are usually derived from natural vasoactive agents can signal through different receptors to increase the permeability of the BBB, like interleukin-2 [154], leukotriene C4 [155], bradykinin [156] histamine, and vascular endothelial growth factor (VEGF) [157, 158], in addition to different viruses that are capable of opening the tight junctions (TJCs) *via* a chemokine upregulation [159]. However, the biological and chemical approaches are both limited due to non-selective BBB disruption giving a non-specific uptake of the drugs with serious side effects [101].

On the other hand, the physical methods include focused ultrasound (FUS), laser, microwave, and an electromagnetic field, which is considered a safer technique due to the high accuracy in creating a local disruption in BCECs by mechanical or hyperthermal effect [100]. Based on these physical approaches, FUS in combination with microbubble is a very promising technology to enhance BBB permeability in a non-invasive and reversible way [160, 161]. In this technique, FUS is applied at a frequency of 220,000 times/second along with intravenously administered microbubbles, causing the microbubbles to expand and contract, which induces physical stress on the endothelial cells and increases the permeability of BBB [162, 163], as shown in Fig. (**3**). The transient and reversible enhancement in BBB permeability might be attributed to the enhanced paracellular diffusion *via* the modified TJCs, or the enhanced endocytosis/ transcytosis pathway [164 - 166]. For this reason, the microbubble-mediated FUS is expected to be a suitable technology that can be administered in combination with a wide range of chemotherapeutics and nanocarriers [80, 167, 168].

Recently, the FUS microbubble technology has been successfully used in combination with magnetic nanoparticles to enhance the localization and immobilization of the chemotherapeutic and diagnostic agents by using an external magnetic field [169, 170]. Furthermore, extensive studies are being performed nowadays using an implantable ultrasound device that can be administered concomitantly with chemotherapeutic agents [171, 172].

Nevertheless, it is important to keep in mind that BBB disruption may cause massive brain injury or inflammation, in addition to the high possibility of passing toxic and harmful molecules into the brain. So, it is important to guarantee an optimal disruption technique with a selective, reversible, specific, and transient effect [80].

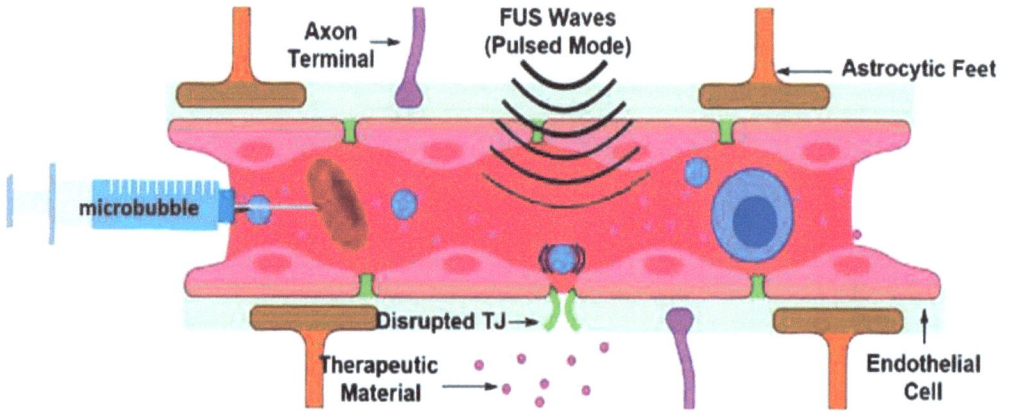

Fig. (3). Microbubble-mediated focused ultrasound (FUS) Technology

Blood-brain Tumor Barrier (BBTB)

Similar to BBB, the blood-brain tumor barrier (BBTB) is located between the abnormal blood vessel and the brain tumor [173, 174]. It results from the modification in the permeability and morphology of the BBB in brain malignancy and differs according to the type, stage, and location of the tumor [175, 176]. During tumor metastasis, high metabolic stress was generated producing a hypoxic environment in the malignant tissue, leading to extensive angiogenesis due to the overexpression of the vascular endothelial growth factor (VEGF) with the formation of abnormal vessels with higher permeability and enhanced permeability and retention effect (EPR), which increases the possibility of drug accumulation in tumor tissue [177 - 179] (Fig. **4**).

However, the BBTB is heterogeneous with three types of endothelial cells, including (i) continuous non-fenestrated (like normal endothelial cells), (ii) fenestrated continuous; and discontinuous epithelial cells [179 - 181]. Consequently, the heterogeneous nature of the BBTB leads to a limited, non-uniform distribution of the chemotherapeutic agent in brain tumors [182, 183]. This is in addition to the higher expression of the efflux transporters including the ABC transporters, especially multidrug resistance receptors (MDR1, ABCB1) in the tumor cells, which adds another challenge to the drug delivery in brain carcinomas [184, 185].

Moreover, the higher expression of certain receptors in the tumor cell offers a good opportunity for targeted drug delivery in brain cancer [177, 179, 186]. Common examples of these receptors are the epidermal growth factor, the adhesion receptor integrin [187, 188], and the epidermal growth factor (EGFR), which is the tyrosine kinase receptor [189 - 191].

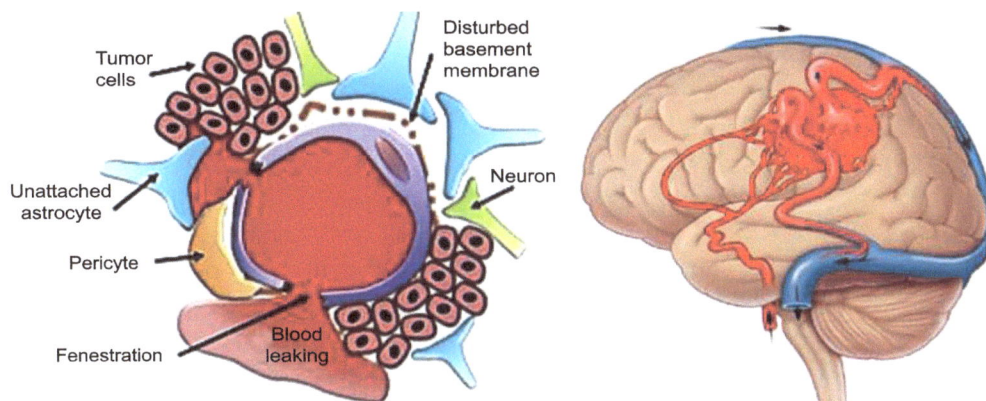

Fig. (4). The basic structure of the blood-brain tumor barrier (BBTB)

Tumor Microenvironment (TME)

The tumor microenvironment (TME) regulates the survival and progression of the tumor (angiogenesis, lymphomagenesis, and inflammation), hence representing the main source of heterogeneity and resistance to conventional chemotherapy. Therefore, understanding the TME composition and role offers good opportunities for new targeting strategies, which ultimately improve therapeutic outcomes [192, 193]. Generally, TME consists of stromal (cellular parts), and non-cellular or extracellular matrix (ECM). The cellular part of the TME involves endothelial cells, pericytes, astrocytes, fibroblasts, and immune cells [194]. Meanwhile the ECM comprises different soluble, and insoluble molecules like collagen, elastin fibers, glycoproteins, proteoglycans, hyaluronic acid, fibronectin, and laminin [195, 196], in addition to various signaling mediators for intercellular communication, including different enzymes (e.g. lipase, protease, and matrix metalloproteinases (MMPs)), growth factors, chemokines, cytokines, and inflammatory mediators, along with their associated receptors (e.g. integrins, CD44) [58, 197]. Recently, many delivery approaches in brain cancer nowadays depend greatly on targeting the endothelial cells, tumor hypoxia, or immune cells.

Generally, during the metastasis of brain cancer, all new cells must be close to the blood vessels to assure their growth by supplying them with necessary nutrients and oxygen [198, 199]. For this reason, studies have demonstrated that primary brain tumors initially grow by cooption adjacent to pre-existing blood vessels, and neovascularization (angiogenesis) is observed later in most situations [200, 201]. Usually, angiogenesis is promoted by hypoxia-induced vascular endothelial growth factors (VEGF), basic fibroblast growth factor (bFGF), and proteases that disrupt the vascular basement membrane [202, 203]. However, vasculogenesis is also observed resulting from the recruitment of the endothelial progenitor cells

(EPCs) from the vasculature, bone marrow, or adipose tissue [204, 205]. Therefore, the high level of VEGF represents a promising approach by targeting angiogenesis in brain tumors using anti-angiogenic therapies like cediranib or bevacizumab, which is an anti-VEGF antibody [206, 207]. Unfortunately, studies show that the use of angiogenesis inhibitors may provoke a further invasion of brain cancer due to cooption near the existing blood vessels [207 - 209]. However, the stabilization and maturation of blood vessels are further accomplished by perivascular cells known as pericytes, which make this type of cell a suitable complementary target for brain cancer to increase vascular destruction when used in combination with the anti-angiogenic therapies [210, 211]. This was proved by Guan et al., who developed a pericyte-targeted drug delivery system by using docetaxel to target the neural/glial antigen 2 (NG2) proteoglycan receptor, which is highly expressed in vascular pericytes of brain cancer [212].

Moreover, the abnormal tumor vasculature in combination with increasing diffusion distance and therapy/or tumor-induced anemia may result in tissue hypoxia [213]. This reduces the level of oxygen and free radicals that are essential in cancer cell destruction by chemotherapy and radiotherapy, which negatively affects brain tumor management [214]. Hypoxia causes the activation of a heterodimeric protein, the hypoxia-inducible transcription factor 1 (HIF-1), which activates the transcription of genes involved in angiogenesis, apoptosis resistance, glucose transport, inflammation, and metastasis [215, 216]. Besides, tissue hypoxia increases the rate of glycolysis causing the formulation and accumulation of carbonic acid, which in turn reduces the extracellular pH to around 5.7–7.2 depending upon the volume, histology, and location of the brain tumor, further increasing the tumor's aggressiveness [217, 218].

Depending on these facts, different targeting strategies could be implemented, such as targeting HIF-1, gene therapy, or targeting various steps in tissue hypoxia [219, 220].

In addition to the abnormal vasculature, immune cells also play an important role in supporting the growth, proliferation, and angiogenesis of brain carcinoma. Different types of immune cells can be observed in TME, including tumor-associated macrophages (TAMs), natural killer T (NKT) cells, T and B lymphocytes, myeloid-derived suppressor cells (MDSCs) dendritic cells (DCs), and tumor-associated fibroblasts (TAFs) [221]. However, TAMs are considered the most abundant immune cell in glioblastoma (30-40% of the cancerous mass) as they have a direct immunosuppressive effect and their accumulation can be used as an indicator of the tumor grade [222, 223]. They reduce immunity by promoting the secretion of soluble factors, which reduce the immune response [224], in addition to the reduced secretion of the inflammatory cytokines and hence a reduction in T-cell activity [225]. In normal conditions, tissue-resident microglia are the main macrophage in the brain. They are developed from embryonic yolk sac progenitor cells and cannot be replaced postnatally [226, 227]. However, in pathological conditions like cancers, macrophages can be recruited from the circulating monocytes and are known as bone marrow-derived macrophages/ monocytes (BMDMs) [228]. Both microglia and BMDMs are present in TME and are referred to as TAM [229, 230]. Two different phenotypes of TAMs are observed in TME exerting two opposite effects, the M1 phenotype with anti-tumor activity, and the M2 phenotype which promotes tumorigenesis [145, 231]. The phenotype of TAM is regulated by the local environment due to the effect of different chemokines, cytokines, and growth factors [232, 233]. The activation by the T_h1-type cytokines IFN_{γ} and LPS produces M1 phenotypes, while the activation by the T_h2-type cytokines IL-4 and IL-13 produces type M2 of TAM that is abundant in most types of cancers [234, 235]. Consequently, targeting the TAM has become an appealing strategy in brain tumor management *via* the use of different nanocarriers [236].

Brain Tumor Stem Cells (BTSCs)

BTSCs are a subpopulation of brain tumor cells with a stem-like property in association with the blood vessel endothelial cells of the TME [237, 238]. Brain tumor stem cells (BTSCs) are capable of proliferation, differentiation, self-renewal, and the induction of tumorigenesis [239, 240]. Consequently, BTSCs are considered to be one of the possible causes of resistance to chemotherapies owing to their long life span, relative quiescence, high expression of ABC transporters, and active DNA repair regulatory systems [241, 242].

In fact, loop-like feedback is noticed between tumor endothelial cells and BTSCs, where the former is responsible for enhancing the self-renewal capacity and tumorigenesis of the BTSCs *via* the secretion of endothelial-derived factors, while the latter hastens the angiogenesis [243, 244]. Nitric oxide (NO) is considered to be an endothelial product that enhances the notch signaling and the stem-like properties of the BTSCs. The NO is secreted by endothelial nitric oxide synthase (eNOS), which is considered a possible target for brain tumor management [254]. Furthermore, the high expression of stem cell markers, especially CD133 and nestin, also provides a very promising target in brain cancer management [246, 247].

TARGETING STRATEGIES OF MICELLAR DRUG DELIVERY IN BRAIN TUMORS

Recently, different delivery technologies have been adapted for the management of brain cancer using local drug delivery, such as implantable biodegradable polymeric wafers [20, 248], intra-arterial delivery [249, 250], convection-enhanced delivery by using locally placed catheters [251, 252], and intranasal drug delivery [253, 254]. However, there are certain restrictions like the invasive and complicated nature of some technologies with the high possibility of brain infection, in addition to the specific dosage and positioning requirement of the intranasal route of administration [80, 255, 256].

Hence, recent studies have focused on the systemic delivery of theranostic agents in brain carcinoma. Consequently, different targeting strategies have been adapted to facilitate its penetration *via* the BBB using nanoparticles like micelles, which are loaded with theranostic molecules by adsorption, encapsulation, or covalent linking, increasing the selectivity and safety of the therapeutic agent and also enhancing the specificity and penetration capacity of many diagnostic agents [257, 258]. These targeting strategies involve passive targeting throughout the leaky vasculature of the tumor, active targeting by attaching different ligand/antibodies that are specific to certain receptors or antigens that are overexpressed cancer cells, and stimuli-responsive targeting, which are affected by special endogenous or exogenous factors [259 - 261].

Passive Targeting

Passive targeting is concerned with theranostic micelle transportation *via* different barriers in brain cancer with respect to various physicochemical and pathological factors. Physicochemical factors involve the effect of shape, size, and surface properties. Ideal drug delivery in brain cancer should have a low-curvature shape with a size around 20-70 nm, and suitable surface chemistry. For this reason, micellar drug delivery is considered a very promising approach in targeting brain cancer owing to their nanosize and hydrophilic shell, which repels the plasma protein and inhibits the clearance by the reticuloendothelial system (RES), an effect enhanced by coating it with a flexible hydrophilic polymer like polyethylene glycol [80, 262 - 264]. Pathological factors are related to the hyper-vascularized, leaky nature of most brain tumors compared to healthy brain tissue, which is referred to as enhanced permeability and retention potential (EPR), as discussed earlier in section 5.2, in addition to poor lymphatic drainage that is observed in most of the cancerous tissues [265, 266].

Active Targeting

Unfortunately, the EPR effect cannot be achieved in all cases owing to the rapid spread of the high-grade brain tumor into the surrounding healthy tissues creating a heterogeneous endothelial cell and TME, which hinders the delivery of nanoparticles by the passive diffusion [178, 267]. Hence, active targeting of the theranostic micelles can be achieved by taking advantage of the different carriers, transporters, or receptors that are overexpressed in brain cancer cells such as transferrin (Tf) receptor, low-density lipoprotein (LDL) receptor, lactoferrin (Lf) receptor, folic acid receptor, insulin receptor, *etc* [268 - 270].

Stimuli-Responsive Targeting

Different internal and external stimuli can be used to achieve optimum control of the release in micellar drug delivery. Internal stimuli include the effect of enzymes, pH, and the reductive nature of brain tumors [271]. The matrix metalloproteinases (MMPs) are one of the more abundant enzymes in TME that can be used for the targeted delivery approach [272, 273]. Moreover, the acidic nature of the TME due to the rapid proliferation of the cancerous cell makes it a suitable candidate for pH-sensitive delivery systems. The changing in the physicochemical properties of these polymers causes conformational changes when they are subjected to the acidic pH of the tumor [274 - 276]. Moreover, the highly reductive nature of the tumor cells owing to the presence of a high concentration of glutathione (GSH) causes the cleavage of the disulfide bond, which can be introduced between the carrier and different theranostic agents, hence controlling their release in the required location [277, 278]. Additionally, external stimuli can also be used, such as temperature/photothermal therapy (PTT), light/photodynamic therapy (PDT), magnetic field, ultrasound, electric pulse, or high levels of radiation [269, 279]. Currently, the combination of internal and external stimuli is preferred to be applied for targeting different cargoes in brain cancer [271, 280].

RECENT RESEARCHES

Nowadays, the theranostic approach has gained great attention in the diagnosis and treatment of brain cancer. However, research dealing with theranostic micelles for brain tumors is still in its infancy and a limited number of research works have been done in this field. Despite this, many studies have been performed on the application of theranostic micelles in breast cancer [281 - 283], liver cancer [284], and neuroendocrine tumors [285].

In 2016, Lova Sun and his colleagues formulated a theranostic micelle loaded with gold and superparamagnetic iron oxide nanoparticles (SPIONs) coated with polyethylene glycol- polycaprolactone (PEG-PCL) polymer. This novel research aims to enhance the selectivity of radiotherapy in case of treatment of glioblastoma-multiform through the radiosensitizing effect of gold nanoparticles, which are capable of propagating free radicals and electron-induced radiation damage to tumor cells. Furthermore, the SPIONs are used as a non-toxic, long-lived contrast agent that can be used in magnetic resonance imaging (MRI) instead of the toxic and rapidly cleared gadolinium. For this reason, SPIONs are applied as T2-weighted MRI contrast agents that are capable of precisely delineating the tumor volume, and can be used to increase the accuracy of diagnosis, in addition to intra-operative imaging and response monitoring after treatment. The results showed a promising result in the mouse model, which can be adapted for further investigation in treating and diagnosing brain cancer in humans [286].

Another study was done later on by Weihua Zhuang and his team, who prepared intelligent theranostic mPEATss micelles of doxorubicin (DOX) equipped with a pH and redox-dual triggered release effect and a two-photon excitable aggregation-induced emission (AIE) fluorescent probe for treating and imaging 4T1 tumor model bearing mice. Two-photon fluorescence imaging (TPFI) is preferred over conventional one-photon imaging due to its deeper penetration ability and minimal damage to biological systems [287, 288]. Furthermore, TPFI possesses a higher resolution compared to the conventional MRI and CT that are commonly applied [289]. However, these two-photon probes have poor aqueous solubility and short half-life, which significantly reduce their bioavailability. For this reason, the incorporation of the two-photon probes into polymeric micelles is considered a suitable solution for their low bioavailability producing high-quality imaging of the tumor tissue. Moreover, the synergistic dual response of the mPEATss micelles produces a better anti-tumor effect of DOX with minimum side effects [290].

Danni Ran *et al.* also recently studied the application of polymeric micelles in all-stage targeting of glioma in mice. This was performed by modifying the surface of the PEG-PLA micelles with a "Y-shaped" well-designed ligand of both GRP78 protein and quorum sensing receptor termed as (^{D}WVAP), followed by loading with parthenolide (PTL) to selectively target glioma stem cells (GSCs) in combination with either paclitaxel (PTX) and temozolomide (TMZ). The results of this study revealed that the application of ^{D}WVAP modified PEG-PLA micelles offers an efficient targeting of both GSCs and glioma when loaded with PTL in combination with either PTL or TMZ without eliciting any cytotoxicity or immunogenicity in mice [291].

CONCLUSION

Brain cancer is widely considered the most fatal disease affecting the CNS due to its rapid metastasis and high relapsing possibilities, accompanied by pronounced resistance to therapy represented by radiotherapy and chemotherapy. In addition, there are difficulties in early diagnosis and with the accurate determination of size and margins of the tumor. For this reason, the theranostic approach was developed using different nanocarriers, such as micelles, offering an optimistic approach for enhancing targeted drug delivery to the affected tissue, while avoiding adverse effects on healthy tissues, as well as facilitating the detection of the tumor and monitoring the therapeutic outcomes. This could be achieved by loading both therapeutic and diagnostic agents in the same polymeric micelle that attaches suitable ligands or proteins to target a specific carrier, transporter, or receptor that is overexpressed in cancer cells. However, research in this field is still in infancy, and further studies need to be performed before translating this technique into clinical studies on humans.

REFERENCES

[1]   Kayode AAA, Shahzadi A, Akram M, Anwar H, Kayode OT, Akinnawo OO, *et al.* 2020.

[2]   Mollah N, Baki A, Afzal N, Hossen A. Clinical and pathological characteristics of brain tumor. Bangabandhu Sheikh Mujib Medical University Journal 2010; 3(2): 68-71.

[3]   Chandana SR, Movva S, Arora M, Singh T. Primary brain tumors in adults. Am Fam Physician 2008; 77(10): 1423-30.
[PMID: 18533376]

[4]   Fox BD, Cheung VJ, Patel AJ, Suki D, Rao G. Epidemiology of metastatic brain tumors. Neurosurg Clin N Am 2011; 22(1): 1-6, v.
[http://dx.doi.org/10.1016/j.nec.2010.08.007] [PMID: 21109143]

[5]   Guzmán-De-Villoria JA, Mateos-Pérez JM, Fernández-García P, Castro E, Desco M. Added value of advanced over conventional magnetic resonance imaging in grading gliomas and other primary brain tumors. Cancer Imaging 2014; 14(1): 35.
[http://dx.doi.org/10.1186/s40644-014-0035-8] [PMID: 25608821]

[6]   Davis FG, Dolecek TA, McCarthy BJ, Villano JL. Toward determining the lifetime occurrence of metastatic brain tumors estimated from 2007 United States cancer incidence data. Neuro-oncol 2012; 14(9): 1171-7.
[http://dx.doi.org/10.1093/neuonc/nos152] [PMID: 22898372]

[7]   Owonikoko TK, Arbiser J, Zelnak A, *et al.* Current approaches to the treatment of metastatic brain tumours. Nat Rev Clin Oncol 2014; 11(4): 203-22.
[http://dx.doi.org/10.1038/nrclinonc.2014.25] [PMID: 24569448]

[8]   Kim W, Novotna K, Amatya B, Khan F. Clinical practice guidelines for the management of brain tumours: A rehabilitation perspective. J Rehabil Med 2019; 51(2): 89-96.
[http://dx.doi.org/10.2340/16501977-2509] [PMID: 30483721]

[9]   Khan I, Bangash M, Baeesa S, *et al.* Epidemiological trends of histopathologically WHO classified CNS tumors in developing countries: systematic review. Asian Pac J Cancer Prev 2015; 16(1): 205-16.
[http://dx.doi.org/10.7314/APJCP.2015.16.1.205] [PMID: 25640353]

[10]   Braganza MZ, Kitahara CM, Berrington de González A, Inskip PD, Johnson KJ, Rajaraman P. Ionizing radiation and the risk of brain and central nervous system tumors: a systematic review. Neuro-oncol 2012; 14(11): 1316-24.
[http://dx.doi.org/10.1093/neuonc/nos208] [PMID: 22952197]

[11]   Strong MJ, Garces J, Vera JC, Mathkour M, Emerson N, Ware ML. Brain tumors: epidemiology and current trends in treatment. Brain Tumors Neurooncol 2015; 1(1): 1-21.

[12]   Castro MG, Cowen R, Williamson IK, *et al.* Current and future strategies for the treatment of malignant brain tumors. Pharmacol Ther 2003; 98(1): 71-108.
[http://dx.doi.org/10.1016/S0163-7258(03)00014-7] [PMID: 12667889]

[13]   Ballabh P, Braun A, Nedergaard M. The blood–brain barrier: an overview. Neurobiol Dis 2004; 16(1):

1-13.
[http://dx.doi.org/10.1016/j.nbd.2003.12.016] [PMID: 15207256]

[14]   Lesniak MS, Brem H. Targeted therapy for brain tumours. Nat Rev Drug Discov 2004; 3(6): 499-508.
[http://dx.doi.org/10.1038/nrd1414] [PMID: 15173839]

[15]   Tamai I, Tsuji A. Transporter-mediated permeation of drugs across the blood-brain barrier. J Pharm Sci 2000; 89(11): 1371-88.
[http://dx.doi.org/10.1002/1520-6017(200011)89:11<1371::AID-JPS1>3.0.CO;2-D]   [PMID: 11015683]

[16]   Deeksha D, Malviya R, Sharma P. Brain Targeted Drug Delivery: Factors, Approaches and Patents. Recent Pat Nanomed 2014; 4(1): 2-14.
[http://dx.doi.org/10.2174/1877912304666140707184721]

[17]   Phanidhar V, Durgabai B. Krishna Chaitanya G, Ramesh M, Sreekanth N. Experimental Pharmacology. magnetic resonance imaging (MRI). 2013; 3(2): 36-42.

[18]   Franceschi E, Tosoni A, Bartolini S, Mazzocchi V, Fioravanti A, Brandes AA. Treatment options for recurrent glioblastoma: pitfalls and future trends. Expert Rev Anticancer Ther 2009; 9(5): 613-9.
[http://dx.doi.org/10.1586/era.09.23] [PMID: 19445578]

[19]   Keles GE, Anderson B, Berger MS. The effect of extent of resection on time to tumor progression and survival in patients with glioblastoma multiforme of the cerebral hemisphere. Surg Neurol 1999; 52(4): 371-9.
[http://dx.doi.org/10.1016/S0090-3019(99)00103-2] [PMID: 10555843]

[20]   Westphal M, Hilt DC, Bortey E, *et al.* A phase 3 trial of local chemotherapy with biodegradable carmustine (BCNU) wafers (Gliadel wafers) in patients with primary malignant glioma. Neuro-oncol 2003; 5(2): 79-88.
[http://dx.doi.org/10.1093/neuonc/5.2.79] [PMID: 12672279]

[21]   Agarwala SS, Kirkwood JM, Gore M, *et al.* Temozolomide for the treatment of brain metastases associated with metastatic melanoma: a phase II study. J Clin Oncol 2004; 22(11): 2101-7.
[http://dx.doi.org/10.1200/JCO.2004.11.044] [PMID: 15169796]

[22]   Jiang X, Xin H, Sha X, *et al.* PEGylated poly(trimethylene carbonate) nanoparticles loaded with paclitaxel for the treatment of advanced glioma: *In vitro* and *in vivo* evaluation. Int J Pharm 2011; 420(2): 385-94.
[http://dx.doi.org/10.1016/j.ijpharm.2011.08.052] [PMID: 21920419]

[23]   Assi H, Candolfi M, Baker G, Mineharu Y, Lowenstein PR, Castro MG. Gene therapy for brain tumors: Basic developments and clinical implementation. Neurosci Lett 2012; 527(2): 71-7.
[http://dx.doi.org/10.1016/j.neulet.2012.08.003] [PMID: 22906921]

[24]   Castro MG, Candolfi M, Wilson TJ, *et al.* Adenoviral vector-mediated gene therapy for gliomas: coming of age. Expert Opin Biol Ther 2014; 14(9): 1241-57.
[http://dx.doi.org/10.1517/14712598.2014.915307] [PMID: 24773178]

[25]   Reszka RC, Jacobs A, Voges J. Liposome-mediated suicide gene therapy in humans. Methods Enzymol 2005; 391: 200-8.
[http://dx.doi.org/10.1016/S0076-6879(05)91012-4] [PMID: 15721383]

[26]   Douglas JT, Kim M, Sumerel LA, Carey DE, Curiel DT. Efficient oncolysis by a replicating adenovirus (ad) *in vivo* is critically dependent on tumor expression of primary ad receptors. Cancer Res 2001; 61(3): 813-7.
[PMID: 11221860]

[27]   Immonen A, Vapalahti M, Tyynelä K, *et al.* AdvHSV-tk gene therapy with intravenous ganciclovir improves survival in human malignant glioma: a randomised, controlled study. Mol Ther 2004; 10(5): 967-72.
[http://dx.doi.org/10.1016/j.ymthe.2004.08.002] [PMID: 15509514]

[28]   Chirmule N, Propert KJ, Magosin SA, Qian Y, Qian R, Wilson JM. Immune responses to adenovirus and adeno-associated virus in humans. Gene Ther 1999; 6(9): 1574-83.
[http://dx.doi.org/10.1038/sj.gt.3300994] [PMID: 10490767]

[29]   Shah AC, Price KH, Parker JN, *et al.* Serial passage through human glioma xenografts selects for a Deltagamma134.5 herpes simplex virus type 1 mutant that exhibits decreased neurotoxicity and prolongs survival of mice with experimental brain tumors. J Virol 2006; 80(15): 7308-15.
[http://dx.doi.org/10.1128/JVI.00725-06] [PMID: 16840311]

[30]   Quirk BJ, Brandal G, Donlon S, *et al.* Photodynamic therapy (PDT) for malignant brain tumors – Where do we stand? Photodiagn Photodyn Ther 2015; 12(3): 530-44.
[http://dx.doi.org/10.1016/j.pdpdt.2015.04.009] [PMID: 25960361]

[31]   Kaneko S, Fujimoto S, Yamaguchi H, Yamauchi T, Yoshimoto T, Tokuda K. Photodynamic therapy of malignant gliomas. Prog Neurol Surg 2018; 32: 1-13.
[http://dx.doi.org/10.1159/000469675] [PMID: 29990969]

[32]   Bechet D, Mordon SR, Guillemin F, Barberi-Heyob MA. Photodynamic therapy of malignant brain tumours: A complementary approach to conventional therapies. Cancer Treat Rev 2014; 40(2): 229-41.
[http://dx.doi.org/10.1016/j.ctrv.2012.07.004] [PMID: 22858248]

[33]   Mahmoudi K, Garvey KL, Bouras A, *et al.* 5-aminolevulinic acid photodynamic therapy for the treatment of high-grade gliomas. J Neurooncol 2019; 141(3): 595-607.
[http://dx.doi.org/10.1007/s11060-019-03103-4] [PMID: 30659522]

[34]   Allison RR, Sibata CH. Oncologic photodynamic therapy photosensitizers: A clinical review. Photodiagn Photodyn Ther 2010; 7(2): 61-75.
[http://dx.doi.org/10.1016/j.pdpdt.2010.02.001] [PMID: 20510301]

[35]   Wang S, Bromley E, Xu L, Chen JC, Keltner L. Talaporfin sodium. Expert Opin Pharmacother 2010; 11(1): 133-40.
[http://dx.doi.org/10.1517/14656560903463893] [PMID: 20001435]

[36]   Kaye AH, Morstyn G, Brownbill D. Adjuvant high-dose photoradiation therapy in the treatment of cerebral glioma: a Phase 1–2 study. J Neurosurg 1987; 67(4): 500-5.
[http://dx.doi.org/10.3171/jns.1987.67.4.0500] [PMID: 3655887]

[37]   Sheline GE. Radiation therapy of brain tumors. Cancer 1977; 39(S2) (Suppl.): 873-81.
[http://dx.doi.org/10.1002/1097-0142(197702)39:2+<873::AID-CNCR2820390725>3.0.CO;2-Y] [PMID: 837351]

[38]   Skowrońska-Gardas A. A literature review of the recent radiotherapy clinical trials in pediatric brain tumors. Rev Recent Clin Trials 2009; 4(1): 42-55.
[http://dx.doi.org/10.2174/157488709787047567] [PMID: 19149762]

[39]   Suh JH. Stereotactic radiosurgery for the management of brain metastases. N Engl J Med 2010; 362(12): 1119-27.
[http://dx.doi.org/10.1056/NEJMct0806951] [PMID: 20335588]

[40]   Doughty A, Hoover A, Layton E, Murray C, Howard E, Chen W. Nanomaterial applications in photothermal therapy for cancer. Materials (Basel) 2019; 12(5): 779.
[http://dx.doi.org/10.3390/ma12050779] [PMID: 30866416]

[41]   Cramer SW, Chen CC. Photodynamic therapy for the treatment of glioblastoma. Front Surg 2020; 6: 81.
[http://dx.doi.org/10.3389/fsurg.2019.00081] [PMID: 32039232]

[42]   Norred SE, Johnson JA. Magnetic resonance-guided laser induced thermal therapy for glioblastoma multiforme: a review 2014.
[http://dx.doi.org/10.1155/2014/761312]

[43]   Grier JT, Batchelor T. Low-grade gliomas in adults. Oncologist 2006; 11(6): 681-93.
[http://dx.doi.org/10.1634/theoncologist.11-6-681] [PMID: 16794247]

[44]   Singhal T, Narayanan TK, Jain V, Mukherjee J, Mantil J. 11C-L-methionine positron emission tomography in the clinical management of cerebral gliomas. Mol Imaging Biol 2008; 10(1): 1-18.
[http://dx.doi.org/10.1007/s11307-007-0115-2] [PMID: 17957408]

[45]   Sharma P, Brown S, Walter G, Santra S, Moudgil B. Nanoparticles for bioimaging. Adv Colloid Interface Sci 2006; 123-126: 471-85.
[http://dx.doi.org/10.1016/j.cis.2006.05.026] [PMID: 16890182]

[46]   Luker GD, Luker KE. Optical imaging: current applications and future directions. J Nucl Med 2008; 49(1): 1-4.
[http://dx.doi.org/10.2967/jnumed.107.045799] [PMID: 18077528]

[47]   Luo S, Zhang E, Su Y, Cheng T, Shi C. A review of NIR dyes in cancer targeting and imaging. Biomaterials 2011; 32(29): 7127-38.
[http://dx.doi.org/10.1016/j.biomaterials.2011.06.024] [PMID: 21724249]

[48]   Mochida Y, Cabral H, Kataoka K. Polymeric micelles for targeted tumor therapy of platinum anticancer drugs. Expert Opin Drug Deliv 2017; 14(12): 1423-38.
[http://dx.doi.org/10.1080/17425247.2017.1307338] [PMID: 28290714]

[49]   Imran M, Shah MR. Amphiphilic block copolymers–based micelles for drug delivery Design and Development of New Nanocarriers. Elsevier 2018; pp. 365-400.

[50]   Adams ML, Lavasanifar A, Kwon GS. Amphiphilic block copolymers for drug delivery. J Pharm Sci 2003; 92(7): 1343-55.
[http://dx.doi.org/10.1002/jps.10397] [PMID: 12820139]

[51]   Tong R, Cheng J. Anticancer polymeric nanomedicines. J Macromol Sci Part C Polym Rev 2007; 47(3): 345-81.

[52]   Trubetskoy VS, Torchilin VP. Use of polyoxyethylene-lipid conjugates as long-circulating carriers for delivery of therapeutic and diagnostic agents. Adv Drug Deliv Rev 1995; 16(2-3): 311-20.
[http://dx.doi.org/10.1016/0169-409X(95)00032-3]

[53]   Jette KK, Law D, Schmitt EA, Kwon GS. Preparation and drug loading of poly(ethylene glycol)-block-poly(ε-caprolactone) micelles through the evaporation of a cosolvent azeotrope. Pharm Res 2004; 21(7): 1184-91.
[http://dx.doi.org/10.1023/B:PHAM.0000033005.25698.9c] [PMID: 15290858]

[54]   Gohy J-F. Block copolymer micelles 2005.
[http://dx.doi.org/10.1007/12_048]

[55]   Lemoine D, Préat V. Polymeric nanoparticles as delivery system for influenza virus glycoproteins. J Control Release 1998; 54(1): 15-27.
[http://dx.doi.org/10.1016/S0168-3659(97)00241-1] [PMID: 9741900]

[56]   Schmidt C, Lamprecht A. Nanocarriers in drug delivery-Design, Manufacture and Physicochemical properties. Nanotherapeutics-drug delivery concepts in nanoscience. 2009; 3-37.

[57]   Soga O, van Nostrum CF, Fens M, *et al.* Thermosensitive and biodegradable polymeric micelles for paclitaxel delivery. J Control Release 2005; 103(2): 341-53.
[http://dx.doi.org/10.1016/j.jconrel.2004.12.009] [PMID: 15763618]

[58]   Mendes M, Sousa JJ, Pais A, Vitorino C. Targeted theranostic nanoparticles for brain tumor treatment. Pharmaceutics 2018; 10(4): 181.
[http://dx.doi.org/10.3390/pharmaceutics10040181] [PMID: 30304861]

[59]   Wei X, Chen X, Ying M, Lu W. Brain tumor-targeted drug delivery strategies. Acta Pharm Sin B 2014; 4(3): 193-201.
[http://dx.doi.org/10.1016/j.apsb.2014.03.001] [PMID: 26579383]

[60]   Dolecek TA, Propp JM, Stroup NE, Kruchko C. CBTRUS statistical report: primary brain and central nervous system tumors diagnosed in the United States in 2005-2009. Neuro-oncol 2012; 14(Suppl 5) (Suppl. 5): v1-v49.
[http://dx.doi.org/10.1093/neuonc/nos218] [PMID: 23095881]

[61]   Obermeier B, Verma A, Ransohoff RM. The blood–brain barrier. Handb Clin Neurol 2016; 133: 39-59.
[http://dx.doi.org/10.1016/B978-0-444-63432-0.00003-7] [PMID: 27112670]

[62]   Ribatti D, Nico B, Crivellato E, Artico M. Development of the blood-brain barrier: A historical point of view. The Anatomical Record Part B: The New Anatomist. An Official Publication of the American Association of Anatomists 2006; 289(1): 3-8.

[63]   Mathiisen TM, Lehre KP, Danbolt NC, Ottersen OP. The perivascular astroglial sheath provides a complete covering of the brain microvessels: An electron microscopic 3D reconstruction. Glia 2010; 58(9): 1094-103.
[http://dx.doi.org/10.1002/glia.20990] [PMID: 20468051]

[64]   Arvanitis CD, Ferraro GB, Jain RK. The blood–brain barrier and blood–tumour barrier in brain tumours and metastases. Nat Rev Cancer 2020; 20(1): 26-41.
[http://dx.doi.org/10.1038/s41568-019-0205-x] [PMID: 31601988]

[65]   Liebner S, Dijkhuizen RM, Reiss Y, Plate KH, Agalliu D, Constantin G. Functional morphology of the blood–brain barrier in health and disease. Acta Neuropathol 2018; 135(3): 311-36.
[http://dx.doi.org/10.1007/s00401-018-1815-1] [PMID: 29411111]

[66]   Engelhardt B, Liebner S. Novel insights into the development and maintenance of the blood–brain barrier. Cell Tissue Res 2014; 355(3): 687-99.
[http://dx.doi.org/10.1007/s00441-014-1811-2] [PMID: 24590145]

[67]   Langen UH, Ayloo S, Gu C. Development and cell biology of the blood-brain barrier. Annu Rev Cell Dev Biol 2019; 35(1): 591-613.
[http://dx.doi.org/10.1146/annurev-cellbio-100617-062608] [PMID: 31299172]

[68]   Daneman R, Engelhardt B. Brain barriers in health and disease. Neurobiol Dis 2017; 107: 1-3.
[http://dx.doi.org/10.1016/j.nbd.2017.05.008] [PMID: 28552387]

[69]   Abbott NJ, Rönnbäck L, Hansson E. Nat Rev Neurosci. Astrocyteendothelial interactions at the blood-brain barrier. 2006; 7(1): 41-53.

[70]   Saunders NR, Habgood MD, Møllgård K, Dziegielewska KM. The biological significance of brain barrier mechanisms: help or hindrance in drug delivery to the central nervous system? F1000 Res 2016; 5: 313.
[http://dx.doi.org/10.12688/f1000research.7378.1] [PMID: 26998242]

[71]   Pardridge WM. Drug transport across the blood-brain barrier. J Cereb Blood Flow Metab 2012; 32(11): 1959-72.
[http://dx.doi.org/10.1038/jcbfm.2012.126] [PMID: 22929442]

[72]   Zhao Z, Nelson AR, Betsholtz C, Zlokovic BV. Establishment and dysfunction of the blood-brain barrier. Cell 2015; 163(5): 1064-78.
[http://dx.doi.org/10.1016/j.cell.2015.10.067] [PMID: 26590417]

[73]   Pardridge WM. The blood-brain barrier: Bottleneck in brain drug development. NeuroRx 2005; 2(1): 3-14.
[http://dx.doi.org/10.1602/neurorx.2.1.3] [PMID: 15717053]

[74]   Pardridge WM. Drug targeting to the brain. Pharm Res 2007; 24(9): 1733-44.
[http://dx.doi.org/10.1007/s11095-007-9324-2] [PMID: 17554607]

[75]   Löscher W, Potschka H. Blood-brain barrier active efflux transporters: ATP-binding cassette gene family. NeuroRx 2005; 2(1): 86-98.

[http://dx.doi.org/10.1602/neurorx.2.1.86] [PMID: 15717060]

[76]   Bart J, Groen HJM, Hendrikse NH, van der Graaf WTA, Vaalburg W, de Vries EGE. The blood-brain barrier and oncology: new insights into function and modulation. Cancer Treat Rev 2000; 26(6): 449-62.
[http://dx.doi.org/10.1053/ctrv.2000.0194] [PMID: 11139374]

[77]   Blakeley J. Drug delivery to brain tumors. Curr Neurol Neurosci Rep 2008; 8(3): 235-41.
[http://dx.doi.org/10.1007/s11910-008-0036-8] [PMID: 18541119]

[78]   Calatozzolo C, Gelati M, Ciusani E, *et al.* Expression of drug resistance proteins Pgp, MRP1, MRP3, MRP5 and GST-π in human glioma. J Neurooncol 2005; 74(2): 113-21.
[http://dx.doi.org/10.1007/s11060-004-6152-7] [PMID: 16193381]

[79]   Szabó D, Keyzer H, Kaiser HE, Molnár J. Reversal of multidrug resistance of tumor cells. Anticancer Res 2000; 20(6B): 4261-74.
[PMID: 11205256]

[80]   Tang W, Fan W, Lau J, Deng L, Shen Z, Chen X. Emerging blood–brain-barrier-crossing nanotechnology for brain cancer theranostics. Chem Soc Rev 2019; 48(11): 2967-3014.
[http://dx.doi.org/10.1039/C8CS00805A] [PMID: 31089607]

[81]   Abdul Razzak R, Florence GJ, Gunn-Moore FJ. Approaches to CNS drug delivery with a focus on transporter-mediated transcytosis. Int J Mol Sci 2019; 20(12): 3108.
[http://dx.doi.org/10.3390/ijms20123108] [PMID: 31242683]

[82]   Uchida Y, Ohtsuki S, Katsukura Y, *et al.* Quantitative targeted absolute proteomics of human blood-brain barrier transporters and receptors. J Neurochem 2011; 117(2): 333-45.
[http://dx.doi.org/10.1111/j.1471-4159.2011.07208.x] [PMID: 21291474]

[83]   Du D, Chang N, Sun S, *et al.* The role of glucose transporters in the distribution of p-aminophenyl-α-d-mannopyranoside modified liposomes within mice brain. J Control Release 2014; 182: 99-110.
[http://dx.doi.org/10.1016/j.jconrel.2014.03.006] [PMID: 24631863]

[84]   Singh I, Swami R, Jeengar MK, Khan W, Sistla R. p-Aminophenyl-α-d-mannopyranoside engineered lipidic nanoparticles for effective delivery of docetaxel to brain. Chem Phys Lipids 2015; 188: 1-9.
[http://dx.doi.org/10.1016/j.chemphyslip.2015.03.003] [PMID: 25819559]

[85]   Ying X, Wen H, Lu WL, *et al.* Dual-targeting daunorubicin liposomes improve the therapeutic efficacy of brain glioma in animals. J Control Release 2010; 141(2): 183-92.
[http://dx.doi.org/10.1016/j.jconrel.2009.09.020] [PMID: 19799948]

[86]   Qin Y, Fan W, Chen H, *et al. In vitro* and *in vivo* investigation of glucose-mediated brain-targeting liposomes. J Drug Target 2010; 18(7): 536-49.
[http://dx.doi.org/10.3109/10611861003587235] [PMID: 20132091]

[87]   Iwao B, Yara M, Hara N, *et al.* Functional expression of choline transporter like-protein 1 (CTL1) and CTL2 in human brain microvascular endothelial cells. Neurochem Int 2016; 93: 40-50.
[http://dx.doi.org/10.1016/j.neuint.2015.12.011] [PMID: 26746385]

[88]   Lockman PR, Allen DD. The transport of choline. Drug Dev Ind Pharm 2002; 28(7): 749-71.
[http://dx.doi.org/10.1081/DDC-120005622] [PMID: 12236062]

[89]   Barar J, Rafi MA, Pourseif MM, Omidi Y. Blood-brain barrier transport machineries and targeted therapy of brain diseases. Bioimpacts 2016; 6(4): 225-48.
[http://dx.doi.org/10.15171/bi.2016.30] [PMID: 28265539]

[90]   Hawkins RA, O'Kane RL, Simpson IA, Viña JR. Structure of the blood-brain barrier and its role in the transport of amino acids. J Nutr 2006; 136(1) (Suppl.): 218S-26S.
[http://dx.doi.org/10.1093/jn/136.1.218S] [PMID: 16365086]

[91]   Smith QR. Transport of glutamate and other amino acids at the blood-brain barrier. J Nutr 2000; 130(4) (Suppl.): 1016S-22S.

[http://dx.doi.org/10.1093/jn/130.4.1016S] [PMID: 10736373]

[92]   Molina-Arcas M, Casado F, Pastor-Anglada M. Nucleoside transporter proteins. Curr Vasc Pharmacol 2009; 7(4): 426-34.
[http://dx.doi.org/10.2174/157016109789043892] [PMID: 19485885]

[93]   Romano A, Koczwara JB, Gallelli CA, *et al.* Fats for thoughts: An update on brain fatty acid metabolism. Int J Biochem Cell Biol 2017; 84: 40-5.
[http://dx.doi.org/10.1016/j.biocel.2016.12.015] [PMID: 28065757]

[94]   Guo D, Bell EH, Chakravarti A. Lipid metabolism emerges as a promising target for malignant glioma therapy. CNS Oncol 2013; 2(3): 289-99.
[http://dx.doi.org/10.2217/cns.13.20] [PMID: 24159371]

[95]   Pérez-Escuredo J, Van Hée VF, Sboarina M, Falces J, Payen VL, Pellerin L, *et al.* Monocarboxylate transporters in the brain and in cancer. Biochimica et Biophysica Acta (BBA)-. Molecular Cell Research 2016; 1863(10): 2481-97.

[96]   Wang YY, Lui PCW, Li JY. Receptor-mediated therapeutic transport across the blood–brain barrier. Immunotherapy 2009; 1(6): 983-93.
[http://dx.doi.org/10.2217/imt.09.75] [PMID: 20635914]

[97]   Fang F, Zou D, Wang W, *et al.* Non-invasive approaches for drug delivery to the brain based on the receptor mediated transport. Mater Sci Eng C 2017; 76: 1316-27.
[http://dx.doi.org/10.1016/j.msec.2017.02.056] [PMID: 28482500]

[98]   Jones AR, Shusta EV. Blood-brain barrier transport of therapeutics *via* receptor-mediation. Pharm Res 2007; 24(9): 1759-71.
[http://dx.doi.org/10.1007/s11095-007-9379-0] [PMID: 17619996]

[99]   Zhou Y, Zhu F, Liu Y, Zheng M, Wang Y, Zhang D, Anraku Y, Zou Y, Li J, Wu H, Pang X. Blood-brain barrier–penetrating siRNA nanomedicine for Alzheimer's disease therapy. Science advances. 2020 Oct 9; 6(41): eabc7031.

[100] Zhang F, xu C, Liu C. Drug delivery strategies to enhance the permeability of the blood–brain barrier for treatment of glioma. Drug Des Devel Ther 2015; 9: 2089-100.
[http://dx.doi.org/10.2147/DDDT.S79592] [PMID: 25926719]

[101] Groothuis DR. The blood-brain and blood-tumor barriers: A review of strategies for increasing drug delivery. Neuro-oncol 2000; 2(1): 45-59.
[http://dx.doi.org/10.1093/neuonc/2.1.45] [PMID: 11302254]

[102] Moos T, Morgan EH. Transferrin and transferrin receptor function in brain barrier systems. Cell Mol Neurobiol 2000; 20(1): 77-95.
[http://dx.doi.org/10.1023/A:1006948027674] [PMID: 10690503]

[103] Prior R, Reifenberger G, Wechsler W. Transferrin receptor expression in tumours of the human nervous system: relation to tumour type, grading and tumour growth fraction. Virchows Arch A Pathol Anat Histopathol 1990; 416(6): 491-6.
[http://dx.doi.org/10.1007/BF01600299] [PMID: 2110696]

[104] Huwyler J, Wu D, Pardridge WM. Brain drug delivery of small molecules using immunoliposomes. Proc Natl Acad Sci USA 1996; 93(24): 14164-9.
[http://dx.doi.org/10.1073/pnas.93.24.14164] [PMID: 8943078]

[105] Liu Z, Zhao H, Shu L, *et al.* Preparation and evaluation of Baicalin-loaded cationic solid lipid nanoparticles conjugated with OX26 for improved delivery across the BBB. Drug Dev Ind Pharm 2015; 41(3): 353-61.
[http://dx.doi.org/10.3109/03639045.2013.861478] [PMID: 25784073]

[106] Fan K, Jia X, Zhou M, *et al.* Ferritin nanocarrier traverses the blood brain barrier and kills glioma. ACS Nano 2018; 12(5): 4105-15.
[http://dx.doi.org/10.1021/acsnano.7b06969] [PMID: 29608290]

[107] Zhang P, Hu L, Yin Q, Zhang Z, Feng L, Li Y. Transferrin-conjugated polyphosphoester hybrid micelle loading paclitaxel for brain-targeting delivery: Synthesis, preparation and *in vivo* evaluation. J Control Release 2012; 159(3): 429-34.
[http://dx.doi.org/10.1016/j.jconrel.2012.01.031] [PMID: 22306333]

[108] Jiang Y, Yang W, Zhang J, Meng F, Zhong Z. Protein toxin chaperoned by LRP-1-targeted virus-mimicking vesicles induces high-efficiency glioblastoma therapy *in vivo*. Adv Mater 2018; 30(30)1800316
[http://dx.doi.org/10.1002/adma.201800316] [PMID: 29893017]

[109] Jiang Y, Zhang J, Meng F, Zhong Z. Apolipoprotein E peptide-directed chimeric polymersomes mediate an ultrahigh-efficiency targeted protein therapy for glioblastoma. ACS Nano 2018; 12(11): 11070-9.
[http://dx.doi.org/10.1021/acsnano.8b05265] [PMID: 30395440]

[110] Sun X, Pang Z, Ye H, *et al.* Co-delivery of pEGFP-hTRAIL and paclitaxel to brain glioma mediated by an angiopep-conjugated liposome. Biomaterials 2012; 33(3): 916-24.
[PMID: 22048008]

[111] Shen Z, Liu T, Li Y, *et al.* Fenton-reaction-acceleratable magnetic nanoparticles for ferroptosis therapy of orthotopic brain tumors. ACS Nano 2018; 12(11): 11355-65.
[http://dx.doi.org/10.1021/acsnano.8b06201] [PMID: 30375848]

[112] Lee HS, Hwang SLB. Kim, JO Kim, KT Oh, ES Lee, H.-G. Choi, and YS Youn. Adv Mater 2017; 291605563
[http://dx.doi.org/10.1002/adma.201605563]

[113] Kumar P, Wu H, McBride JL, *et al.* Transvascular delivery of small interfering RNA to the central nervous system. Nature 2007; 448(7149): 39-43.
[http://dx.doi.org/10.1038/nature05901] [PMID: 17572664]

[114] Pardridge WM, Kang YS, Buciak JL, Yang J. Human insulin receptor monoclonal antibody undergoes high affinity binding to human brain capillaries *in vitro* and rapid transcytosis through the blood-brain barrier *in vivo* in the primate. Pharm Res 1995; 12(6): 807-16.
[http://dx.doi.org/10.1023/A:1016244500596] [PMID: 7667183]

[115] Ulbrich K, Knobloch T, Kreuter J. Targeting the insulin receptor: nanoparticles for drug delivery across the blood–brain barrier (BBB). J Drug Target 2011; 19(2): 125-32.
[http://dx.doi.org/10.3109/10611861003734001] [PMID: 20387992]

[116] Hervé F, Ghinea N, Scherrmann JM. CNS delivery *via* adsorptive transcytosis. AAPS J 2008; 10(3): 455-72.
[http://dx.doi.org/10.1208/s12248-008-9055-2] [PMID: 18726697]

[117] Lu W, Zhang Y, Tan YZ, Hu KL, Jiang XG, Fu SK. Cationic albumin-conjugated pegylated nanoparticles as novel drug carrier for brain delivery. J Control Release 2005; 107(3): 428-48.
[http://dx.doi.org/10.1016/j.jconrel.2005.03.027] [PMID: 16176844]

[118] Zou LL, Ma JL, Wang T, Yang TB, Liu CB. Cell-penetrating Peptide-mediated therapeutic molecule delivery into the central nervous system. Curr Neuropharmacol 2013; 11(2): 197-208.
[http://dx.doi.org/10.2174/1570159X11311020006] [PMID: 23997754]

[119] Soares S, Sousa J, Pais A, Vitorino C. Nanomedicine: principles, properties, and regulatory issues. Front Chem 2018; 6: 360.
[http://dx.doi.org/10.3389/fchem.2018.00360] [PMID: 30177965]

[120] Forest V, Pourchez J. Preferential binding of positive nanoparticles on cell membranes is due to electrostatic interactions: A too simplistic explanation that does not take into account the nanoparticle protein corona. Mater Sci Eng C 2017; 70(Pt 1): 889-96.
[http://dx.doi.org/10.1016/j.msec.2016.09.016] [PMID: 27770966]

[121] Song E, Gaudin A, King AR, *et al.* Surface chemistry governs cellular tropism of nanoparticles in the

brain. Nat Commun 2017; 8(1): 15322.
[http://dx.doi.org/10.1038/ncomms15322] [PMID: 28524852]

[122] Lu W, Tan YZ, Hu KL, Jiang XG. Cationic albumin conjugated pegylated nanoparticle with its transcytosis ability and little toxicity against blood–brain barrier. Int J Pharm 2005; 295(1-2): 247-60.
[http://dx.doi.org/10.1016/j.ijpharm.2005.01.043] [PMID: 15848009]

[123] Lu W, Sun Q, Wan J, She Z, Jiang XG. Cationic albumin-conjugated pegylated nanoparticles allow gene delivery into brain tumors *via* intravenous administration. Cancer Res 2006; 66(24): 11878-87.
[http://dx.doi.org/10.1158/0008-5472.CAN-06-2354] [PMID: 17178885]

[124] Gupta B, Levchenko T, Torchilin V. Intracellular delivery of large molecules and small particles by cell-penetrating proteins and peptides. Adv Drug Deliv Rev 2005; 57(4): 637-51.
[http://dx.doi.org/10.1016/j.addr.2004.10.007] [PMID: 15722168]

[125] Mäe M, Langel U. Cell-penetrating peptides as vectors for peptide, protein and oligonucleotide delivery. Curr Opin Pharmacol 2006; 6(5): 509-14.
[http://dx.doi.org/10.1016/j.coph.2006.04.004] [PMID: 16860608]

[126] Qin Y, Chen H, Zhang Q, *et al.* Liposome formulated with TAT-modified cholesterol for improving brain delivery and therapeutic efficacy on brain glioma in animals. Int J Pharm 2011; 420(2): 304-12.
[http://dx.doi.org/10.1016/j.ijpharm.2011.09.008] [PMID: 21945185]

[127] Wang S, Chen R. PH-responsive, lysine-based, hyperbranched polymers mimicking endosomolytic cell-penetrating peptides for efficient intracellular delivery. Chem Mater 2017; 29(14): 5806-15.
[http://dx.doi.org/10.1021/acs.chemmater.7b00054]

[128] Yoo J, Sanoj Rejinold N, Lee D, Jon S, Kim YC. Protease-activatable cell-penetrating peptide possessing ROS-triggered phase transition for enhanced cancer therapy. J Control Release 2017; 264: 89-101.
[http://dx.doi.org/10.1016/j.jconrel.2017.08.026] [PMID: 28842316]

[129] Yang Y, Yang Y, Xie X, Cai X, Mei X. Preparation and characterization of photo-responsive cell-penetrating peptide-mediated nanostructured lipid carrier. J Drug Target 2014; 22(10): 891-900.
[http://dx.doi.org/10.3109/1061186X.2014.940589] [PMID: 25045925]

[130] Wang D, Guo M, Yu J, *et al.* Glioma targeting peptide in combination with the P53 C terminus inhibits glioma cell proliferation *in vitro*. Cytotechnology 2018; 70(1): 153-61.
[http://dx.doi.org/10.1007/s10616-017-0122-3] [PMID: 28879517]

[131] Eriste E, Kurrikoff K, Suhorutšenko J, *et al.* Peptide-based glioma-targeted drug delivery vector gHoPe2. Bioconjug Chem 2013; 24(3): 305-13.
[http://dx.doi.org/10.1021/bc300370w] [PMID: 23350661]

[132] Joshi S, Cooke JRN, Ellis JA, Emala CW, Bruce JN. Targeting brain tumors by intra-arterial delivery of cell-penetrating peptides: a novel approach for primary and metastatic brain malignancy. J Neurooncol 2017; 135(3): 497-506.
[http://dx.doi.org/10.1007/s11060-017-2615-5] [PMID: 28875440]

[133] Wang H, Moon C, Shin MC, *et al.* Heparin-regulated prodrug-type macromolecular theranostic systems for cancer therapy. Nanotheranostics 2017; 1(1): 114-30.
[http://dx.doi.org/10.7150/ntno.18292] [PMID: 29071181]

[134] Stalmans S, Bracke N, Wynendaele E, *et al.* Cell-penetrating peptides selectively cross the blood-brain barrier *in vivo*. PLoS One 2015; 10(10)e0139652
[http://dx.doi.org/10.1371/journal.pone.0139652] [PMID: 26465925]

[135] Petersen S, Barchanski A, Taylor U, Klein S, Rath D, Barcikowski S. Penetratin-conjugated gold nanoparticles– design of cell-penetrating nanomarkers by femtosecond laser ablation. J Phys Chem C 2011; 115(12): 5152-9.
[http://dx.doi.org/10.1021/jp1093614]

[136] Yang Y, Yang Y, Xie X, *et al.* PEGylated liposomes with NGR ligand and heat-activable cell-

penetrating peptide–doxorubicin conjugate for tumor-specific therapy. Biomaterials 2014; 35(14): 4368-81.
[http://dx.doi.org/10.1016/j.biomaterials.2014.01.076] [PMID: 24565519]

[137] Dunkin CM, Pokorny A, Almeida PF, Lee HS. Molecular dynamics studies of transportan 10 (tp10) interacting with a POPC lipid bilayer. J Phys Chem B 2011; 115(5): 1188-98.
[http://dx.doi.org/10.1021/jp107763b] [PMID: 21194203]

[138] Opačak-Bernardi T, Ryu JS, Raucher D. Effects of cell penetrating Notch inhibitory peptide conjugated to elastin-like polypeptide on glioblastoma cells. J Drug Target 2017; 25(6): 523-31.
[http://dx.doi.org/10.1080/1061186X.2017.1289537] [PMID: 28140690]

[139] Walker L, Perkins E, Kratz F, Raucher D. Cell penetrating peptides fused to a thermally targeted biopolymer drug carrier improve the delivery and antitumor efficacy of an acid-sensitive doxorubicin derivative. Int J Pharm 2012; 436(1-2): 825-32.
[http://dx.doi.org/10.1016/j.ijpharm.2012.07.043] [PMID: 22850291]

[140] Clavreul A, Lautram N, Franconi F, *et al.* Targeting and treatment of glioblastomas with human mesenchymal stem cells carrying ferrociphenol lipid nanocapsules. Int J Nanomedicine 2015; 10: 1259-71.
[http://dx.doi.org/10.2147/IJN.S69175] [PMID: 25709447]

[141] Qiao Y, Gumin J, MacLellan CJ, *et al.* Magnetic resonance and photoacoustic imaging of brain tumor mediated by mesenchymal stem cell labeled with multifunctional nanoparticle introduced *via* carotid artery injection. Nanotechnology 2018; 29(16)165101
[http://dx.doi.org/10.1088/1361-6528/aaaf16] [PMID: 29438105]

[142] Cheng Y, Morshed R, Cheng SH, *et al.* Nanoparticle-programmed self-destructive neural stem cells for glioblastoma targeting and therapy. Small 2013; 9(24): 4123-9.
[http://dx.doi.org/10.1002/smll.201301111] [PMID: 23873826]

[143] Gutova M, Frank JA, D'Apuzzo M, *et al.* Magnetic resonance imaging tracking of ferumoxytol-labeled human neural stem cells: studies leading to clinical use. Stem Cells Transl Med 2013; 2(10): 766-75.
[http://dx.doi.org/10.5966/sctm.2013-0049] [PMID: 24014682]

[144] Li TF, Li K, Wang C, *et al.* Harnessing the cross-talk between tumor cells and tumor-associated macrophages with a nano-drug for modulation of glioblastoma immune microenvironment. J Control Release 2017; 268: 128-46.
[http://dx.doi.org/10.1016/j.jconrel.2017.10.024] [PMID: 29051064]

[145] Ngambenjawong C, Gustafson HH, Pun SH. Progress in tumor-associated macrophage (TAM)-targeted therapeutics. Adv Drug Deliv Rev 2017; 114: 206-21.
[http://dx.doi.org/10.1016/j.addr.2017.04.010] [PMID: 28449873]

[146] Jia G, Han Y, An Y, *et al.* NRP-1 targeted and cargo-loaded exosomes facilitate simultaneous imaging and therapy of glioma *in vitro* and *in vivo*. Biomaterials 2018; 178: 302-16.
[http://dx.doi.org/10.1016/j.biomaterials.2018.06.029] [PMID: 29982104]

[147] Yuan D, Zhao Y, Banks WA, *et al.* Macrophage exosomes as natural nanocarriers for protein delivery to inflamed brain. Biomaterials 2017; 142: 1-12.
[http://dx.doi.org/10.1016/j.biomaterials.2017.07.011] [PMID: 28715655]

[148] Brenner JS, Pan DC, Myerson JW, *et al.* Red blood cell-hitchhiking boosts delivery of nanocarriers to chosen organs by orders of magnitude. Nat Commun 2018; 9(1): 2684.
[http://dx.doi.org/10.1038/s41467-018-05079-7] [PMID: 29992966]

[149] Su Y, Wang T, Su Y, *et al.* A neutrophil membrane-functionalized black phosphorus riding inflammatory signal for positive feedback and multimode cancer therapy. Mater Horiz 2020; 7(2): 574-85.
[http://dx.doi.org/10.1039/C9MH01068H]

[150] Ho YJ, Chiang YJ, Kang ST, Fan CH, Yeh CK. Camptothecin-loaded fusogenic nanodroplets as ultrasound theranostic agent in stem cell-mediated drug-delivery system. J Control Release 2018; 278: 100-9.
[http://dx.doi.org/10.1016/j.jconrel.2018.04.001] [PMID: 29630986]

[151] Liu Y, Lu W. Recent advances in brain tumor-targeted nano-drug delivery systems. Expert Opin Drug Deliv 2012; 9(6): 671-86.
[http://dx.doi.org/10.1517/17425247.2012.682726] [PMID: 22607535]

[152] Rapoport SI, Thompson HK. Osmotic opening of the blood-brain barrier in the monkey without associated neurological deficits. Science 1973; 180(4089): 971.
[http://dx.doi.org/10.1126/science.180.4089.971] [PMID: 4196324]

[153] Han L, Kong DK, Zheng M, *et al.* Increased nanoparticle delivery to brain tumors by autocatalytic priming for improved treatment and imaging. ACS Nano 2016; 10(4): 4209-18.
[http://dx.doi.org/10.1021/acsnano.5b07573] [PMID: 26967254]

[154] Gutman M, Laufer R, Eisenthal A, *et al.* Increased microvascular permeability induced by prolonged interleukin-2 administration is attenuated by the oxygen-free-radical scavenger dimethylthiourea. Cancer Immunol Immunother 1996; 43(4): 240-4.
[http://dx.doi.org/10.1007/s002620050328] [PMID: 9003470]

[155] Black KL, Chio CC. Increased opening of blood-tumour barrier by leukotriene C$_4$ is dependent on size of molecules. Neurol Res 1992; 14(5): 402-4.
[http://dx.doi.org/10.1080/01616412.1992.11740093] [PMID: 1282688]

[156] Inamura T, Black KL. Bradykinin selectively opens blood-tumor barrier in experimental brain tumors. J Cereb Blood Flow Metab 1994; 14(5): 862-70.
[http://dx.doi.org/10.1038/jcbfm.1994.108] [PMID: 8063881]

[157] Kumar P, Shen Q, Pivetti CD, Lee ES, Wu MH, Yuan SY. Molecular mechanisms of endothelial hyperpermeability: implications in inflammation. Expert Rev Mol Med 2009; 11e19
[http://dx.doi.org/10.1017/S1462399409001112] [PMID: 19563700]

[158] Abbott NJ. Inflammatory mediators and modulation of blood-brain barrier permeability. Cell Mol Neurobiol 2000; 20(2): 131-47.
[http://dx.doi.org/10.1023/A:1007074420772] [PMID: 10696506]

[159] Kuang Y, Lackay SN, Zhao L, Fu ZF. Role of chemokines in the enhancement of BBB permeability and inflammatory infiltration after rabies virus infection. Virus Res 2009; 144(1-2): 18-26.
[http://dx.doi.org/10.1016/j.virusres.2009.03.014] [PMID: 19720239]

[160] Fan CH, Cheng YH, Ting CY, *et al.* Ultrasound/magnetic targeting with SPIO-DOX-microbubble complex for image-guided drug delivery in brain tumors. Theranostics 2016; 6(10): 1542-56.
[http://dx.doi.org/10.7150/thno.15297] [PMID: 27446489]

[161] Hynynen K, McDannold N, Vykhodtseva N, Jolesz FA. Noninvasive MR imaging-guided focal opening of the blood-brain barrier in rabbits. Radiology 2001; 220(3): 640-6.
[http://dx.doi.org/10.1148/radiol.2202001804] [PMID: 11526261]

[162] Wu SK, Tsai CL, Huang Y, Hynynen K. Focused Ultrasound and Microbubbles-Mediated Drug Delivery to Brain Tumor. Pharmaceutics 2020; 13(1): 15.
[http://dx.doi.org/10.3390/pharmaceutics13010015] [PMID: 33374205]

[163] Dasgupta A, Liu M, Ojha T, Storm G, Kiessling F, Lammers T. Ultrasound-mediated drug delivery to the brain: principles, progress and prospects. Drug Discov Today Technol 2016; 20: 41-8.
[http://dx.doi.org/10.1016/j.ddtec.2016.07.007] [PMID: 27986222]

[164] Burgess A, Shah K, Hough O, Hynynen K. Focused ultrasound-mediated drug delivery through the blood–brain barrier. Expert Rev Neurother 2015; 15(5): 477-91.
[http://dx.doi.org/10.1586/14737175.2015.1028369] [PMID: 25936845]

[165]   Evans DGR, Salvador H, Chang VY, *et al.* Cancer and central nervous system tumor surveillance in pediatric neurofibromatosis 2 and related disorders. Clin Cancer Res 2017; 23(12): e54-61.
[http://dx.doi.org/10.1158/1078-0432.CCR-17-0590] [PMID: 28620005]

[166]   Yoon YI, Yoon TJ, Lee HJ. Optimization of ultrasound parameters for microbubble-nanoliposome complex-mediated delivery. Ultrasonography 2015; 34(4): 297-303.
[http://dx.doi.org/10.14366/usg.15009] [PMID: 26044281]

[167]   Etame AB, Diaz RJ, O'Reilly MA, *et al.* Enhanced delivery of gold nanoparticles with therapeutic potential into the brain using MRI-guided focused ultrasound. Nanomedicine 2012; 8(7): 1133-42.
[http://dx.doi.org/10.1016/j.nano.2012.02.003] [PMID: 22349099]

[168]   Etame AB, Diaz RJ, Smith CA, Mainprize TG, Hynynen K, Rutka JT. Focused ultrasound disruption of the blood-brain barrier: a new frontier for therapeutic delivery in molecular neurooncology. Neurosurg Focus 2012; 32(1)E3
[http://dx.doi.org/10.3171/2011.10.FOCUS11252] [PMID: 22208896]

[169]   Chen PY, Liu HL, Hua MY, *et al.* Novel magnetic/ultrasound focusing system enhances nanoparticle drug delivery for glioma treatment. Neuro-oncol 2010; 12(10): 1050-60.
[http://dx.doi.org/10.1093/neuonc/noq054] [PMID: 20663792]

[170]   Liu HL, Hua MY, Yang HW, *et al.* Magnetic resonance monitoring of focused ultrasound/magnetic nanoparticle targeting delivery of therapeutic agents to the brain. Proc Natl Acad Sci USA 2010; 107(34): 15205-10.
[http://dx.doi.org/10.1073/pnas.1003388107] [PMID: 20696897]

[171]   Carpentier A, Canney M, Vignot A, Reina V, Beccaria K, Horodyckid C, *et al.* Clinical trial of blood-brain barrier disruption by pulsed ultrasound 2016.
[http://dx.doi.org/10.1126/scitranslmed.aaf6086]

[172]   Idbaih A, Canney M, Belin L, *et al.* Safety and feasibility of repeated and transient blood–brain barrier disruption by pulsed ultrasound in patients with recurrent glioblastoma. Clin Cancer Res 2019; 25(13): 3793-801.
[http://dx.doi.org/10.1158/1078-0432.CCR-18-3643] [PMID: 30890548]

[173]   Ningaraj NS, Rao M, Hashizume K, Asotra K, Black KL. Regulation of blood-brain tumor barrier permeability by calcium-activated potassium channels. J Pharmacol Exp Ther 2002; 301(3): 838-51.
[http://dx.doi.org/10.1124/jpet.301.3.838] [PMID: 12023511]

[174]   Yin L, Li H, Liu W, *et al.* A highly potent CDK4/6 inhibitor was rationally designed to overcome blood brain barrier in gliobastoma therapy. Eur J Med Chem 2018; 144: 1-28.
[http://dx.doi.org/10.1016/j.ejmech.2017.12.003] [PMID: 29247857]

[175]   Hardee ME, Zagzag D. Mechanisms of glioma-associated neovascularization. Am J Pathol 2012; 181(4): 1126-41.
[http://dx.doi.org/10.1016/j.ajpath.2012.06.030] [PMID: 22858156]

[176]   Nir I, Levanon D, Iosilevsky G. Permeability of blood vessels in experimental gliomas: uptake of 99mTc-glucoheptonate and alteration in blood-brain barrier as determined by cytochemistry and electron microscopy. Neurosurgery 1989; 25(4): 523-32.
[http://dx.doi.org/10.1227/00006123-198910000-00004] [PMID: 2797390]

[177]   Berghoff AS, Preusser M. Role of the blood–brain barrier in metastatic disease of the central nervous system. Handb Clin Neurol 2018; 149: 57-66.
[http://dx.doi.org/10.1016/B978-0-12-811161-1.00004-9] [PMID: 29307361]

[178]   Karim R, Palazzo C, Evrard B, Piel G. Nanocarriers for the treatment of glioblastoma multiforme: Current state-of-the-art. J Control Release 2016; 227: 23-37.
[http://dx.doi.org/10.1016/j.jconrel.2016.02.026] [PMID: 26892752]

[179]   van Tellingen O, Yetkin-Arik B, de Gooijer MC, Wesseling P, Wurdinger T, de Vries HE. Overcoming the blood–brain tumor barrier for effective glioblastoma treatment. Drug Resist Updat

2015; 19: 1-12.
[http://dx.doi.org/10.1016/j.drup.2015.02.002] [PMID: 25791797]

[180] Schlageter KE, Molnar P, Lapin GD, Groothuis DR. Microvessel organization and structure in experimental brain tumors: microvessel populations with distinctive structural and functional properties. Microvasc Res 1999; 58(3): 312-28.
[http://dx.doi.org/10.1006/mvre.1999.2188] [PMID: 10527772]

[181] Belykh E, Shaffer KV, Lin C, Byvaltsev VA, Preul MC, Chen L. Blood-brain barrier, blood-brain tumor barrier, and fluorescence-guided neurosurgical oncology: delivering optical labels to brain tumors. Front Oncol 2020; 10: 739.
[http://dx.doi.org/10.3389/fonc.2020.00739] [PMID: 32582530]

[182] Zhan C, Lu W. The blood-brain/tumor barriers: challenges and chances for malignant gliomas targeted drug delivery. Curr Pharm Biotechnol 2012; 13(12): 2380-7.
[http://dx.doi.org/10.2174/138920112803341798] [PMID: 23016643]

[183] Yuan F, Salehi HA, Boucher Y, Vasthare US, Tuma RF, Jain RK. Vascular permeability and microcirculation of gliomas and mammary carcinomas transplanted in rat and mouse cranial windows. Cancer Res 1994; 54(17): 4564-8.
[PMID: 8062241]

[184] Bronger H, König J, Kopplow K, *et al.* ABCC drug efflux pumps and organic anion uptake transporters in human gliomas and the blood-tumor barrier. Cancer Res 2005; 65(24): 11419-28.
[http://dx.doi.org/10.1158/0008-5472.CAN-05-1271] [PMID: 16357150]

[185] Wijaya J, Fukuda Y, Schuetz J. Obstacles to brain tumor therapy: key ABC transporters. Int J Mol Sci 2017; 18(12): 2544.
[http://dx.doi.org/10.3390/ijms18122544] [PMID: 29186899]

[186] Pardridge WM. CSF, blood-brain barrier, and brain drug delivery. Expert Opin Drug Deliv 2016; 13(7): 963-75.
[http://dx.doi.org/10.1517/17425247.2016.1171315] [PMID: 27020469]

[187] Brooks PC, Clark RAF, Cheresh DA. Requirement of Vascular Integrin $\alpha_v \beta_3$ for Angiogenesis. Science 1994; 264(5158): 569-71.
[http://dx.doi.org/10.1126/science.7512751] [PMID: 7512751]

[188] Kim S, Bell K, Mousa SA, Varner JA. Regulation of angiogenesis *in vivo* by ligation of integrin $\alpha5\beta1$ with the central cell-binding domain of fibronectin. Am J Pathol 2000; 156(4): 1345-62.
[http://dx.doi.org/10.1016/S0002-9440(10)65005-5] [PMID: 10751360]

[189] Alifieris C, Trafalis DT. Glioblastoma multiforme: Pathogenesis and treatment. Pharmacol Ther 2015; 152: 63-82.
[http://dx.doi.org/10.1016/j.pharmthera.2015.05.005] [PMID: 25944528]

[190] Tsutsui Y, Tomizawa K, Nagita M, *et al.* Development of bionanocapsules targeting brain tumors. J Control Release 2007; 122(2): 159-64.
[http://dx.doi.org/10.1016/j.jconrel.2007.06.019] [PMID: 17692421]

[191] Feng B, Tomizawa K, Michiue H, *et al.* Delivery of sodium borocaptate to glioma cells using immunoliposome conjugated with anti-EGFR antibodies by ZZ-His. Biomaterials 2009; 30(9): 1746-55.
[http://dx.doi.org/10.1016/j.biomaterials.2008.12.010] [PMID: 19121537]

[192] Perus LJM, Walsh LA. Microenvironmental heterogeneity in brain malignancies. Front Immunol 2019; 10: 2294.
[http://dx.doi.org/10.3389/fimmu.2019.02294] [PMID: 31632393]

[193] Lorger M. Tumor microenvironment in the brain. Cancers (Basel) 2012; 4(1): 218-43.
[http://dx.doi.org/10.3390/cancers4010218] [PMID: 24213237]

[194] Quail DF, Joyce JA. The microenvironmental landscape of brain tumors. Cancer Cell 2017; 31(3):

326-41.
[http://dx.doi.org/10.1016/j.ccell.2017.02.009] [PMID: 28292436]

[195] Shimizu T, Kurozumi K, Ishida J, Ichikawa T, Date I. Adhesion molecules and the extracellular matrix as drug targets for glioma. Brain Tumor Pathol 2016; 33(2): 97-106.
[http://dx.doi.org/10.1007/s10014-016-0261-9] [PMID: 26992378]

[196] Jahanban-Esfahlan R, Seidi K, Banimohamad-Shotorbani B, Jahanban-Esfahlan A, Yousefi B. Combination of nanotechnology with vascular targeting agents for effective cancer therapy. J Cell Physiol 2018; 233(4): 2982-92.
[http://dx.doi.org/10.1002/jcp.26051] [PMID: 28608554]

[197] Baghban R, Roshangar L, Jahanban-Esfahlan R, et al. Tumor microenvironment complexity and therapeutic implications at a glance. Cell Commun Signal 2020; 18(1): 59.
[http://dx.doi.org/10.1186/s12964-020-0530-4] [PMID: 32264958]

[198] Carbonell WS, Ansorge O, Sibson N, Muschel R. The vascular basement membrane as "soil" in brain metastasis. PLoS One 2009; 4(6)e5857
[http://dx.doi.org/10.1371/journal.pone.0005857] [PMID: 19516901]

[199] Lorger M, Felding-Habermann B. Capturing changes in the brain microenvironment during initial steps of breast cancer brain metastasis. Am J Pathol 2010; 176(6): 2958-71.
[http://dx.doi.org/10.2353/ajpath.2010.090838] [PMID: 20382702]

[200] Bernstein JJ, Woodard CA. Glioblastoma cells do not intravasate into blood vessels. Neurosurgery 1995; 36(1): 124-32.
[http://dx.doi.org/10.1227/00006123-199501000-00016] [PMID: 7708148]

[201] Holash J, Maisonpierre PC, Compton D, et al. Vessel cooption, regression, and growth in tumors mediated by angiopoietins and VEGF. Science 1999; 284(5422): 1994-8.
[http://dx.doi.org/10.1126/science.284.5422.1994] [PMID: 10373119]

[202] Baeriswyl V, Christofori G, Eds. The angiogenic switch in carcinogenesis. Elsevier 2009.
[http://dx.doi.org/10.1016/j.semcancer.2009.05.003]

[203] Iruela-Arispe LM, Dvorak HF. Angiogenesis: a dynamic balance of stimulators and inhibitors. Thromb Haemost 1997; 78(1): 672-7.
[http://dx.doi.org/10.1055/s-0038-1657610] [PMID: 9198237]

[204] Chao H, Hirschi KK. Hemato-vascular origins of endothelial progenitor cells? Microvasc Res 2010; 79(3): 169-73.
[http://dx.doi.org/10.1016/j.mvr.2010.02.003] [PMID: 20149806]

[205] Dome B, Dobos J, Tovari J, et al. Circulating bone marrow-derived endothelial progenitor cells: Characterization, mobilization, and therapeutic considerations in malignant disease. Cytometry A 2008; 73A(3): 186-93.
[http://dx.doi.org/10.1002/cyto.a.20480] [PMID: 18000872]

[206] Pàez-Ribes M, Allen E, Hudock J, et al. Antiangiogenic therapy elicits malignant progression of tumors to increased local invasion and distant metastasis. Cancer Cell 2009; 15(3): 220-31.
[http://dx.doi.org/10.1016/j.ccr.2009.01.027] [PMID: 19249680]

[207] JuanYin J, Tracy K, Zhang L, et al. Noninvasive imaging of the functional effects of anti-VEGF therapy on tumor cell extravasation and regional blood volume in an experimental brain metastasis model. Clin Exp Metastasis 2009; 26(5): 403-14.
[http://dx.doi.org/10.1007/s10585-009-9238-y] [PMID: 19277878]

[208] Kienast Y, von Baumgarten L, Fuhrmann M, et al. Real-time imaging reveals the single steps of brain metastasis formation. Nat Med 2010; 16(1): 116-22.
[http://dx.doi.org/10.1038/nm.2072] [PMID: 20023634]

[209] Leenders WPJ, Küsters B, Verrijp K, et al. Antiangiogenic therapy of cerebral melanoma metastases results in sustained tumor progression via vessel co-option. Clin Cancer Res 2004; 10(18): 6222-30.

[http://dx.doi.org/10.1158/1078-0432.CCR-04-0823] [PMID: 15448011]

[210] Bergers G, Song S. The role of pericytes in blood-vessel formation and maintenance. Neuro-oncol 2005; 7(4): 452-64.
[http://dx.doi.org/10.1215/S1152851705000232] [PMID: 16212810]

[211] Loi M, Marchiò S, Becherini P, *et al.* Combined targeting of perivascular and endothelial tumor cells enhances anti-tumor efficacy of liposomal chemotherapy in neuroblastoma. J Control Release 2010; 145(1): 66-73.
[http://dx.doi.org/10.1016/j.jconrel.2010.03.015] [PMID: 20346382]

[212] Guan YY, Luan X, Xu JR, *et al.* Selective eradication of tumor vascular pericytes by peptide-conjugated nanoparticles for antiangiogenic therapy of melanoma lung metastasis. Biomaterials 2014; 35(9): 3060-70.
[http://dx.doi.org/10.1016/j.biomaterials.2013.12.027] [PMID: 24393268]

[213] Vaupel P, Kelleher DK, Höckel M, Eds. Oxygenation status of malignant tumors: pathogenesis of hypoxia and significance for tumor therapy. Elsevier 2001.

[214] Vaupel P, Mayer A, Höckel M. Tumor hypoxia and malignant progression. Methods Enzymol 2004; 381: 335-54.
[http://dx.doi.org/10.1016/S0076-6879(04)81023-1] [PMID: 15063685]

[215] Masoud GN, Li W. HIF-1α pathway: role, regulation and intervention for cancer therapy. Acta Pharm Sin B 2015; 5(5): 378-89.
[http://dx.doi.org/10.1016/j.apsb.2015.05.007] [PMID: 26579469]

[216] Tafani M, Di Vito M, Frati A, *et al.* Pro-inflammatory gene expression in solid glioblastoma microenvironment and in hypoxic stem cells from human glioblastoma. J Neuroinflammation 2011; 8(1): 32.
[http://dx.doi.org/10.1186/1742-2094-8-32] [PMID: 21489226]

[217] Damaghi M, Wojtkowiak JW, Gillies RJ. pH sensing and regulation in cancer. Front Physiol 2013; 4: 370.
[http://dx.doi.org/10.3389/fphys.2013.00370] [PMID: 24381558]

[218] Zhang X, Lin Y, Gillies RJ. Tumor pH and its measurement. J Nucl Med 2010; 51(8): 1167-70.
[http://dx.doi.org/10.2967/jnumed.109.068981] [PMID: 20660380]

[219] Wigerup C, Påhlman S, Bexell D. Therapeutic targeting of hypoxia and hypoxia-inducible factors in cancer. Pharmacol Ther 2016; 164: 152-69.
[http://dx.doi.org/10.1016/j.pharmthera.2016.04.009] [PMID: 27139518]

[220] Lee ES, Gao Z, Bae YH. Recent progress in tumor pH targeting nanotechnology. J Control Release 2008; 132(3): 164-70.
[http://dx.doi.org/10.1016/j.jconrel.2008.05.003] [PMID: 18571265]

[221] Razavi SM, Lee KE, Jin BE, Aujla PS, Gholamin S, Li G. Immune evasion strategies of glioblastoma. Front Surg 2016; 3: 11.
[http://dx.doi.org/10.3389/fsurg.2016.00011] [PMID: 26973839]

[222] Hambardzumyan D, Bergers G. Glioblastoma: defining tumor niches. Trends Cancer 2015; 1(4): 252-65.
[http://dx.doi.org/10.1016/j.trecan.2015.10.009] [PMID: 27088132]

[223] Ginhoux F, Schultze JL, Murray PJ, Ochando J, Biswas SK. New insights into the multidimensional concept of macrophage ontogeny, activation and function. Nat Immunol 2016; 17(1): 34-40.
[http://dx.doi.org/10.1038/ni.3324] [PMID: 26681460]

[224] Wurdinger T, Deumelandt K, van der Vliet HJ, Wesseling P, de Gruijl TD. Mechanisms of intimate and long-distance cross-talk between glioma and myeloid cells: how to break a vicious cycle. Biochim Biophys Acta 2014; 1846(2): 560-75.
[PMID: 25453365]

[225] Hussain SF, Yang D, Suki D, Aldape K, Grimm E, Heimberger AB. The role of human glioma-infiltrating microglia/macrophages in mediating antitumor immune responses1. Neuro-oncol 2006; 8(3): 261-79.
[http://dx.doi.org/10.1215/15228517-2006-008] [PMID: 16775224]

[226] Ginhoux F, Greter M, Leboeuf M, *et al.* Fate mapping analysis reveals that adult microglia derive from primitive macrophages. Science 2010; 330(6005): 841-5.
[http://dx.doi.org/10.1126/science.1194637] [PMID: 20966214]

[227] Gomez Perdiguero E, Klapproth K, Schulz C, *et al.* Tissue-resident macrophages originate from yolk-sac-derived erythro-myeloid progenitors. Nature 2015; 518(7540): 547-51.
[http://dx.doi.org/10.1038/nature13989] [PMID: 25470051]

[228] Shi C, Pamer EG. Monocyte recruitment during infection and inflammation. Nat Rev Immunol 2011; 11(11): 762-74.
[http://dx.doi.org/10.1038/nri3070] [PMID: 21984070]

[229] Tomaszewski W, Sanchez-Perez L, Gajewski TF, Sampson JH. Brain tumor microenvironment and host state: implications for immunotherapy. Clin Cancer Res 2019; 25(14): 4202-10.
[http://dx.doi.org/10.1158/1078-0432.CCR-18-1627] [PMID: 30804019]

[230] Bowman RL, Klemm F, Akkari L, *et al.* Macrophage ontogeny underlies differences in tumor-specific education in brain malignancies. Cell Rep 2016; 17(9): 2445-59.
[http://dx.doi.org/10.1016/j.celrep.2016.10.052] [PMID: 27840052]

[231] Chanmee T, Ontong P, Konno K, Itano N. Tumor-associated macrophages as major players in the tumor microenvironment. Cancers (Basel) 2014; 6(3): 1670-90.
[http://dx.doi.org/10.3390/cancers6031670] [PMID: 25125485]

[232] Gordon S, Taylor PR. Monocyte and macrophage heterogeneity. Nat Rev Immunol 2005; 5(12): 953-64.
[http://dx.doi.org/10.1038/nri1733] [PMID: 16322748]

[233] Gordon S. Alternative activation of macrophages. Nat Rev Immunol 2003; 3(1): 23-35.
[http://dx.doi.org/10.1038/nri978] [PMID: 12511873]

[234] Mantovani A, Sica A. Macrophages, innate immunity and cancer: balance, tolerance, and diversity. Curr Opin Immunol 2010; 22(2): 231-7.
[http://dx.doi.org/10.1016/j.coi.2010.01.009] [PMID: 20144856]

[235] Mills CD, Kincaid K, Alt JM, Heilman MJ, Hill AM. M-1/M-2 macrophages and the Th1/Th2 paradigm. J Immunol 2000; 164(12): 6166-73.
[http://dx.doi.org/10.4049/jimmunol.164.12.6166] [PMID: 10843666]

[236] Chen Z, Feng X, Herting CJ, *et al.* Cellular and molecular identity of tumor-associated macrophages in glioblastoma. Cancer Res 2017; 77(9): 2266-78.
[http://dx.doi.org/10.1158/0008-5472.CAN-16-2310] [PMID: 28235764]

[237] Charles NA, Holland EC. The perivascular niche microenvironment in brain tumor progression. Cell Cycle 2010; 9(15): 3084-93.
[http://dx.doi.org/10.4161/cc.9.15.12710] [PMID: 20714216]

[238] Pietras A, Katz AM, Ekström EJ, *et al.* Osteopontin-CD44 signaling in the glioma perivascular niche enhances cancer stem cell phenotypes and promotes aggressive tumor growth. Cell Stem Cell 2014; 14(3): 357-69.
[http://dx.doi.org/10.1016/j.stem.2014.01.005] [PMID: 24607407]

[239] Yuan X, Wu H, Xu H, *et al.* Notch signaling: An emerging therapeutic target for cancer treatment. Cancer Lett 2015; 369(1): 20-7.
[http://dx.doi.org/10.1016/j.canlet.2015.07.048] [PMID: 26341688]

[240] Zanotti S, Canalis E. Notch signaling and the skeleton. Endocr Rev 2016; 37(3): 223-53.

[http://dx.doi.org/10.1210/er.2016-1002] [PMID: 27074349]

[241] Bao S, Wu Q. McLendon rE, Hao y, Shi Q, Hjelmeland AB, Dewhirst MW, Bigner DD and Rich JN: Glioma stem cells promote radioresistance by preferential activation of the DnA damage response. Nature. 2006; 444: 756-60.

[242] Dean M, Fojo T, Bates S. Tumour stem cells and drug resistance. Nat Rev Cancer 2005; 5(4): 275-84.
[http://dx.doi.org/10.1038/nrc1590] [PMID: 15803154]

[243] Calabrese C, Poppleton H, Kocak M, *et al.* A perivascular niche for brain tumor stem cells. Cancer Cell 2007; 11(1): 69-82.
[http://dx.doi.org/10.1016/j.ccr.2006.11.020] [PMID: 17222791]

[244] Charles N, Ozawa T, Squatrito M, *et al.* Perivascular nitric oxide activates notch signaling and promotes stem-like character in PDGF-induced glioma cells. Cell Stem Cell 2010; 6(2): 141-52.
[http://dx.doi.org/10.1016/j.stem.2010.01.001] [PMID: 20144787]

[245] Charles NA, Holland EC, Gilbertson R, Glass R, Kettenmann H. The brain tumor microenvironment. Glia 2011; 59(8): 1169-80.
[http://dx.doi.org/10.1002/glia.21136] [PMID: 21446047]

[246] Sun J, Zhang C, Liu G, *et al.* A novel mouse CD133 binding-peptide screened by phage display inhibits cancer cell motility *in vitro*. Clin Exp Metastasis 2012; 29(3): 185-96.
[http://dx.doi.org/10.1007/s10585-011-9440-6] [PMID: 22228571]

[247] Beck S, Jin X, Yin J, *et al.* Identification of a peptide that interacts with Nestin protein expressed in brain cancer stem cells. Biomaterials 2011; 32(33): 8518-28.
[http://dx.doi.org/10.1016/j.biomaterials.2011.07.048] [PMID: 21880363]

[248] Chowdhary SA, Ryken T, Newton HB. Survival outcomes and safety of carmustine wafers in the treatment of high-grade gliomas: a meta-analysis. J Neurooncol 2015; 122(2): 367-82.
[http://dx.doi.org/10.1007/s11060-015-1724-2] [PMID: 25630625]

[249] Joshi S, Ellis JA, Ornstein E, Bruce JN. Intraarterial drug delivery for glioblastoma mutiforme. J Neurooncol 2015; 124(3): 333-43.
[http://dx.doi.org/10.1007/s11060-015-1846-6] [PMID: 26108656]

[250] Fortin D, Desjardins A, Benko A, Niyonsega T, Boudrias M. Enhanced chemotherapy delivery by intraarterial infusion and blood-brain barrier disruption in malignant brain tumors. Cancer 2005; 103(12): 2606-15.
[http://dx.doi.org/10.1002/cncr.21112] [PMID: 15880378]

[251] Lonser RR, Sarntinoranont M, Morrison PF, Oldfield EH. Convection-enhanced delivery to the central nervous system. J Neurosurg 2015; 122(3): 697-706.
[http://dx.doi.org/10.3171/2014.10.JNS14229] [PMID: 25397365]

[252] Bobo RH, Laske DW, Akbasak A, Morrison PF, Dedrick RL, Oldfield EH. Convection-enhanced delivery of macromolecules in the brain. Proc Natl Acad Sci USA 1994; 91(6): 2076-80.
[http://dx.doi.org/10.1073/pnas.91.6.2076] [PMID: 8134351]

[253] Sood S, Jain K, Gowthamarajan K. Intranasal therapeutic strategies for management of Alzheimer's disease. J Drug Target 2014; 22(4): 279-94.
[http://dx.doi.org/10.3109/1061186X.2013.876644] [PMID: 24404923]

[254] Pires A, Fortuna A, Alves G, Falcão A. Intranasal drug delivery: how, why and what for? J Pharm Pharm Sci 2009; 12(3): 288-311.
[http://dx.doi.org/10.18433/J3NC79] [PMID: 20067706]

[255] Mu F, Lucas JT Jr, Watts JM, *et al.* Tumor resection with carmustine wafer placement as salvage therapy after local failure of radiosurgery for brain metastasis. J Clin Neurosci 2015; 22(3): 561-5.
[http://dx.doi.org/10.1016/j.jocn.2014.08.020] [PMID: 25560387]

[256] Oller-Salvia B, Sánchez-Navarro M, Giralt E, Teixidó M. Blood–brain barrier shuttle peptides: an

emerging paradigm for brain delivery. Chem Soc Rev 2016; 45(17): 4690-707.
[http://dx.doi.org/10.1039/C6CS00076B] [PMID: 27188322]

[257]   Zhao M, van Straten D, Broekman MLD, Préat V, Schiffelers RM. Nanocarrier-based drug combination therapy for glioblastoma. Theranostics 2020; 10(3): 1355-72.
[http://dx.doi.org/10.7150/thno.38147] [PMID: 31938069]

[258]   Francis GE, Delgado C. Drug targeting: strategies, principles, and applications. Springer 2000.
[http://dx.doi.org/10.1385/1592590756]

[259]   Rana S, Bhattacharjee J, Barick KC, Verma G, Hassan PA, Yakhmi JV. Interfacial engineering of nanoparticles for cancer therapeutics Nanostructures for Cancer Therapy. Elsevier 2017; pp. 177-209.
[http://dx.doi.org/10.1016/B978-0-323-46144-3.00007-6]

[260]   Pinto MP, Arce M, Yameen B, Vilos C. Targeted brain delivery nanoparticles for malignant gliomas. Nanomedicine (Lond) 2017; 12(1): 59-72.
[http://dx.doi.org/10.2217/nnm-2016-0307] [PMID: 27876436]

[261]   Sato Y, Sakurai Y, Kajimoto K, *et al.* Innovative technologies in nanomedicines: from passive targeting to active targeting/from controlled pharmacokinetics to controlled intracellular pharmacokinetics. Macromol Biosci 2017; 17(1)1600179
[http://dx.doi.org/10.1002/mabi.201600179] [PMID: 27797146]

[262]   Salmaso S, Caliceti P. Stealth properties to improve therapeutic efficacy of drug nanocarriers 2013.
[http://dx.doi.org/10.1155/2013/374252]

[263]   Kim S, Shi Y, Kim JY, Park K, Cheng JX. Overcoming the barriers in micellar drug delivery: loading efficiency, *in vivo* stability, and micelle–cell interaction. Expert Opin Drug Deliv 2010; 7(1): 49-62.
[http://dx.doi.org/10.1517/17425240903380446] [PMID: 20017660]

[264]   Blanco E, Shen H, Ferrari M. Principles of nanoparticle design for overcoming biological barriers to drug delivery. Nat Biotechnol 2015; 33(9): 941-51.
[http://dx.doi.org/10.1038/nbt.3330] [PMID: 26348965]

[265]   Moghimi SM, Hunter AC, Murray JC. Long-circulating and target-specific nanoparticles: theory to practice. Pharmacol Rev 2001; 53(2): 283-318.
[PMID: 11356986]

[266]   Fang J, Nakamura H, Maeda H. The EPR effect: Unique features of tumor blood vessels for drug delivery, factors involved, and limitations and augmentation of the effect. Adv Drug Deliv Rev 2011; 63(3): 136-51.
[http://dx.doi.org/10.1016/j.addr.2010.04.009] [PMID: 20441782]

[267]   Danhier F. To exploit the tumor microenvironment: Since the EPR effect fails in the clinic, what is the future of nanomedicine? J Control Release 2016; 244(Pt A): 108-21.
[http://dx.doi.org/10.1016/j.jconrel.2016.11.015] [PMID: 27871992]

[268]   Ferraris C, Cavalli R, Panciani PP, Battaglia L. Overcoming the Blood–Brain Barrier: Successes and Challenges in Developing Nanoparticle-Mediated Drug Delivery Systems for the Treatment of Brain Tumours. Int J Nanomedicine 2020; 15: 2999-3022.
[http://dx.doi.org/10.2147/IJN.S231479] [PMID: 32431498]

[269]   Li J, Zhao J, Tan T, *et al.* Nanoparticle drug delivery system for glioma and its efficacy improvement strategies: a comprehensive review. Int J Nanomedicine 2020; 15: 2563-82.
[http://dx.doi.org/10.2147/IJN.S243223] [PMID: 32368041]

[270]   Thomas TP, Majoros IJ, Kotlyar A, *et al.* Targeting and inhibition of cell growth by an engineered dendritic nanodevice. J Med Chem 2005; 48(11): 3729-35.
[http://dx.doi.org/10.1021/jm040187v] [PMID: 15916424]

[271]   Lu N, Huang P, Fan W, *et al.* Tri-stimuli-responsive biodegradable theranostics for mild hyperthermia enhanced chemotherapy. Biomaterials 2017; 126: 39-48.
[http://dx.doi.org/10.1016/j.biomaterials.2017.02.025] [PMID: 28254692]

[272] Ke W, Zha Z, Mukerabigwi JF, *et al.* Matrix metalloproteinase-responsive multifunctional peptide-linked amphiphilic block copolymers for intelligent systemic anticancer drug delivery. Bioconjug Chem 2017; 28(8): 2190-8.
[http://dx.doi.org/10.1021/acs.bioconjchem.7b00330] [PMID: 28661654]

[273] Yang X, Lv S, Liu Y, *et al.* RETRACTED ARTICLE: The Clinical Utility of Matrix Metalloproteinase 9 in Evaluating Pathological Grade and Prognosis of Glioma Patients: A Meta-Analysis. Mol Neurobiol 2015; 52(1): 38-44.
[http://dx.doi.org/10.1007/s12035-014-8850-2] [PMID: 25108671]

[274] Yin Y, Fu C, Li M, *et al.* A pH-sensitive hyaluronic acid prodrug modified with lactoferrin for glioma dual-targeted treatment. Mater Sci Eng C 2016; 67: 159-69.
[http://dx.doi.org/10.1016/j.msec.2016.05.012] [PMID: 27287110]

[275] Zheng XC, Ren W, Zhang S, *et al.* The theranostic efficiency of tumor-specific, pH-responsive, peptide-modified, liposome-containing paclitaxel and superparamagnetic iron oxide nanoparticles. Int J Nanomedicine 2018; 13: 1495-504.
[http://dx.doi.org/10.2147/IJN.S157082] [PMID: 29559778]

[276] Xu HL, Fan ZL, ZhuGe DL, *et al.* Ratiometric delivery of two therapeutic candidates with inherently dissimilar physicochemical property through pH-sensitive core–shell nanoparticles targeting the heterogeneous tumor cells of glioma. Drug Deliv 2018; 25(1): 1302-18.
[http://dx.doi.org/10.1080/10717544.2018.1474974] [PMID: 29869524]

[277] Zhu Y, Zhang J, Meng F, *et al.* cRGD-functionalized reduction-sensitive shell-sheddable biodegradable micelles mediate enhanced doxorubicin delivery to human glioma xenografts *in vivo*. J Control Release 2016; 233: 29-38.
[http://dx.doi.org/10.1016/j.jconrel.2016.05.014] [PMID: 27178807]

[278] Chen F, Zhang J, He Y, Fang X, Wang Y, Chen M. Glycyrrhetinic acid-decorated and reduction-sensitive micelles to enhance the bioavailability and anti-hepatocellular carcinoma efficacy of tanshinone IIA. Biomater Sci 2016; 4(1): 167-82.
[http://dx.doi.org/10.1039/C5BM00224A] [PMID: 26484363]

[279] Movahedi F, Hu RG, Becker DL, Xu C. Stimuli-responsive liposomes for the delivery of nucleic acid therapeutics. Nanomedicine 2015; 11(6): 1575-84.
[http://dx.doi.org/10.1016/j.nano.2015.03.006] [PMID: 25819885]

[280] Kim J, Lee YM, Kim H, Park D, Kim J, Kim WJ. Phenylboronic acid-sugar grafted polymer architecture as a dual stimuli-responsive gene carrier for targeted anti-angiogenic tumor therapy. Biomaterials 2016; 75: 102-11.
[http://dx.doi.org/10.1016/j.biomaterials.2015.10.022] [PMID: 26491998]

[281] Guo J, Hong H, Chen G, *et al.* Image-guided and tumor-targeted drug delivery with radiolabeled unimolecular micelles. Biomaterials 2013; 34(33): 8323-32.
[http://dx.doi.org/10.1016/j.biomaterials.2013.07.085] [PMID: 23932288]

[282] Muthu MS, Kutty RV, Luo Z, Xie J, Feng SS. Theranostic vitamin E TPGS micelles of transferrin conjugation for targeted co-delivery of docetaxel and ultra bright gold nanoclusters. Biomaterials 2015; 39: 234-48.
[http://dx.doi.org/10.1016/j.biomaterials.2014.11.008] [PMID: 25468374]

[283] Shi X, Hou M, Bai S, *et al.* Acid-activatable theranostic unimolecular micelles composed of amphiphilic star-like polymeric prodrug with high drug loading for enhanced cancer therapy. Mol Pharm 2017; 14(11): 4032-41.
[http://dx.doi.org/10.1021/acs.molpharmaceut.7b00704] [PMID: 28980818]

[284] Lin W, Zhang X, Qian L, Yao N, Pan Y, Zhang L. Doxorubicin-loaded unimolecular micelle-stabilized gold nanoparticles as a theranostic nanoplatform for tumor-targeted chemotherapy and computed tomography imaging. Biomacromolecules 2017; 18(12): 3869-80.
[http://dx.doi.org/10.1021/acs.biomac.7b00810] [PMID: 29032674]

[285] Chen G, Jaskula-Sztul R, Esquibel CR, *et al.* Neuroendocrine tumor-targeted upconversion nanoparticle-based micelles for simultaneous nir-controlled combination chemotherapy and photodynamic therapy, and fluorescence imaging. Adv Funct Mater 2017; 27(8)1604671
[http://dx.doi.org/10.1002/adfm.201604671] [PMID: 28989337]

[286] Sun L, Joh DY, Al-Zaki A, *et al.* Theranostic application of mixed gold and superparamagnetic iron oxide nanoparticle micelles in glioblastoma multiforme. J Biomed Nanotechnol 2016; 12(2): 347-56.
[http://dx.doi.org/10.1166/jbn.2016.2173] [PMID: 27305768]

[287] Ebina T, Masamizu Y, Tanaka YR, *et al.* Two-photon imaging of neuronal activity in motor cortex of marmosets during upper-limb movement tasks. Nat Commun 2018; 9(1): 1879.
[http://dx.doi.org/10.1038/s41467-018-04286-6] [PMID: 29760466]

[288] Zheng Z, Zhang T, Liu H, *et al.* Bright near-infrared aggregation-induced emission luminogens with strong two-photon absorption, excellent organelle specificity, and efficient photodynamic therapy potential. ACS Nano 2018; 12(8): 8145-59.
[http://dx.doi.org/10.1021/acsnano.8b03138] [PMID: 30074773]

[289] Chen B, Feng G, He B, *et al.* Silole-Based Red Fluorescent Organic Dots for Bright Two-Photon Fluorescence *In vitro* Cell and *In vivo* Blood Vessel Imaging. Small 2016; 12(6): 782-92.
[http://dx.doi.org/10.1002/smll.201502822] [PMID: 26701147]

[290] Zhuang W, Ma B, Hu J, *et al.* Two-photon AIE luminogen labeled multifunctional polymeric micelles for theranostics. Theranostics 2019; 9(22): 6618-30.
[http://dx.doi.org/10.7150/thno.33901] [PMID: 31588239]

[291] Ran D, Zhou J, Chai Z, *et al.* All-stage precisional glioma targeted therapy enabled by a well-designed D-peptide. Theranostics 2020; 10(9): 4073-87.
[http://dx.doi.org/10.7150/thno.41382] [PMID: 32226540]

CHAPTER 8

Theranostics Inorganic Nano-particles for Brain Tumor Diagnosis and Treatment

Krishna Yadav[1], Swati Dubey[2], Shalini Singh[2], Geetika Sharma[2], Madhulika Pradhan[3], Narayana Subbiah Hari Narayana Moorthy[2] and Sunita Minz[2,*]

[1] *University Institute of Pharmacy, Pt. Ravishankar Shukla University, Raipur, Chhattisgarh 492010, India*

[2] *Department of Pharmacy, Indira Gandhi National Tribal University, Amarkantak, Madhya Pradesh, India*

[3] *Rungta College of Pharmaceutical Sciences and Research, Kohka, Kurud Road, Bhilai, Chhattisgarh, India*

Abstract: Brain tumors pose a major threat to human health due to difficult treatment, rapid progression, and poor prognosis, resulting in a terrible fatality rate that has remained high over the years. As arteries have limited drug permeability into brain tumor tissue, the success rate of chemotherapy remains low. Considering the anatomic concerns of brain tumors and the interaction between the blood-brain barrier (BBB) and nano-particles (NPs), nanotechnology is deemed an attractive approach as it has the potential to increase brain drug distribution. Theranostic strategies have also been proposed in recent years and they are seen promising. NPs are considered ideal due to their size, ease of surface modification and, adaptability to integrating several functional components in one system. In lieu of this, the design of nano-particles with therapeutic and diagnostic uses has increased tremendously, particularly in cancer treatment. This two-pronged technique aids in understanding tumor tissue location, treatment progress, nanoparticle's bio-distribution and, its efficacy as it is particularly valuable for personalized medicine-based treatments. In this chapter, we will focus on the properties of the blood-brain barrier and the blood-brain tumor barrier (BBTB), two important hurdles in brain-tumor targeted delivery, and the targeting strategies that aim at different stages of brain tumor growth and development as well as their recent advances in brain tumor-targeted novel nano-drug delivery systems.

Keywords: Blood-brain barrier, Brain targeting, Brain tumor, Inorganic nano-particles.

---

* **Corresponding author Sunita Minz:** Department of Pharmacy, Indira Gandhi National Tribal University, Amarkantak, Madhya Pradesh, India; E-mail id-sunita.minz@igntu.ac.in

Ram Kumar Sahu (Ed.)

INTRODUCTION

Cancer is often regarded as one of the major causes of death worldwide. It is estimated that more than 10 million instances of cancer are discovered each year, with this figure projected to increase approximately to 28.4 million by 2040. As a result, it is critical to obtain early diagnosis and treatment of this fatal illness. The options for cancer treatment include surgery, radiation and chemotherapy which the latter is the most commonly utilized treatment modality in both early and advanced-stage malignancies [1]. Chemotherapeutic drugs, on the other hand, have disadvantages such as low stability, difficulty to penetrate the cell membrane, non-specific distribution, and vulnerability to drug resistance [2].

As a result, new methods to improve the care of patients with malignant brain tumors are required, including early detection, monitoring therapy response as well as more effective medicines. In terms of therapeutics, medication delivery to the brain is a significant problem due to its strong resistance to foreign molecules' entrance. Many compounds were reported effective for brain diseases yet they had failed therapeutic trials due to their inability to pass the blood-brain barrier [3]. This necessitates the development of more effective drug transport methods. Nanostructured delivery systems have gained the attention of researchers in both treatment and diagnosis, claiming two uses simultaneously due to their ability to transport a variety of therapeutic substances including drugs, proteins, peptides and, nucleic acids [4].

In this context, theranostic nano-particles (NPs) would promote systems that offer opportunities for a controlled and specific release of the drug by overcoming the limitations of current brain tumor treatment/diagnosis options at the clinic, protecting the drug from metabolism and simultaneously transporting two or more drugs to exert a synergist effect [5].

In creating theranostic nano-particles, a thorough understanding of the treatment and detection process is required. This expertise comprises a grasp of many aspects such as chemical compatibility, synthesis parameters with special regard to the chemicals used, toxicity concerns, biocompatibility and biodegradability of formulation ingredients, pharmacokinetics, and dynamic parameters. An ideal theranostic nanoparticle should possess several characteristics such as a selective and fast gathering of NPs in cancerous cells, effective administration of the optimal dosage of medication, minimal harm to nearby non-cancerous cells, rapid removal from the body or metabolism into non-toxic metabolites [6].

Nanoscale compounds that are utilized in cancer therapy can be classified as organic and inorganic. Polymeric NPs, liposomes, dendrimers, and solid-lipid NPs are some examples of organic materials. Inorganic NPs on the other hand, are either metal-based, semiconductor-based or magnetic material-based nano-particles. Inorganic NPs provide a greater potential as drug carriers than organic NPs due to high quantum yields, simple surface modification, controlled drug release, safety concern, enhanced bioavailability, high loading capacity, extended lifespan, high stability against light, and wide surface area [7, 8]. Of late, most research on inorganic NPs has focused on cancer detection, diagnosis, and treatment. Inorganic NPs have received quite an attention due to their exclusive physicochemical (material and size-dependent) characteristics, which organic NPs do not possess. In general, inorganic NPs are constituted of a core and a shell region, where the former is composed of inorganic materials such as gold, iron oxide or, silica while the latter consists of organic polymers such as proteins or complex sugars. Furthermore, the shell region would protect the inner core from undesirable physicochemical interactions. Gold NPs, quantum Dots, mesoporous silica NPs, superparamagnetic iron-oxide NPs, and hybrid nanocarriers are the most frequently utilized inorganic NPs for therapy and diagnosis of cancer as they possess high stability, ease of fabrication, surface modification, inertness, and magnetic properties. Therefore, they are considered as the most appropriate modality for imaging, and removal of cancerous cells. Moreover, inorganic NPs also possess higher quantum yield, longer lifespan and better photostability than organic NPs [9, 10].

This chapter focuses on the various methods of brain targeting, uptake and processing of NPs in the brain, and the role and applications of inorganic nano-particles as theranostic systems for cancer therapy.

BARRIERS TO TARGETED DRUG DELIVERY STRATEGIES IN BLOOD BRAIN BARRIER

Brain tumors pose a significant threat to human health due to their rapid growth, poor prognosis, and difficult treatment which would result in persisting terrible mortality rate. Due to poor drug permeability from the vessels into brain tumor tissue, chemotherapy has made limited progress to date. The effectiveness of a brain tumor-targeted nano-drug delivery system is evaluated based on the accuracy of the drug delivery to the exact foci. Moreover, a reduction in the accumulated drugs in the peripheral tissue and normal brain has been observed in recent decades [11]. There are certain barriers that prevent various targeted drug delivery systems from reaching to the brain (Fig. **1**).

Blood-Brain Barrier Targeting Methods and Related Mechanisms

Neurological disorders such as infections, psychiatric disorders, pain, cancers, neurodegenerative diseases, *etc.* are the most common causes of mortality, morbidity, and disability, affecting people around the world and the numbers are still predicted to increase until treatments are discovered. The blood-brain barrier ensures the majority of the curative agents out of the brain thus making it difficult to deliver drugs to the brain. Poor brain delivery continues to be a bottleneck throughout the production of central nervous system (CNS) therapies as it takes longer time than expected, therefore, resulting in a high rate of failure in clinical trials and drug development [12].

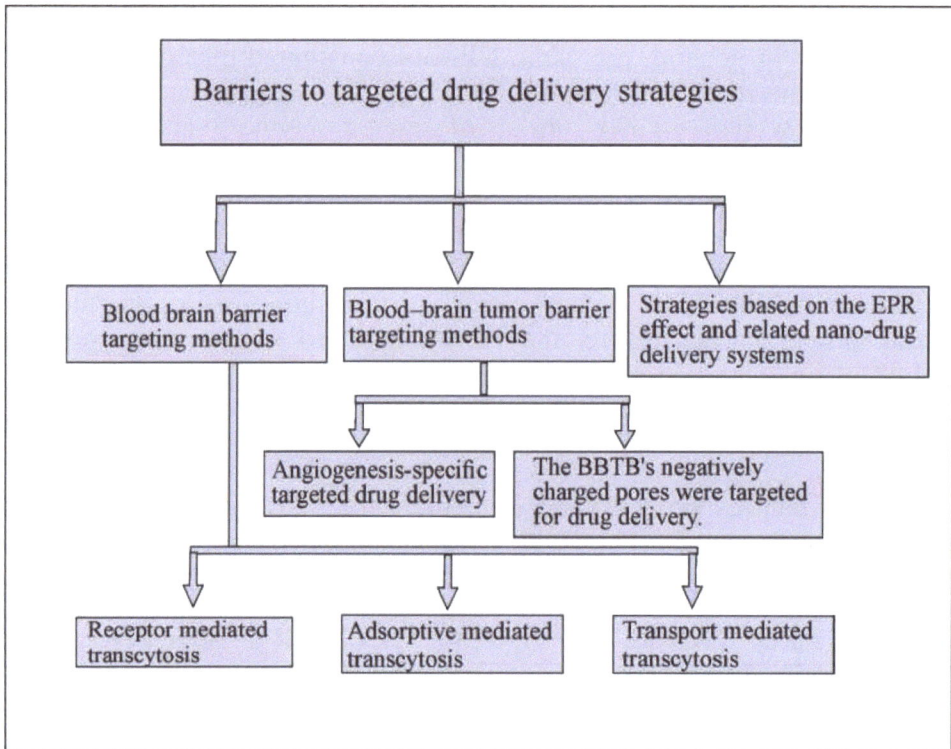

Fig. (1). Types of barriers to targeted drug delivery strategies

The blood–brain barrier remains intact throughout the early stages of development of brain tumors. The main obstacle in administering drugs to brain tumors is the blood-brain barrier (BBB) [13]. The BBB has a capillary endothelial cells system that is specialized and it is protected by basement membrane and pericytes. It is almost completely encircled by astrocytes, preventing the entrance of about 100% of large molecules and nearly 98% of the small molecules together with genes and recombinant proteins to the neoplasm sites. Thus, the blood-brain barrier serves as a physical and immunological barrier that would limit drug transportation into the brain [14]. Many different active targeting strategies have been utilized to build successful drug carriers for the brain to overcome this particular issue. RMT (receptor-mediated endocytosis), AMT (adsorptive-mediated transcytosis), and

TMT (transporter-mediated transcytosis) are the most common active targeting systems (Fig. **2**) [15].

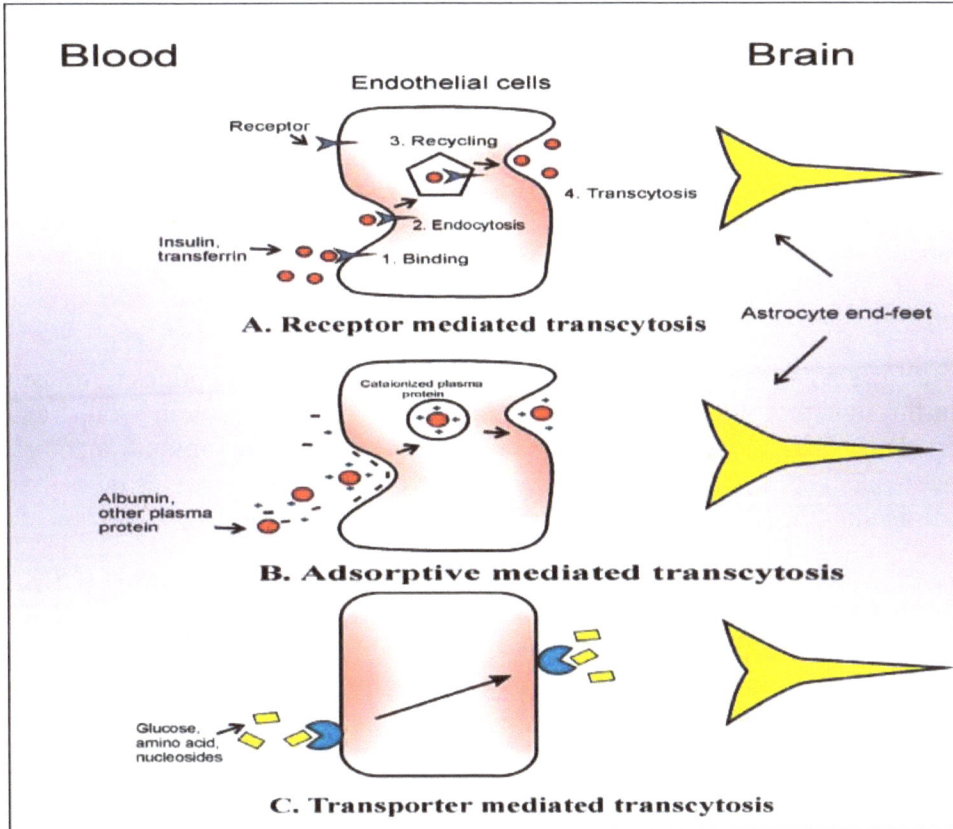

Fig. (2). Transport mechanisms across the BBB.

Receptor-Mediated Transcytosis (RMT)

Most plasma proteins are unable to reach the brain due to the hydrogen-bonding efficiency, hydrophilicity, and size, as evident by the cerebral spinal fluid (CSF). Endocytosis allows macromolecules like proteins, peptides, particulate formulations (functionalized nano-particles drug conjugates, chimeric proteins, antibody conjugates), and large-molecular-weight compounds to cross the BBB through RMT [12]. Even though the mechanism of action is unidentified, the process involves a unique ligand attachment to its receptor of membrane on the cell surface which causes the receptor protein to be modified. This would cause the development of invaginations that are able to be clathrin-coated. Furthermore, the endosomes are able to fuse with these endocytotic vesicles, allowing the ligand to be dissociated from the receptor and a free receptor which will be recycled to the surface of the cell [16].

There are several receptor proteins available for the purpose of transportation. Once they are bonded to their ligand, the transferrin receptors would migrate to the coated pits and cross across the plasma membrane by diffusion mechanism. Low-density lipoprotein receptors with the coated pits can be found even if there is no ligand bound to them while the low-density lipoprotein receptors (LRP1) can transport compounds in both directions. Ligand-containing vesicles may be exocytosed and transported through the BBB that is fused with a lysosome and degraded inside the cell [3].

Adsorptive-Mediated Transcytosis (AMT)

AMT allows positively charged proteins and cell-penetrating peptides to transport drugs through the blood-brain barrier. Positively charged protein would cause electrostatic interactions as the brain endothelial cells have an anionic membrane surface area. The absorptive-mediated transcytosis of nano-particles is mediated by cationic bovine serum albumin, which is a good example of AMT.

Lu *et al.* were the first to describe cationic bovine serum albumin (CBSA)-modified polyethylene glycol–polylactic acid (PEG-PLA) nanoparticle (CBSA NP) that could be used for brain delivery. The study discovered that by increasing the nanoparticle's surface CBSA density, it would increase the permeability of BBB, decrease blood area under curve (AUC), and speed up blood clearance. CBSA-modified tumor necrosis factor-related apoptosis-inducing ligand (hTRAIL)-loaded nano-particles achieved strong transfection, which occurred both *in vitro* and *in vivo* post loading plasmid open reading frame (pORF) hTRAIL plasmid DNA (pDNA) for gene therapy of gliomas. In contrast to unmodified nanoparticle hTRAIL, which was stuck in the endolysosomal compartment, it was first internalized by C6 glioma cells and found in the cytoplasm for 30 minutes after transfection. Apoptosis was triggered by releasing pDNA in the nucleus 6 and 48 hours after transfection. After 30 minutes i.v. administration to nude mice with intravenous administration of C6 gliomas, cationic bovine serum albumin-modified hTRAIL loaded nano-particles colocalized with tumor microvasculature and glycoproteins in brain and tumor was accumulated in the cells through AMT. After one and two days, the cationic bovine serum albumin-modified hTRAIL-loaded nano-particles were administered by the intravenous route, and protein and hTRAIL mRNA were identified in both tumors and healthy brain tissue. In addition, continuous intravenous administration of cationic bovine serum albumin-modified hTRAIL loaded nano-particles triggered *in vivo* apoptosis and greatly inhibited brain tumor enlargement [11, 14].

Transport Mediated Transcytosis (TMT)

The cerebral endothelium contains a variety of transport mechanisms that supply the brain with endogenous substances and essential nutrients. The use of TMT as a brain-targeting approach has the advantages of these mechanisms. However, only drugs with high similarity with endogenous substrates can be delivered into the brain *via* TMT [17]. Glucose transporters, which help glucose to move from the bloodstream to the brain, offer a lot of potential uses in brain targeting. The glucose transporter 1 (GLUT1) allows liposomes containing a mannose derivative to cross the BBB in the brain of a mouse [18].

Blood-Brain Tumor Barrier (BBTB) Targeting Methods and Related Mechanism

The BBB and BBTB observed between microvessels and brain tumor tissues are formed by endothelial cells with a high level of specialization and would prevent most hydrophilic molecules from reaching tumor tissue *via* paracellular delivery. The *BBB* will be weakened and the development of >blood tumor tissue will occur after the tumor cell clusters have reached a specific size. Solid malignant tumors that form in the peripheral region have high permeable BBTB than those which originate in the brain [3].

Researchers have combined both trans-blood brain barrier targeting and BBTB with an aim to improve brain tumor delivery by using the following two principles:

1. Modification with a dual-targeting moiety, for example, mannopyranoside plus transferrin (Tf), wheat germ agglutinin (WGA) plus Tf, *etc.*

2. Modification with a single targeting moiety, for example, angiopep2, lactoferrin (Lf) and transferrin which target both BBB, and brain tumor cells [19].

BBTB becomes the primary barrier for nanocarriers as brain tumors form, angiogenesis begins and the BBB gradually deteriorates. To date, there are only two techniques of BBTB targeting proposed.

Angiogenesis-Specific Targeted Drug Delivery

Integrins which are cell adhesion molecules found in the neovasculature, are common targets for angiogenesis. The role of $\alpha v \beta 3$ integrin, particularly in cancer progression is well-known and it is typically overexpressed in the sprouting endothelium cells and brain tumor cells but not in the quiescent endothelium cells or normal brain cells. Arginine-glycine-aspartic acid (RGD) sequence has been extensively explored as an integrin ligand to disrupt tumor angiogenesis and kill the tumor cells following passage through the neovasculature [20].

The BBTB's Negatively Charged Pores were Targeted for Drug Delivery

Nanofibers in the luminal glycocalyx layer which are overlying the anatomic flaws inside the BBTB are thought to be responsible for BBTB resistance to nano-particles larger than 12nm. This negatively charged barrier is sensitive to the charge of small molecules, peptides, and nano-drug delivery systems, especially long-circulating nano-particles that circulate *in vivo* for a long period and can fully interact with the inner surface of microvessels. Sarin *et al.* used positively charged terminal amines to attach rhodamine B dye to dendrimers. The study had suggested that the glycocalyx of the previously porous blood tumor cell and the normally nonporous blood-brain barrier were disrupted, resulting in increased rhodamine B-conjugated dendrimers to extravasate across the blood tumor tissue barrier. However, research on positively charged nano-particles that are smaller than 12nm for trans-BBB transport is yet to be explored for the purpose of drug administration therefore, more experimental validation is needed [21, 22].

Strategies based on the Enhanced Permeability and Retention Effect (EPR) Effect and Related Nano-Drug Delivery Systems

Theoretically, the high resistance of BBB and BBTB to passively targeted nano vehicles should limit the entrance of passively targeted nano vehicles to the brain tumor. However, when tumors grow bigger, the enhanced permeability and retention effect (EPR) would arise, particularly in brain tumor tissues. Although it is considerably weaker than in peripheral tumors, it allows nanosystems to penetrate the brain tumor through the endothelial gaps in the brain cancer microvessels with proper particle sizes. This could explain the success of numerous nanocarriers that did not require any particular trans-BBB transport modifications. Even without active-targeting alteration, liposomes with proper diameters (100 nm) can be passively targeted to tumors *via* the EPR effect [11].

INORGANIC NANO-PARTICLES (NPS) AS THERANOSTIC SYSTEMS AND THEIR APPLICATIONS

One of the most exciting potential characteristics of nanomedicine is its multifaceted use in each given application. It is a potent approach to enhance the existing drug delivery efforts by incorporating both diagnostic and therapeutic technologies onto the same NP. This has contributed further to the word "theranostic," which is attributed to Funkhouser [23].

Theranostics is developed as a targeted, secure and effective pharmacotherapy that primarily concentrates on patient-centered treatment. It is essentially a fusion of diagnostic and treatment possibilities. It serves as a bridge between traditional treatment and customized therapy. The word "theranostics" refers to the utilization of one irradiated substance to detect (diagnose) along with another substance to provide therapy to treat the primary tumor together with metastatic cancers [23, 5]. Theranostics emphasizes on the appropriate treatment of cancer or other diseases and improve patients' survival rates by lowering the detrimental consequences of treatment or imparting additional therapeutic modules.

Quantum dots (QDs), ceramic, magnetic, polystyrene and metallic NPs consist of an inorganic basic structure that determines their electrical, fluorescent, optical, and magnetic features. Aside from having the capacity to modulate drug release profiles, inorganic NPs also will safeguard the therapeutics against decomposition and lower recurrence of drug delivery and dose, ensuring a considerable decline in drug toxicity, specifically for tumor/ cancer therapeutics. Therefore, inorganic NPs offer a lot of potential for theranostic research [23].

Brain Tumor Imaging and Therapy Utilizing NPs

While NPs may serve as delivery vehicles that are customizable in size, shape, surface and targeting moieties, they also may act as drug reservoirs by adding multiple medicines or as an *in vivo* imaging probe [24, 22, 25, 26]. Additionally, NPs possess intrinsic benefits due to their composition. There are a few techniques that can be used to accomplish thermal ablation of tumors in which the NPs can be heated by light or radio frequencies or by a magnetic field [27, 28]. Another contrast enhancement method to accomplish the imaging can be done through magnetic NPs for magnetic resonance imaging (MRI) and gold NPs (AuNPs) for computed tomography (CT). Inorganic NPs have had limited usage in clinical applications for cancer [27 - 30]. Nonetheless, they are still under-researched and further study is needed to properly understand their clearance and safety [31, 32]. MRI contrast agents such as iron oxide (Fe_3O_4) and gadolinium (Gd_3O_4) are used to treat inorganic NPs that are found to have therapeutic usage. GdNPs (with sizes ranging from 50 to 80 nm) have shown to be well-tolerated in the clinical setting. Despite that, certain incidences of toxicity have occurred for Fe_3O_4 NPs, especially in nephrogenic systemic fibrosis [33, 34]. Numerous industrial research studies focusing on ultra-tiny particles with diameters less than 100 nm have been conducted. However, an industrial study that is focusing on all inorganic NPs is yet to be established [24, 32]. As a result, the material used; size, and the method in which it is coated or protected, are important considerations in taking an inorganic NPs based therapy from the bench to the bedside. In general, selecting an inert material is more advantageous than picking a material with intrinsic negative effects [33, 35]. Nonbiodegradable polymers such as polyethylene and polypropylene can only be ejected if their diameter is less than the renal filtration cutoff of roughly 5–6 nm. It is often recognized that most biodegradable polymeric NPs are well-tolerated in clinical studies [36]. However, research on the long-term persistence and toxicity of polymers in neuronal cells remains limited [37]. The vast majority of inorganic NPs are layered with an organic polymer to improve circulation half-life, shield the particle from the body and body from particles [23, 38]. Uncoated inorganic NPs present numerous problems in their long-term delivery and safety. Therefore, it can be suggested that there is a lot more work to be done. However, due to the risks associated with brain cancer and its low median survival, the potential advantages of the aforementioned NPs may overshadow their negative consequences [39 - 41]. As previously demonstrated with Gd and Fe_3O_4 NPs, the new materials could be developed prior to the toxicity of all NPs being completely understood. Due to their intrinsic magnetic properties, Gd and Fe_3O_4 NPs have been extensively researched and they are currently utilized as contrast agents in MRI for the diagnosis and tracing of brain cancers. The hydrophilic Fe_3O_4 NPs would induce MRI contrast enhancement for predominantly T2-weighted images, which aids in the visualization of blood vessels and other tissues with higher water content [42, 43]. T1-weighted pictures provide the best contrast enhancement for fatty tissues and they are also capable to provide superior contrast enhancement between white and gray matter or between cancerous tissue types [44, 45]. In comparison to the newer GdNPs, Gd ions require a longer duration to leave tumors therefore, they are utilized for clinical usage over non-nanoparticulate Gd. Furthermore, the non-nanoparticulate Gd might also display toxicity in certain individuals due to the outflow of the Gd from the chelating agent [24, 44, 46]. However, there are no documented reports of tissue injury or pathologic alterations due to the biodegradability of these particles in the brain of mice studied [24, 42, 43]. Similarly, QDs are tremendously beneficial as they can be tuned for fluorescence emission spectra from 400 to 2000 nm. The theoretical modeling studies have shown that the spectral windows of 700–900 and 1200–1600 nm are optimum for *in vivo* imaging [36]. However, without a separate polymer coating, QDs might be collected in the body due to their heavy metal composition, therefore making them harmful if they are collected in normal tissues [36]. The long-term effects on *in vivo* toxicity and degradation of QDs are yet to be determined in which more research is required. In the last few years, AuNPs have garnered a lot of interest in the biomedical sciences and are frequently utilized as they possess several possible applications in delivering medicines to the brain as well as brain cancer treatment [38, 47 - 51]. They have an ease of synthesis, simple surface functionalization, tiny sizes, corresponding excretion in the body, and little toxicity [47, 49, 51 - 53]. Of late, the extent of evidence on the biodistribution and toxicity of AuNPs has dramatically increased while nanosized particles have been evaluated by the USA National Institute of Standards and Technology as a prospective standard for research [23, 47, 49, 51 - 53]. The previous research has indicated that AuNPs have a diameter of up to 50 nm therefore, they are acceptable for the transportation of molecules over the BBB. The latest findings also have indicated that particles with diameters of up to 50 nm are able to pass across the BBB [23, 47, 49, 51 - 53].

In addition to the utilization of these effective inorganic NPs, the organic-based delivery vehicles have exhibited great potential as well. Approximately, 80% of the medicinal items that have been licensed for clinical use are made of polymers. The inorganic NPs do not usually have an organic polymer to increase the circulation half-life and allow the incorporation of targeting agents or imaging probes. Therefore, imparting a polymeric layer over inorganic NPs is essential [23, 47, 49, 51 - 53]. Studies have indicated an impressive range of polymer compositions, with poly (lactic-co-glycolic acid), polysorbate 80-coated poly (butyl cyanoacrylate), and poly (ε-caprolactone) are the most common core compositions for such purposes. However, most of these NPs are still in the trial phase in regards to the treatment of brain cancer [23, 47, 49, 51 - 53].

Inorganic NPs for Diagnostic and Therapeutic Purposes

Gd (III) MRI contrast agents are becoming the accepted practice as it is the only ion with the highest T_1 magnetization; hence, NPs that are enclosed with this ion are extensively utilized. Both relaxation and contrast enhancement are said to be boosted by nanoscale GdNPs [44, 45]. The Gd would chelate thus, excrete into the brain tissue during the surgical breakdown of the BBB and leak into the surrounding tissues. This would result in the significant contrast of other tissue and make tumors indistinguishable from the normal tissue, therefore, causing MRI-guided surgical reassignment to be more difficult [44 - 46]. The studies also have exhibited contrast augmentation of rat brain tumors within a few hours by GdNPs, along with a lack of toxicity *in vitro* [44].

Ultra-tiny superparamagnetic Fe_3O_4 NPs are currently in Phase III clinical studies for the lymphographic application as blood pool whereas dextran-coated superparamagnetic Fe_3O_4 NPs are FDA-approved for hepatic reticuloendothelial cell imaging [54]. Monocrystal-line Fe_3O_4 NPs, which have been linked to tumor-explicit monoclonal antibodies are the leading NPs which are designed for brain tumor imaging [24, 55]. However, they have only achieved success when the targeted particles are phagocytosed by the brain tumor cells. The MRI imaging of brain tumors could be enhanced by phagocytosis of these particles over a considerable long period of about one to two days [24, 56]. As Fe_3O_4 NPs must be administered up to a day before surgery with an objective of no enrichment in normal tissues, surgeons have to ensure the safety and complete clearance of all contrast-compound form tissue after an MRI [24]. This substance is yet to be utilized on its own in brain tumors but often used with other contrast agents such as Gd in the treatment of other conditions, including macular degeneration [35, 57, 58]. In one research, QDs were reported to facilitate tumor-infiltrating tissue macrophage phagocytosis and delivery of NPs to tumors, causing an optical delineation of the brain tumor infiltrative margination [58]. AuNPs also have found success in the treatment of brain cancer as well as in diagnostics. Moreover, AuNPs also have been used to inject Gd as well as the photoacoustic and Raman imaging agents as potential theranostic in regards to MRI detection and surgical applications (Fig. **3**) [59]. Although this is merely a diagnostic device, it is quite possible to imagine the incorporation of additional therapies such as systemic treatments that use chemotherapeutics for localized treatments. Additionally, fluorescent imaging agents also may be added to AuNPs for diagnostic reasons [47].

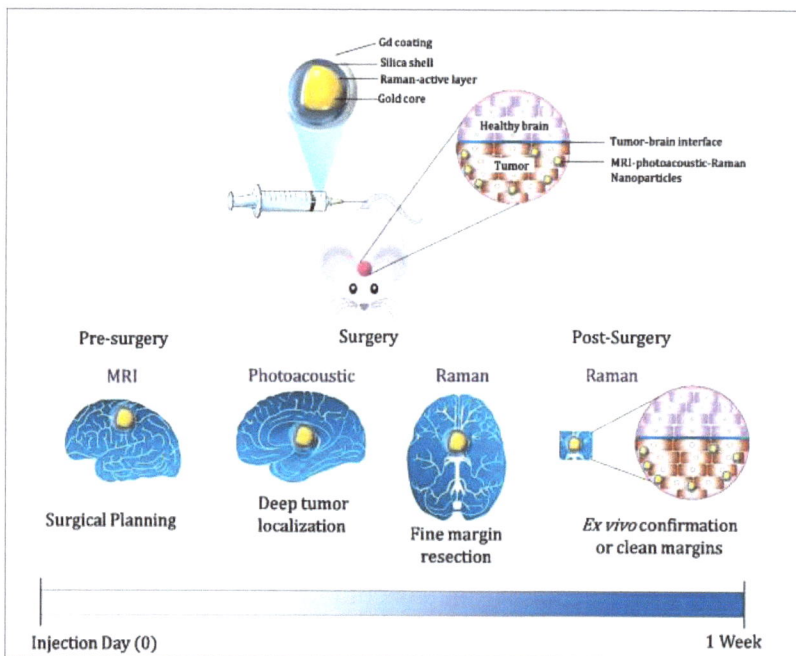

Fig. (3). A delivery method based on AuNPs in identifying brain tumor regions and improving surgical removal. Adopted from [59].

Fe_3O_4 and Au as inorganic NPs have correspondingly been examined as the therapy for brain cancer. The efficacy of antibody therapies as well as thermotherapy treatment using an oscillating magnetic field has been highlighted in studies on Fe_3O_4 NPs [27, 28, 42]. Another good feature of AuNPs is their capability to deliver noncovalent medications *in vivo* without AuNPs being taken up by tumor cells [47, 53, 60, 61]. Thermotherapy with visual, infrared, or radiofrequency pulses could also be used to apply heat to the gold to produce localized tumor destruction [62]. Although this sort of approach for AuNPs is yet to be utilized in brain tumors, it is predicted to have a desirable outcome in doing so.

Theranostic Potential of Inorganic NPs

An attractive possibility for future study in brain cancer imaging and treatment arises when there is a possibility of creating a "theranostic NP" by utilizing a "multimodal drug". Magnetic NPs are excellent examples of NP therapeutic agents as they are useful for MRI applications due to their intrinsic magnetic properties. Polymer-coated magnetic NPs were used to transport the anticancer medication epirubicin and acted as an MRI contrast compound in brain tissue. Despite using ultra-sound to manufacture microbubbles, the scientists had demonstrated that these bubbles had affected the BBB's permeability and made it possible for the magnetic NPs to go through it. To achieve better brain tumor uptake and accumulation of the NPs, Dilnawaz *et al.* reported the delivery of paclitaxel with glyceryl monooleate-coated magnetic NPs and found that the drug could be taken up by brain tumor tissue and there were significantly more NPs to be used as an MRI contrast agent in rats. Magnetic NP-based theranostics also have been seen in other research investigations [63 - 65]. MRI and drug delivery are often seen in non-prescription organic NP systems because they often have a magnetic contrast agent that is covalently bonded to the polymer structure. In the case of investigation by Reddy *et al.*, they described the use of a contrast agent that comprised a fluorescent drug cargo in combination with a polymer NP [66]. A significant development in theranostics is highlighted by them due to the contributions of diagnostic and therapeutic properties by the NPs which include the use of photodynamic therapy (PDT) as Photofrin® [66]. Since PDT agents are often capable of generating singlet oxygen and emitting fluorescence, it is possible to apply PDT and imaging at the same time. The distribution of medications relative to their NP carrier may be investigated by using medicines that can be photographed. A small group of researchers explored the application of metallic NPs to administer the PDT medication, phthalocyanine to brain tumors while the fluorescence of the drug was used as a potent tool to evaluate the amount of medication that reached the tumor [47]. Following biodistribution, further research by the same authors discovered substantial discrepancies in the biodistribution of the NPs and the drug, presumably due to the reversible hydrophobic adsorption of the therapeutic to the NPs [67, 68].

QDs, Fe_3O_4 NPs, and AuNPs have been proven effective as theranostic NPs. Each of these substances has been utilized to carry the therapeutic activities and imaging agents to the patients [23]. While Fe_3O_4 and AuNPs may act as theranostic NPs on their own, they also have the capacity to perform all the functions as theranostic. As the Fe_3O_4 NPs comprise magnetic resonance tracers and the AuNPs can function as CT diagnostic fluorescent probes due to their concentration, both can be used in successful theranostic application [43, 44, 47]. Theranostic delivery vehicles that employ QDs as an integrated delivery platform possess several assets that include targeted, multimodal tracing, and efficacious conveyance of siRNA-based chemotherapeutics [69]. Fe_3O_4 NPs are proven to be successful in targeting cancer by utilizing an externally induced magnetic field and increasing Fe_3O_4 nanoparticle delivery in tumors. In the future, this technology will be employed for brain cancer treatments progressively as it displays the ability to improve the administration of MRI contrast compounds, optical fluorescence imaging compounds and cancer chemotherapeutics by using external magnetic field applied [70, 71]. The potential of this MRI contrast compound delivery system to enhance the administration of optical fluorescence imaging agents and cancer therapies for brain tumors is indeed promising [29]. PDT medicines containing AuNPs have been verified to be effective and they are perfectly capable of drug distribution. Infrared radiation also can be used to initiate PDT which aids in the annihilation of tumor cells [47]. The MRI contrast of polymeric NPs has risen significantly when the encapsulation of Fe_3O_4 and PDT (or PDT medicines) are introduced [72]. Drugs are transported to tumor locations to aid in the identification of tumors inside the brain parenchyma, as well as the potential of delivering intraoperative PDT therapy, further improving the probability of successful tumor removal during surgery.

The NP application seems to depend extensively on single and multimodal systems. The treatments and detection have ensured no substantial decrease in brain tumor-related mortality rates in the last decade. The tumor's heterogeneity, lack of specificity in drug delivery and diagnostic failure in early-stage detection are all factors that have led to treatment ineffectiveness. Through the concept of theranostics, a strategy to improve brain tumor treatment is devised, enabling earlier sickness identification and more precise disease targeting [73]. Theranostic approaches also can be used to diagnose, detect and monitor the course of brain tumors which would help in the management of brain tumors.

Preclinical Stages and Clinical Studies of Theranostic NPs

Based on past hypotheses, theranostic NPs (ThNPs) are ideal for cancer theranostics due to their great affinity and specificity for tumor cells. Eventually, they can be adjusted to improve their functions such as circulation periods and target-delivering ligands. The utilization of imaging agents in a single formulation has been highlighted in recent researches. However, despite the advancements in ThNPs, it poses a challenge to convert them into the market [73]. ThNPs toxicity, pharmacodynamics, and safety factors have all been investigated in the preclinical investigations. The information on the different dosages of NPs that will be evaluated is established in this essential research, which concentrates on cell culture and animal testing. It is possible to examine the biocompatibility and behavior of NPs by analyzing their cytocompatibility in relation to animals. The goal of this preclinical research is to get ThNPs contenders into clinical trials. Inorganic NPs (such as QDs, AuNPs, and silica NPs) and organic NPs (such as liposomes, micelles/polymeric micelles, lipid NPs, and protein-based NPs) have been employed for medication co-delivery, as well as for imaging contrast [73]. The challenges of clinical translation and regulatory approval that come with growing complexity and tenuous reproducibility will be significant. There are several inorganic NPs, including FerahemeTM (Ferumoxytol), DexIron®/Dexferrum Feridex®, NanoTherm®, INFeD®, AuroLase Therapy, Venofer®, and AuNPs-nanosensor currently utilized in clinical research or have been approved for medicinal use [73, 74]. The treatment is conducted by using NanoTherm, a method in which magnetic NPs are transfused into the tumor and subsequently heated with an alternating magnetic field. Post the additional, minimally invasive operation to transfer magnetic fluid to the tumor, a thermometry catheter is used to assess the temperature in the treatment location, allowing direct heat management [73]. Although the relations between *in vitro* and *in vivo* data are yet to be discovered, there are still a number of ThNPs at various phases of development.

CONCLUSION

The treatment of cancer with existing methods is difficult and complex due to drug resistance, tumor heterogeneity, and poor selectivity. Meticulous diagnostics and treatment planning are needed to develop novel cancer management and treatment methods. Through real-time monitoring of medication accumulation, theranostics would provide possibilities for customized medicine. Theranostic nano-particles have the potential to change illness management. Inorganic NPs, given their inherent characteristics, have been extensively utilized to create theranostic systems of drug transport. In the past decade, such theranostic nano-particles were developed to optimize output from a range of inorganic materials in diverse combinations for particular purposes. However, factors such as toxicity, immunogenicity and adverse effects of these particles must be recognized, and examined thoroughly before they are brought into the clinic. The creation of tailored inorganic NPs would also allow for a comprehensive knowledge of each molecule of each kind of cancer in the future. These inorganic NPs would be able to identify cancer cells efficiently, observe their position throughout the body, distribute drugstores to transforming cells and bypass chemoresistance. The functions of inorganic NPs in cancer treatment are increasing and the development of efficient inorganic multi-targeting NPs will significantly overcome the physiological effects of different disease conditions and improve the accuracy of cancer treatment.

REFERENCES

[1]   Sung H, Ferlay J, Siegel RL, *et al.* Global cancer statistics 2020: GLOBOCAN estimates of incidence and mortality worldwide for 36 cancers in 185 countries. CA Cancer J Clin 2021; 71(3): 209-49.
[http://dx.doi.org/10.3322/caac.21660] [PMID: 33538338]

[2]   Zhao CY, Cheng R, Yang Z, Tian ZM. Nanotechnology for cancer therapy based on chemotherapy. Molecules 2018; 23(4): 826.
[http://dx.doi.org/10.3390/molecules23040826] [PMID: 29617302]

[3]   Belhadj Z, Zhan C, Ying M, *et al.* Multifunctional targeted liposomal drug delivery for efficient glioblastoma treatment. Oncotarget 2017; 8(40): 66889-900.
[http://dx.doi.org/10.18632/oncotarget.17976] [PMID: 28978003]

[4]   Brasnjevic I, Steinbusch HWM, Schmitz C, Martinez-Martinez P. Delivery of peptide and protein drugs over the blood–brain barrier. Prog Neurobiol 2009; 87(4): 212-51.
[http://dx.doi.org/10.1016/j.pneurobio.2008.12.002] [PMID: 19395337]

[5]   Kelkar SS, Reineke TM. Theranostics: combining imaging and therapy. Bioconjug Chem 2011; 22(10): 1879-903.
[http://dx.doi.org/10.1021/bc200151q] [PMID: 21830812]

[6]   Patra JK, Das G, Fraceto LF, *et al.* Nano based drug delivery systems: recent developments and future prospects. J Nanobiotechnology 2018; 16(1): 71.
[http://dx.doi.org/10.1186/s12951-018-0392-8] [PMID: 30231877]

[7]   Lombardo D, Kiselev MA, Caccamo MT. Smart nano-particles for drug delivery application: development of versatile nanocarrier platforms in biotechnology and nanomedicine. J Nanomater 2019; 2019: 1-26.
[http://dx.doi.org/10.1155/2019/3702518]

[8]   Khan MA, Singh D, Ahmad A, Siddique HR. Revisiting inorganic nano-particles as promising therapeutic agents: A paradigm shift in oncological theranostics. Eur J Pharm Sci 2021; 164: 105892-8.
[http://dx.doi.org/10.1016/j.ejps.2021.105892] [PMID: 34052295]

[9]   Vakili-Ghartavol R, Momtazi-Borojeni AA, Vakili-Ghartavol Z, *et al.* Toxicity assessment of superparamagnetic iron oxide nano-particles in different tissues. Artif Cells Nanomed Biotechnol 2020; 48(1): 443-51.
[http://dx.doi.org/10.1080/21691401.2019.1709855] [PMID: 32024389]

[10]   Bakshi S, Zakharchenko A, Minko S, Kolpashchikov D, Katz E. Towards nanomaterials for cancer theranostics: A system of DNA-modified magnetic nano-particles for detection and suppression of RNA marker in cancer cells. Magnetochemistry 2019; 5(2): 24.
[http://dx.doi.org/10.3390/magnetochemistry5020024]

[11]   Liu Y, Lu W. Recent advances in brain tumor-targeted nano-drug delivery systems. Expert Opin Drug Deliv 2012; 9(6): 671-86.
[http://dx.doi.org/10.1517/17425247.2012.682726] [PMID: 22607535]

[12]   Lalatsa A, Butt AM. Physiology of the blood–brain barrier and mechanisms of transport across the BBB. 2018.

[http://dx.doi.org/10.1016/B978-0-12-812218-1.00003-8]

[13]   Chen L, Zeng D, Xu N, *et al.* Blood–Brain Barrier- and Blood–Brain Tumor Barrier-Penetrating Peptide-Derived Targeted Therapeutics for Glioma and Malignant Tumor Brain Metastases. ACS Appl Mater Interfaces 2019; 11(45): 41889-97.
[http://dx.doi.org/10.1021/acsami.9b14046] [PMID: 31615203]

[14]   Pang Z, Gao H, Chen J, *et al.* Intracellular delivery mechanism and brain delivery kinetics of biodegradable cationic bovine serum albumin-conjugated polymersomes. Int J Nanomedicine 2012; 7(7): 3421-32.
[PMID: 22848168]

[15]   Wong AD, Ye M, Levy AF, Rothstein JD, Bergles DE, Searson PC. The blood-brain barrier: an engineering perspective. Front Neuroeng 2013; 6(7): 7.
[PMID: 24009582]

[16]   Sahu KK, Minz S, Kaurav M, Pandey RS. Proteins and peptides: The need to improve them as promising therapeutics for ulcerative colitis. Artif Cells Nanomed Biotechnol 2016; 44(2): 642-53.
[http://dx.doi.org/10.3109/21691401.2014.975239] [PMID: 25379956]

[17]   de Boer AG, Gaillard PJ. Drug targeting to the brain. Annu Rev Pharmacol Toxicol 2007; 47(1): 323-55.
[http://dx.doi.org/10.1146/annurev.pharmtox.47.120505.105237] [PMID: 16961459]

[18]   Fenart L, Casanova A, Dehouck B, *et al.* Evaluation of effect of charge and lipid coating on ability of 60-nm nano-particles to cross an *in vitro* model of the blood-brain barrier. J Pharmacol Exp Ther 1999; 291(3): 1017-22.
[PMID: 10565819]

[19]   Fischer D, Kissel T. Histochemical characterization of primary capillary endothelial cells from porcine brains using monoclonal antibodies and fluorescein isothiocyanate-labelled lectins: implications for drug delivery. Eur J Pharm Biopharm 2001; 52(1): 1-11.
[http://dx.doi.org/10.1016/S0939-6411(01)00159-X] [PMID: 11438418]

[20]   Zako T, Nagata H, Terada N, *et al.* Cyclic RGD peptide-labeled upconversion nanophosphors for tumor cell-targeted imaging. Biochem Biophys Res Commun 2009; 381(1): 54-8.
[http://dx.doi.org/10.1016/j.bbrc.2009.02.004] [PMID: 19351594]

[21]   Squire JM, Chew M, Nneji G, Neal C, Barry J, Michel C. Quasi-periodic substructure in the microvessel endothelial glycocalyx: a possible explanation for molecular filtering? J Struct Biol 2001; 136(3): 239-55.
[http://dx.doi.org/10.1006/jsbi.2002.4441] [PMID: 12051903]

[22]   Sarin H, Kanevsky AS, Wu H, *et al.* Effective transvascular delivery of nano-particles across the blood-brain tumor barrier into malignant glioma cells. J Transl Med 2008; 6(1): 80.
[http://dx.doi.org/10.1186/1479-5876-6-80] [PMID: 19094226]

[23]   Meyers JD, Doane T, Burda C, Basilion JP. Nano-particles for imaging and treating brain cancer. Nanomedicine (Lond) 2013; 8(1): 123-43.
[http://dx.doi.org/10.2217/nnm.12.185] [PMID: 23256496]

[24]   Orringer DA, Koo YE, Chen T, Kopelman R, Sagher O, Philbert MA. Small solutions for big problems: the application of nano-particles to brain tumor diagnosis and therapy. Clin Pharmacol Ther 2009; 85(5): 531-4.
[http://dx.doi.org/10.1038/clpt.2008.296] [PMID: 19242401]

[25]   Doane T, Burda C. Nanoparticle mediated non-covalent drug delivery. Adv Drug Deliv Rev 2013; 65(5): 607-21.
[http://dx.doi.org/10.1016/j.addr.2012.05.012] [PMID: 22664231]

[26]   Sampson JH, Archer GE, Mitchell DA, Heimberger AB, Bigner DD. Tumor-specific immunotherapy targeting the EGFRvIII mutation in patients with malignant glioma. Semin Immunol 2008; 20(5): 267-

75.
[http://dx.doi.org/10.1016/j.smim.2008.04.001] [PMID: 18539480]

[27]   Jordan A, Scholz R, Maier-Hauff K, *et al.* The effect of thermotherapy using magnetic nano-particles on rat malignant glioma. J Neurooncol 2006; 78(1): 7-14.
[http://dx.doi.org/10.1007/s11060-005-9059-z] [PMID: 16314937]

[28]   Maier-Hauff K, Rothe R, Scholz R, *et al.* Intracranial thermotherapy using magnetic nano-particles combined with external beam radiotherapy: results of a feasibility study on patients with glioblastoma multiforme. J Neurooncol 2007; 81(1): 53-60.
[http://dx.doi.org/10.1007/s11060-006-9195-0] [PMID: 16773216]

[29]   Popovtzer R, Agrawal A, Kotov NA, *et al.* Targeted gold nano-particles enable molecular CT imaging of cancer. Nano Lett 2008; 8(12): 4593-6.
[http://dx.doi.org/10.1021/nl8029114] [PMID: 19367807]

[30]   Kumar M, Medarova Z, Pantazopoulos P, Dai G, Moore A. Novel membrane-permeable contrast agent for brain tumor detection by MRI. Magn Reson Med 2010; 63(3): 617-24.
[http://dx.doi.org/10.1002/mrm.22216] [PMID: 20146231]

[31]   Dickson M, Gagnon JP. Key factors in the rising cost of new drug discovery and development. Nat Rev Drug Discov 2004; 3(5): 417-29.
[http://dx.doi.org/10.1038/nrd1382] [PMID: 15136789]

[32]   Gwinn MR, Vallyathan V. Nano-particles: health effects--pros and cons. Environ Health Perspect 2006; 114(12): 1818-25.
[http://dx.doi.org/10.1289/ehp.8871] [PMID: 17185269]

[33]   Khurana A, Runge VM, Narayanan M, Greene JF Jr, Nickel AE. Nephrogenic systemic fibrosis: a review of 6 cases temporally related to gadodiamide injection (omniscan). Invest Radiol 2007; 42(2): 139-45.
[http://dx.doi.org/10.1097/01.rli.0000253505.88945.d5] [PMID: 17220732]

[34]   Bernd H, De Kerviler E, Gaillard S, Bonnemain B. Safety and tolerability of ultrasmall superparamagnetic iron oxide contrast agent: comprehensive analysis of a clinical development program. Invest Radiol 2009; 44(6): 336-42.
[http://dx.doi.org/10.1097/RLI.0b013e3181a0068b] [PMID: 19661843]

[35]   Gao X, Yang L, Petros JA, Marshall FF, Simons JW, Nie S. *In vivo* molecular and cellular imaging with quantum dots. Curr Opin Biotechnol 2005; 16(1): 63-72.
[http://dx.doi.org/10.1016/j.copbio.2004.11.003] [PMID: 15722017]

[36]   Soo Choi H, Liu W, Misra P, *et al.* Renal clearance of quantum dots. Nat Biotechnol 2007; 25(10): 1165-70.
[http://dx.doi.org/10.1038/nbt1340] [PMID: 17891134]

[37]   Costantino L, Boraschi D. Is there a clinical future for polymeric nano-particles as brain-targeting drug delivery agents? Drug Discov Today 2012; 17(7-8): 367-78.
[http://dx.doi.org/10.1016/j.drudis.2011.10.028] [PMID: 22094246]

[38]   Khlebtsov N, Dykman L. Biodistribution and toxicity of engineered gold nano-particles: a review of *in vitro* and *in vivo* studies. Chem Soc Rev 2011; 40(3): 1647-71.
[http://dx.doi.org/10.1039/C0CS00018C] [PMID: 21082078]

[39]   Ullrich NJ, Pomeroy SL. Pediatric brain tumors. Neurol Clin 2003; 21(4): 897-913.
[http://dx.doi.org/10.1016/S0733-8619(03)00014-8] [PMID: 14743655]

[40]   Pardridge WM. The blood-brain barrier: Bottleneck in brain drug development. NeuroRx 2005; 2(1): 3-14.
[http://dx.doi.org/10.1602/neurorx.2.1.3] [PMID: 15717053]

[41]   Wen PY, Kesari S. Malignant gliomas in adults. N Engl J Med 2008; 359(5): 492-507.
[http://dx.doi.org/10.1056/NEJMra0708126] [PMID: 18669428]

[42]   Hadjipanayis CG, Machaidze R, Kaluzova M, *et al.* EGFRvIII antibody-conjugated iron oxide nano-particles for magnetic resonance imaging-guided convection-enhanced delivery and targeted therapy of glioblastoma. Cancer Res 2010; 70(15): 6303-12.
[http://dx.doi.org/10.1158/0008-5472.CAN-10-1022] [PMID: 20647323]

[43]   Muldoon LL, Sàndor M, Pinkston KE, Neuwelt EA. Imaging, distribution, and toxicity of superparamagnetic iron oxide magnetic resonance nano-particles in the rat brain and intracerebral tumor. Neurosurgery 2005; 57(4): 785-96.
[http://dx.doi.org/10.1227/01.NEU.0000175731.25414.4c] [PMID: 16239893]

[44]   Park JY, Baek MJ, Choi ES, *et al.* Paramagnetic ultrasmall gadolinium oxide nano-particles as advanced T1 MRI contrast agent: account for large longitudinal relaxivity, optimal particle diameter, and *in vivo* T1 MR images. ACS Nano 2009; 3(11): 3663-9.
[http://dx.doi.org/10.1021/nn900761s] [PMID: 19835389]

[45]   Faucher L, Guay-Bégin AA, Lagueux J, Côté MF, Petitclerc E, Fortin MA. Ultra-small gadolinium oxide nano-particles to image brain cancer cells *in vivo* with MRI. Contrast Media Mol Imaging 2011; 6(4): 209-18.
[PMID: 21861281]

[46]   Veiseh O, Sun C, Fang C, *et al.* Specific targeting of brain tumors with an optical/magnetic resonance imaging nanoprobe across the blood-brain barrier. Cancer Res 2009; 69(15): 6200-7.
[http://dx.doi.org/10.1158/0008-5472.CAN-09-1157] [PMID: 19638572]

[47]   Cheng Y, Meyers JD, Agnes RS, *et al.* Addressing brain tumors with targeted gold nano-particles: a new gold standard for hydrophobic drug delivery? Small 2011; 7(16): 2301-6.
[http://dx.doi.org/10.1002/smll.201100628] [PMID: 21630446]

[48]   Sousa F, Mandal S, Garrovo C, *et al.* Functionalized gold nano-particles: a detailed *in vivo* multimodal microscopic brain distribution study. Nanoscale 2010; 2(12): 2826-34.
[http://dx.doi.org/10.1039/c0nr00345j] [PMID: 20949211]

[49]   Lasagna-Reeves C, Gonzalez-Romero D, Barria MA, *et al.* Bioaccumulation and toxicity of gold nano-particles after repeated administration in mice. Biochem Biophys Res Commun 2010; 393(4): 649-55.
[http://dx.doi.org/10.1016/j.bbrc.2010.02.046] [PMID: 20153731]

[50]   Jong WHD, Burger MC, Verheijen MA, Geertsma RE. Detection of the presence of gold nano-particles in organs by transmission electron microscopy. Materials (Basel) 2010; 3(9): 4681-94.
[http://dx.doi.org/10.3390/ma3094681] [PMID: 28883347]

[51]   Sonavane G, Tomoda K, Makino K. Biodistribution of colloidal gold nano-particles after intravenous administration: Effect of particle size. Colloids Surf B Biointerfaces 2008; 66(2): 274-80.
[http://dx.doi.org/10.1016/j.colsurfb.2008.07.004] [PMID: 18722754]

[52]   Han G, Ghosh P, Rotello VM. Functionalized gold nano-particles for drug delivery. Nanomedicine (Lond) 2007; 2(1): 113-23.
[http://dx.doi.org/10.2217/17435889.2.1.113] [PMID: 17716197]

[53]   Cheng Y, Meyers JD, Broome AM, Kenney ME, Basilion JP, Burda C. Deep penetration of a PDT drug into tumors by noncovalent drug-gold nanoparticle conjugates. J Am Chem Soc 2011; 133(8): 2583-91.
[http://dx.doi.org/10.1021/ja108846h] [PMID: 21294543]

[54]   Frank JA, Miller BR, Arbab AS, *et al.* Clinically applicable labeling of mammalian and stem cells by combining superparamagnetic iron oxides and transfection agents. Radiology 2003; 228(2): 480-7.
[http://dx.doi.org/10.1148/radiol.2281020638] [PMID: 12819345]

[55]   Remsen LG, McCormick CI, Roman-Goldstein S, *et al.* MR of carcinoma-specific monoclonal antibody conjugated to monocrystalline iron oxide nano-particles: the potential for noninvasive diagnosis. AJNR Am J Neuroradiol 1996; 17(3): 411-8.

[PMID: 8881233]

[56]   Anderson SA, Glod J, Arbab AS, *et al.* Noninvasive MR imaging of magnetically labeled stem cells to directly identify neovasculature in a glioma model. Blood 2005; 105(1): 420-5.
[http://dx.doi.org/10.1182/blood-2004-06-2222] [PMID: 15331444]

[57]   Oostendorp M, Douma K, Hackeng TM, Post MJ, van Zandvoort MAMJ, Backes WH. Gadolinium-labeled quantum dots for molecular magnetic resonance imaging: R1 versus R2 mapping. Magn Reson Med 2010; 64(1): 291-8.
[http://dx.doi.org/10.1002/mrm.22342] [PMID: 20572132]

[58]   Jackson H, Muhammad O, Daneshvar H, *et al.* Quantum dots are phagocytized by macrophages and colocalize with experimental gliomas. Neurosurgery 2007; 60(3): 524-30.
[http://dx.doi.org/10.1227/01.NEU.0000255334.95532.DD] [PMID: 17327798]

[59]   Kircher MF, de la Zerda A, Jokerst JV, *et al.* A brain tumor molecular imaging strategy using a new triple-modality MRI-photoacoustic-Raman nanoparticle. Nat Med 2012; 18(5): 829-34.
[http://dx.doi.org/10.1038/nm.2721] [PMID: 22504484]

[60]   Cheng Y, Samia AC, Meyers JD, Panagopoulos I, Fei B, Burda C. Highly efficient drug delivery with gold nanoparticle vectors for *in vivo* photodynamic therapy of cancer. J Am Chem Soc 2008; 130(32): 10643-7.
[http://dx.doi.org/10.1021/ja801631c] [PMID: 18642918]

[61]   Cheng Y, Samia AC, Li J, Kenney ME, Resnick A, Burda C. Delivery and efficacy of a cancer drug as a function of the bond to the gold nanoparticle surface. Langmuir 2010; 26(4): 2248-55.
[http://dx.doi.org/10.1021/la902390d] [PMID: 19719162]

[62]   Letfullin RR, Iversen CB, George TF. Modeling nanophotothermal therapy: kinetics of thermal ablation of healthy and cancerous cell organelles and gold nano-particles. Nanomedicine 2011; 7(2): 137-45.
[http://dx.doi.org/10.1016/j.nano.2010.06.011] [PMID: 20732456]

[63]   Hua MY, Liu HL, Yang HW, *et al.* The effectiveness of a magnetic nanoparticle-based delivery system for BCNU in the treatment of gliomas. Biomaterials 2011; 32(2): 516-27.
[http://dx.doi.org/10.1016/j.biomaterials.2010.09.065] [PMID: 21030073]

[64]   Mejías R, Pérez-Yagüe S, Roca AG, *et al.* Liver and brain imaging through dimercaptosuccinic acid-coated iron oxide nano-particles. Nanomedicine (Lond) 2010; 5(3): 397-408.
[http://dx.doi.org/10.2217/nnm.10.15] [PMID: 20394533]

[65]   Kievit FM, Veiseh O, Fang C, *et al.* Chlorotoxin labeled magnetic nanovectors for targeted gene delivery to glioma. ACS Nano 2010; 4(8): 4587-94.
[http://dx.doi.org/10.1021/nn1008512] [PMID: 20731441]

[66]   Reddy GR, Bhojani MS, McConville P, *et al.* Vascular targeted nano-particles for imaging and treatment of brain tumors. Clin Cancer Res 2006; 12(22): 6677-86.
[http://dx.doi.org/10.1158/1078-0432.CCR-06-0946] [PMID: 17121886]

[67]   Liu HL, Hua MY, Yang HW, *et al.* Magnetic resonance monitoring of focused ultrasound/magnetic nanoparticle targeting delivery of therapeutic agents to the brain. Proc Natl Acad Sci USA 2010; 107(34): 15205-10.
[http://dx.doi.org/10.1073/pnas.1003388107] [PMID: 20696897]

[68]   Dilnawaz F, Singh A, Mewar S, Sharma U, Jagannathan NR, Sahoo SK. The transport of non-surfactant based paclitaxel loaded magnetic nano-particles across the blood brain barrier in a rat model. Biomaterials 2012; 33(10): 2936-51.
[http://dx.doi.org/10.1016/j.biomaterials.2011.12.046] [PMID: 22264522]

[69]   Jung J, Solanki A, Memoli KA, *et al.* Selective inhibition of human brain tumor cells through multifunctional quantum-dot-based siRNA delivery. Angew Chem Int Ed 2010; 49(1): 103-7.
[http://dx.doi.org/10.1002/anie.200905126] [PMID: 19950159]

[70] Sharma R, Saini S, Ros PR, *et al.* Safety profile of ultrasmall superparamagnetic iron oxide ferumoxtran-10: Phase II clinical trial data. J Magn Reson Imaging 1999; 9(2): 291-4.
[http://dx.doi.org/10.1002/(SICI)1522-2586(199902)9:2<291::AID-JMRI21>3.0.CO;2-#] [PMID: 10077027]

[71] Jung CW, Jacobs P. Physical and chemical properties of superparamagnetic iron oxide MR contrast agents: Ferumoxides, ferumoxtran, ferumoxsil. Magn Reson Imaging 1995; 13(5): 661-74.
[http://dx.doi.org/10.1016/0730-725X(95)00024-B] [PMID: 8569441]

[72] Foy SP, Manthe RL, Foy ST, Dimitrijevic S, Krishnamurthy N, Labhasetwar V. Optical imaging and magnetic field targeting of magnetic nano-particles in tumors. ACS Nano 2010; 4(9): 5217-24.
[http://dx.doi.org/10.1021/nn101427t] [PMID: 20731413]

[73] Mendes M, Sousa JJ, Pais A, Vitorino C. Targeted theranostic nano-particles for brain tumor treatment. Pharmaceutics 2018; 10(4): 181.
[http://dx.doi.org/10.3390/pharmaceutics10040181] [PMID: 30304861]

[74] Maier-Hauff K, Ulrich F, Nestler D, *et al.* Efficacy and safety of intratumoral thermotherapy using magnetic iron-oxide nano-particles combined with external beam radiotherapy on patients with recurrent glioblastoma multiforme. J Neurooncol 2011; 103(2): 317-24.
[http://dx.doi.org/10.1007/s11060-010-0389-0] [PMID: 20845061]

SUBJECT INDEX

A

www.ingramcontent.com/pod-product-compliance
Lightning Source LLC
Chambersburg PA
CBHW050831220326

41598CB00006B/350